KATRINA ELLIS N.D.

NATUROPATH, IRIDOLOGIST, HERBALIST, AUTHOR

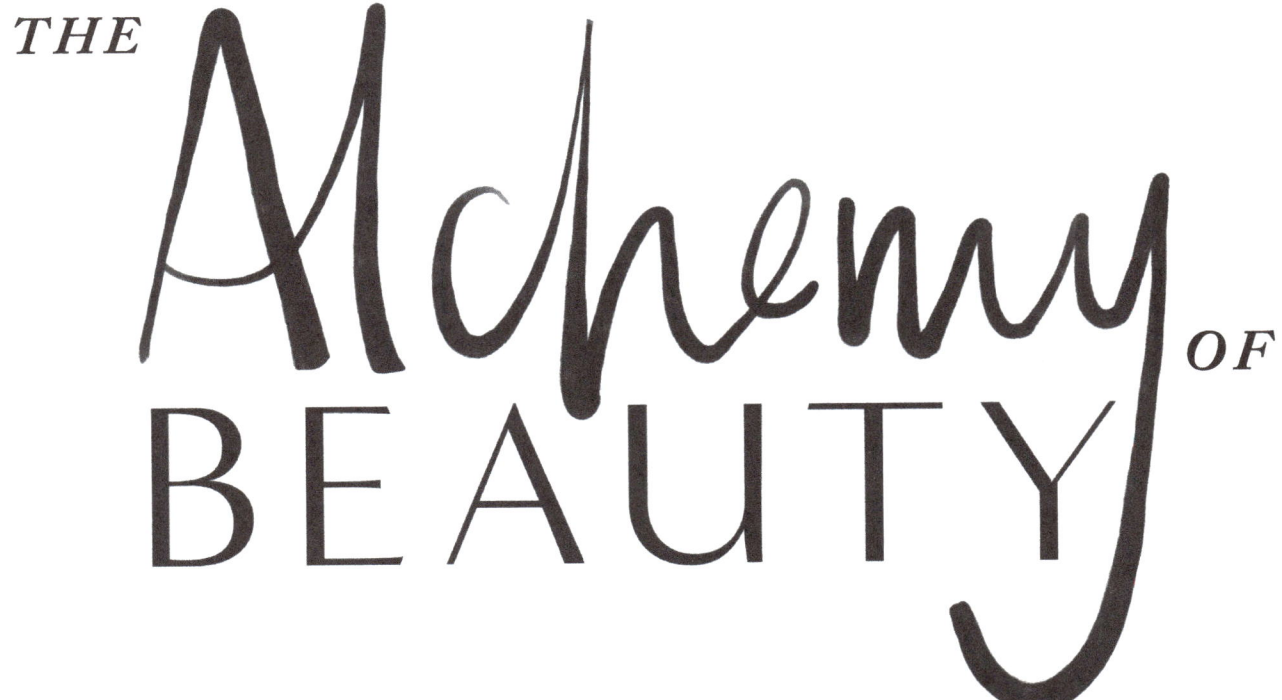

THE *Alchemy* OF BEAUTY

THE ULTIMATE
GUIDE TO NATURAL
BEAUTY AND
COMPLETE WELLNESS

OVER 100 DELICIOUS,
HEALING RECIPES TO
BOOST GUT, IMMUNE &
COLLAGEN HEALTH

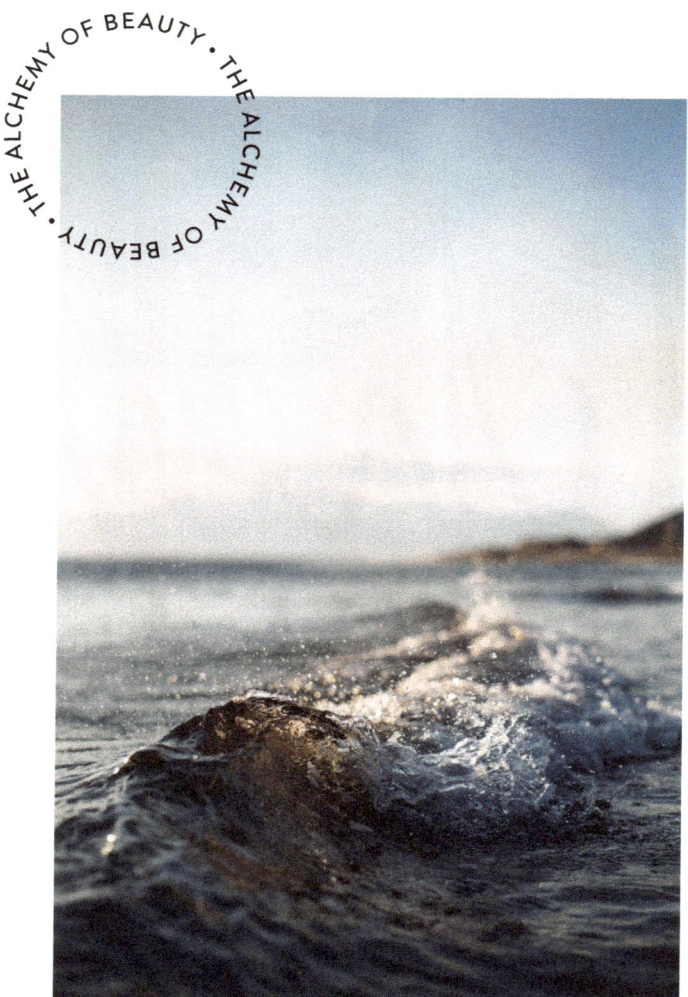

I BELIEVE THAT EVERY SOUL IN THIS WORLD IS UNIQUELY BEAUTIFUL IN THEIR OWN WAY.

In writing this book I want every child, including my own, and every human being to appreciate the perfection of the beauty inside them and to understand how important it is to celebrate this. For supporting me and offering their patience and wisdom in the creation of this book, I wish to thank the following beautiful souls:

The man who always looks good, even when he goes to bed, Clay; my beautiful daughter Evie-Ray for her unharnessed love and honesty; my son Carter who was born beautiful and continues to be beautiful everyday; my gorgeous mum who has had my back through every lifetime; my dad who guides me every day from the spirit world; my nineteen-year-old Husky dog Keeta who let me test all of my anti-ageing remedies on him (obviously some of them worked); and my gorgeous brothers Larry and Brett.

I also want to thank my BFF Sabby for taking me on mad shopping sprees to research natural products, 007 for showing me that EVERYTHING is possible, my moon sister Amy for her hilarious, wise words of wisdom, Casey (luv ya – told you I would shout out), Amy Mills, Marissa Bowden, Sarah of Hazel Haus, Tara of Mercer Makeup and Styling, Brian from Ocean Road Magazine for his incredible pictures, The Edit Suite, the gorgeous models Christina Macpherson and Georgia Ansell, my amazing friends, talented work colleagues and incredible clients and each soul that has taken the time to read my books. I am eternally grateful from the bottom of my heart.

In love, happiness, peace and beauty,

Katrina (AKA–to anyone who knows me–KAIA xxx)

Katrina Ellis

Contents

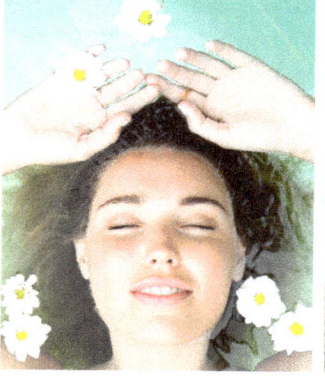
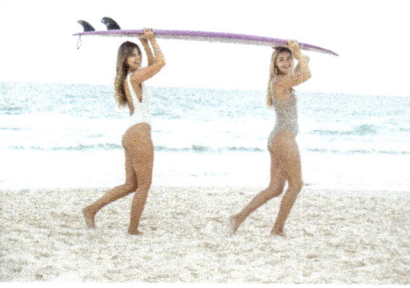

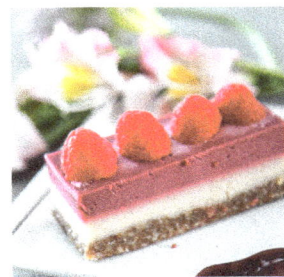

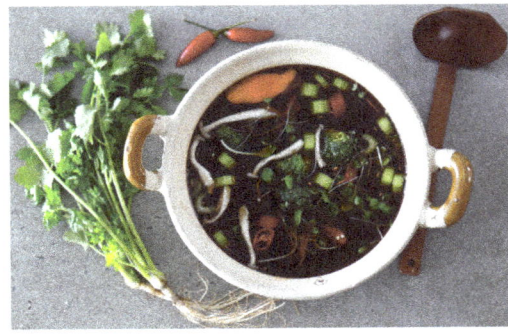

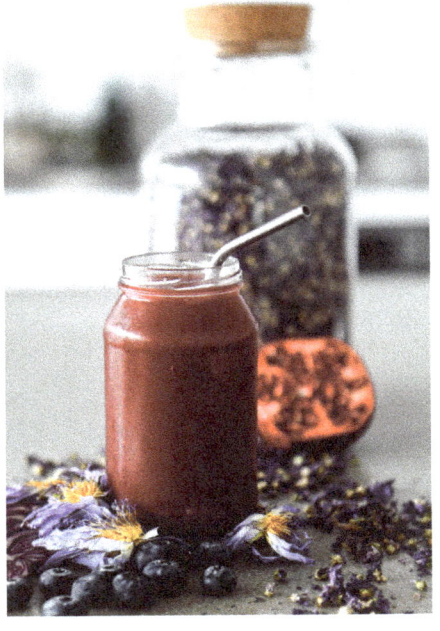

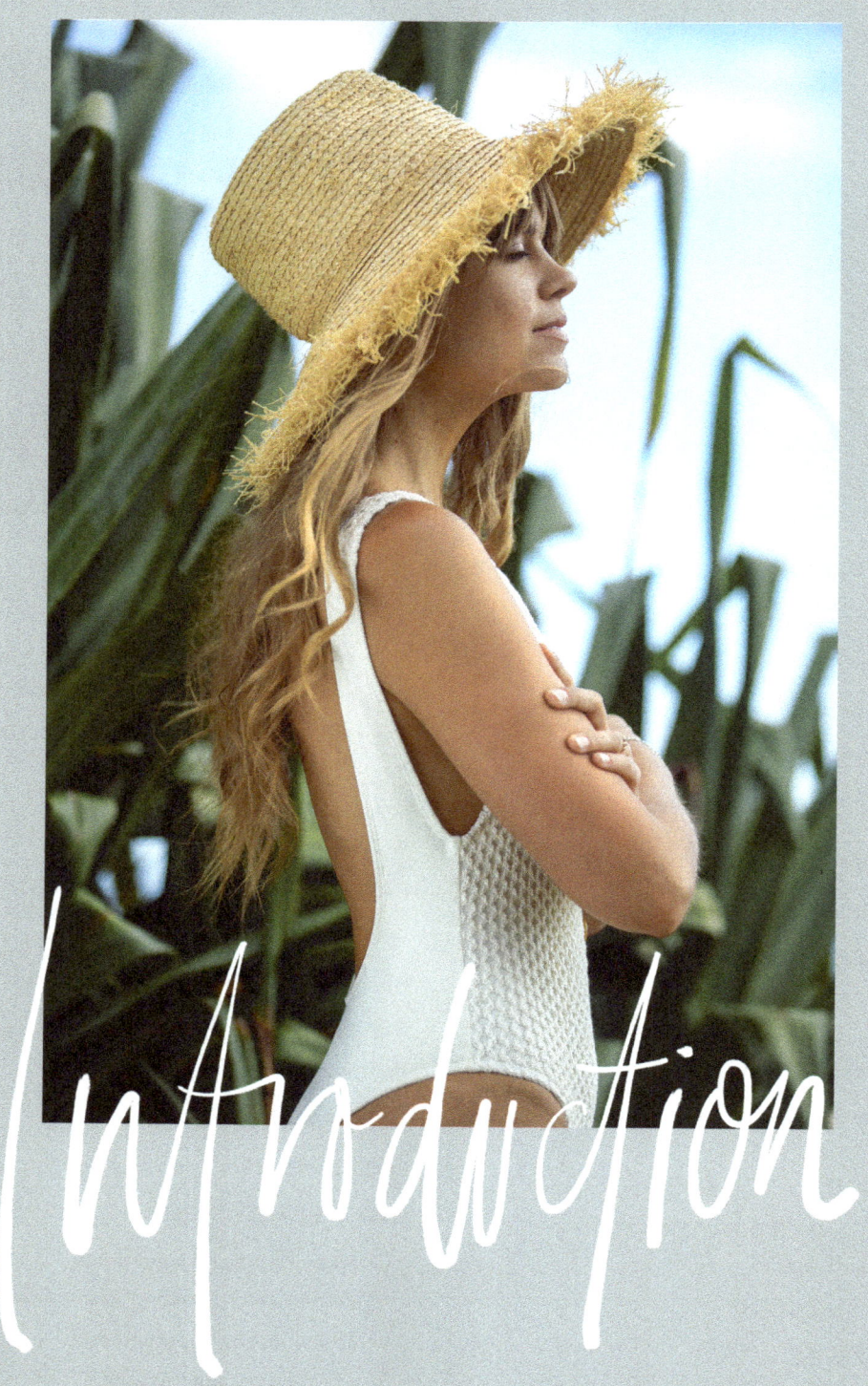

Introduction

'WHAT IS 'BEAUTY?'' AND WHAT IS THE
REAL DEFINITION OF THIS WORD?

SINCE I WAS A LITTLE GIRL, I HAVE BEEN FASCINATED BY BEAUTY IN ALL ITS FORMS. I REMEMBER EXPERIMENTING WITH MY MUM, MAKING FACE MASKS FROM BANANA, AVOCADO, PINEAPPLE, EGG WHITES AND OTHER FOODS. I EVEN REMEMBER PUTTING MASHED AVOCADO AND EGG IN MY HAIR (YUK, THE SMELL!) IN AN ATTEMPT TO KEEP MY HAIR SHINY AND LUSTROUS. WHAT WAS I THINKING? TO UNDERSTAND WHY I AND MILLIONS OF OTHER WOMEN WOULD DO SOMETHING LIKE THIS, I TO ASK THE QUESTION: WHAT IS BEAUTY? AND WHAT IS THE REAL DEFINITION OF THIS WORD?

'Beauty' was originally defined as: 'a combination of qualities, such as shape, colour or form, that pleased the aesthetic senses, especially the sight.' However, this original meaning was too restrictive. Eventually another term was added to this definition that specified: 'and a personality in which high spiritual qualities manifest'. The original meaning only focused on external beauty, but never took any internal qualities of beauty into consideration. Now we understand through studying the neuroscience of the mind that authentic beauty is not just about having symmetrical features – it is so much more than that! True beauty encompasses a beautiful mind, an empathetic heart and a benevolent soul that shows kindness and compassion for others.

Because I understand that authentic beauty is not purely about symmetry, I have not focused this book only on physical methods to enhance beauty – although there are many clever tools that may be used for this within these pages. The message within this book is about restoring health and harmony at a deep, cellular level, both physically, mentally and spiritually, enhancing one's inner and outer beauty and in doing so, becoming the most beautiful versions of ourselves, like we were always meant to be.

The desire to be more beautiful is not a new concept. The Ancient Greeks practiced methods of enhancing beauty with the use of hydrotherapy and herbs. The Ancient Greeks loved crushing berries to stain cheeks and lips and they even used ox hair to recreate eyebrows.

The Romans had some of the most beautiful bathhouses in the world where they used hydrotherapy in their beauty rituals. They even crushed oyster shells to whiten their skin, and created false teeth from ivory, bones and pastes in the hope of having more beautiful smiles. The Egyptians, too, were masters of beauty, creating Dead Sea salt scrubs, and honey and milk masks. They even used burnt almonds to make the first eyebrow pencils. In fact, every known culture since time began has incorporated some form of beauty ritual to enhance attractiveness.

Even in today's world, most of us have endured some sort of process aimed at enhancing our outer image in some way, whether it be slapping hot wax onto a sensitive bikini line in order to look more glamorous in our swimwear, or sitting through fake eyelashes being applied with glue in the hope that someone will comment on our genetically inherited 'natural lashes'. But why? If we were truly happy with ourselves on the inside, would we care if a few sun speckles peppered our nose or if our eyelashes were not as long as a Kardashian's? The attempt to enhance our beauty by enriching the human form is genetically imprinted into our DNA and remains an innate part of our soul's desire to increase our sexual appeal and, in many cultures, our social status. In following this ancient quest, many of us may believe that we will attract a better life partner (and therefore genetically stronger children), more financial security and hopefully find the inner happiness we all secretly desire.

The ability to appreciate our own individual beauty in today's world has become more difficult to achieve. Hectic schedules, financial pressures, poor-quality food and constant barrages of photoshopped images of beauty have made many of us feel that inner and outer beauty is constantly beyond our reach. Many of us are now caught up in seeking out only external methods to enhance beauty. This isn't surprising as visual images of modern beauty are posted on social media and on television, magazines and billboards. Everywhere you look, pictures of 'perfect' men and women with no fat, cellulite, imperfections or wrinkles are making many women feel unworthy, unloved and not beautiful enough. Yet what many of us do not realise is that these images are airbrushed, giving the illusion of 'perfection' in order to make us believe that this look is easily achievable by using chemical-filled face creams or expensive cosmetic procedures.

I want to express that I am not against anyone getting plastic surgery or cosmetic procedures for the right reasons. I also think that some of today's surgical techniques for enhancing beauty are quite amazing. For people that have been born with bodily disfigurations that they are not happy with and it is affecting their confidence and ability to be happy in life, then I completely understand. But when a twenty-year-old client tells me she is having muscle-relaxing injections to stop her from getting wrinkles when she gets older, it is alarming to me on a deep level. At that age cells and tissues are still regenerating, not breaking down. It is also sad when the real reason for a person's lack of confidence about their external beauty is not being addressed from the inside.

I absolutely love natural beauty treatments, and as I mentioned I have many of my own beauty rituals which I started in my teens. But as I travelled the world and pursued my love for natural medicine, I became aware that many of these outer beauty rituals will only work short-term, unless you repair and nourish yourself from the inside with the correct foods and the emotions of joy, purpose, compassion, fulfillment and freedom. And this is where AUTHENTIC BEAUTY resonates from. REAL, AUTHENTIC BEAUTY is easy to attain by performing selfless actions, thinking kind thoughts about others, living your passion in life, eating the right beautifying foods and water, and charging your cells with nature's superfoods to radiate beauty on the outside. Foods are important as every food has a different, healing vibration and can work not only on renewing elastin, hyaluronic acid and collagen in the skin, but also on improving mental health, so we can attain a more beautiful self-image and appreciation of our own beauty.

The answer to attaining authentic beauty is not found in a spray can, a chemical injection or in a magic pill. It is something that is captured as you develop techniques to refine yourself into a more beautiful soul internally, which then radiates an attractive image externally.

Natural beauty is directly connected to your actions, to your ability to feel empathy and to consciously choose the right foods and nutrients for your wellbeing.

When you eat cleanly and all of your internal systems are working beautifully, this harmony is reflected in your outer image in the form of radiant, youthful skin, thick and shiny hair, strong nails and sparkling eyes.

> *The answer to attaining authentic beauty is not found in a spray can, a chemical injection or in a magic pill. It is something that is captured as you develop techniques to refine yourself into a more beautiful soul internally, which then radiates an attractive image externally."*

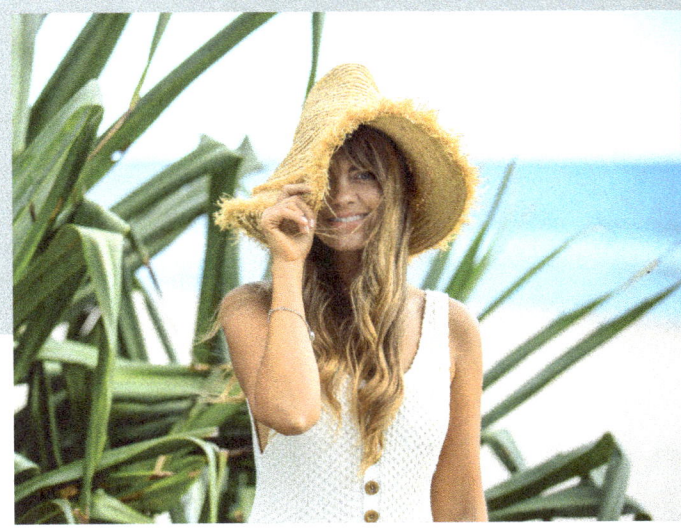

As you delve through these pages I will reveal modern and age-old tools which can be used to enhance your own natural beauty and wellness. I will also uncover nature's beauty secrets and how natural substances can protect you against the cumulative effects of chemical fillers, as well as mimicking the actions of these if you choose to go in a more natural direction. I am offering safer, natural and more effective support tools and alternatives which will allow you to maintain a youthful appearance and graceful ageing on a deep and spiritual level.

This book is divided into two important sections. The first section explores modern day beauty thieves like free radicals and telomeres. It also addresses the most magnetic beauty foods, how to achieve perfect digestion, how to purify your insides and all of the key elements of increasing your attractiveness and happiness. The second section contains delicious and beautifying recipes to enhance weight loss, improve collagen turnover, beautify your hair, skin and nails and so much more. Every recipe has been designed to be a perfect balance of beauty-electrifying minerals, vitamins and phytonutrients. In the back of this book you will find unique beauty tables to help boost collagen, hyalauronic acid, natural tanning and so much more.

This book was intended to provide you with the physical and spiritual tools to help you rejuvenate your insides and, in doing so, improve the beauty of your connective tissues, skin, hair, eyes and nails. Anyone who knows me understands how passionate I am about healing and about helping every soul achieve the greatest level of happiness. I also believe it is important to protect the earth. By using more of earth's natural tools in an ethical way it will we help to preserve our planet's health as well. The beauty tools in this book are magical, and in alignment with nature, and they will help you to live life more richly and more harmoniously. In doing this you will radiate your beautiful, magnetic soul out to others, allowing others in your life to feel your magic. Natural beauty and wellness is found within these pages!!!

Please read on to discover the secrets that it took me over twenty-five years of consistent natural medicine practice to learn, but which I believe every individual has a right to know.

In love, health, freedom and happiness and of course 'natural beauty'.

Katrina
Ellis

CHAPTER ONE

Nature's Secrets

TO RADIANT BEAUTY

BEAUTY THIEVES and YOUTH BENEFACTORS

DNA BEAUTY CODE –
Unlocking your Genes

I am sure you know at least one person who can eat anything they want and their skin stays flawless, their metabolism perfect and their tummy as flat as a board. And yet, someone else can eat the smallest amount of sugar and suddenly their hips begin to bulge and their skin erupts in protest. The beauty of genetics! Flawless skin, a fast metabolism, thick luscious hair and other youth-promoting attributes definitely have a lot to do with the genetics we are given. If you feel you were handed the curse of 'bad genetics', luckily, not all is lost. This can be rectified. Yes, it is true!

Gene expression can be altered in both a positive and negative way by the foods and nutrients you eat, as well as by the emotions you express. This phenomenon is known as 'epigenetics'. Epigenetics is the study of changes in gene activity that is not caused by changes in the actual DNA line-up. Epigenetic responses to physical factors like stress, diet and exercise can occur within just a few hours, so whatever you choose to eat, think or even feel can alter the expression of your genes either in a good or bad way.

But are genetics the only reason why we age?

Scientists believe ageing has to do with a decline in important biological and metabolic functions. This decline is driven by many factors that emerge from not only heredity, but also from our environments, lifestyles and diets. Ageing is a multi-faceted process, involving a large number of functions including genetic instability, telomere shrinking, poor nutrient absorption, free radical attack and senescence.

Of course, good genetics can have a beneficial impact on skin health and ageing; however, lifestyle and environmental factors can definitely uproot this potential either in a negative or positive way. Our genetic material provides an important backbone to help protect against advanced ageing – however, it is constantly under assault from external factors like sunlight, air pollution, chemical-filled cosmetics, illness and inflammation, and also from internal factors like stress, a high alcohol intake, toxic foods, smoking, poor cooking methods and even the passage of time. If a person's DNA is not repaired, this can lead to advanced ageing and disease. When we are young, the body's cells repair quickly, but as we age, this process slows down. Longevity and beauty research looks at ways to reduce cell damage while speeding up new cell turnover. To understand how to do this, it is important to understand what the 'free radical theory' is.

Quick Tip

DID YOU KNOW THAT YOUR 100 TRILLION CELLS UNDERGO UP TO 100,000 DAMAGING ATTACKS PER DAY?

Luckily our cells are programmed to die so that new ones can regenerate,
effectively rebuilding our body's tissues over and over again.

When we are babies, cell renewal occurs every	When we become a teenager it occurs every	In middle-age it occurs every	When we are over fifty it occurs every
14 DAYS	**21-28** DAYS	**28-42** DAYS	**42-84** DAYS

WITH CELL TURNOVER IT IS POSSIBLE TO GET:

A NEW STOMACH LINING	A NEW LIVER	NEW NAILS	NEW HEAD OF HAIR
every five days.	every five months.	every six to ten months.	every three to six years.

Cell regeneration is programmed into our DNA, but luckily nature has some cell-regenerating superheroes to speed this up.

MY FAV'S ARE:

HERBAL HEROES

withania, rosemary, Green tea, turmeric, burdock root and milk thistle.

FOOD SUPERHEROES

broccoli, sprouts, asparagus, artichokes, pomegranate, berries, parsley, coriander, shiitake mushrooms, maitake, garlic, ginger and cruciferous vegetables.

FREE RADICALS
are MASTER THIEVES

Free radicals are dangerous little predators that roam around taking bites out of our cells and DNA, creating stress and advanced ageing. They are oxygen molecules that have lost an electron, which is why they are nicknamed Reactive Oxygen Species (ROS). This makes them dangerous and unstable. In the search to repair themselves, they steal electrons from healthy molecules, creating more free radicals and a great deal of damage to other cells. Free radicals are extremely damaging to the health of our DNA, skin, tissues and cells. Over sixty different diseases, including advanced ageing, are linked to free radical attack.

Free radicals can be made internally from poor food breakdown, but they can also be found roaming in the environment in the form of cigarette smoke, pesticides, herbicides, toxins, heavy metals, pollution and sunlight. Overexposure from harmful UV rays is the worst ageing culprit. As soon as we step out into the bright, midday sun our skin draws in these rays, activating free radicals. Collagen, the yummy substance that keeps our skin looking young, is extremely vulnerable to free radical damage. These free radicals activate molecules that travel to the DNA, turning on a chemical called AP-1 that creates collagen-dissolving enzymes, and you guessed it, like a fire they melt away the collagen matrix, causing wrinkles.

Luckily, nature has gifted us with some fire-fighting superheroes known as antioxidants. Antioxidants selflessly offer an electron to break the free radical chain, stopping the ageing chaos. Antioxidant superheroes are abundantly found in living foods. There are many different types. Some antioxidants, like the flavonoids found in berries, act like a shield, giving direct protection. Non-enzymatic antioxidants, found in foods rich in Vitamin A, C, E, manganese, selenium, zinc, carotenes and polyphenols, stop breakdown by disrupting the free radical chain. Enzymatic antioxidants stop DNA damage by converting free radicals into hydrogen peroxide and then into water.

MY FAV BEAUTY ANTIOXIDANTS INCLUDE:

*   Superoxide dismutase (SOD) – this breaks down superoxide into hydrogen peroxide and oxygen with the aid of copper, zinc, manganese and iron.

*   Catalase (CAT) works by converting hydrogen peroxide into water and oxygen.

*   Glutathione peroxidase (GSH) – selenium-containing enzymes that break down hydrogen peroxide into alcohols.

By eating a nutritious, antioxidant-rich diet, you can easily defend against modern day free radical predators which destroy natural beauty and create ageing chaos.

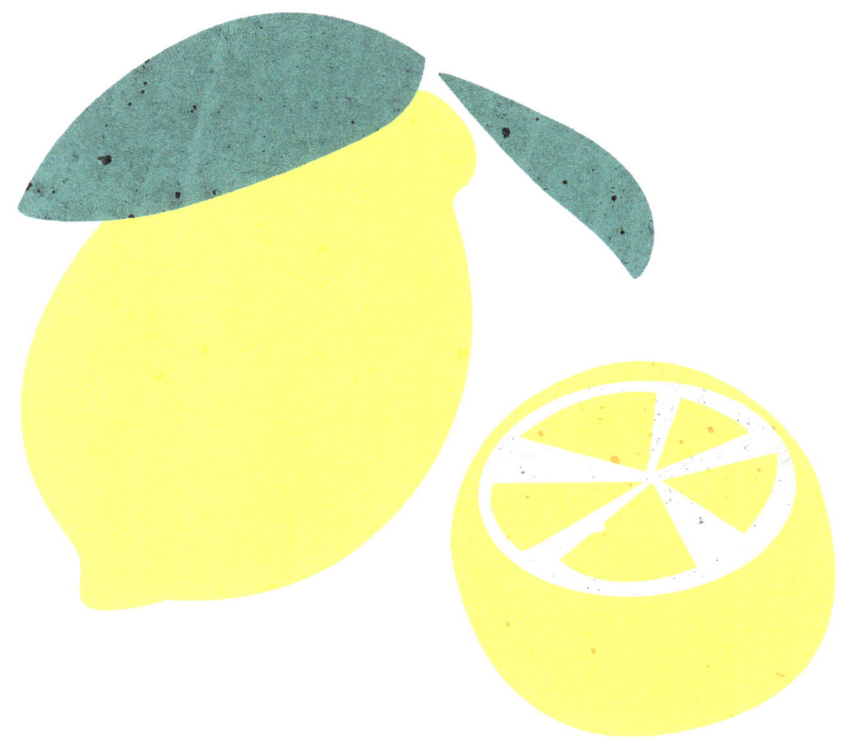

Youth-Promoting Antioxidants

Glutathione-rich foods like grass-fed meats, raw dairy and eggs, protein, turmeric, avocado, artichokes and oily fish.

Resveratrol, found in dark grapes, berries and red wine.

Carotenoids, found in carrots, sweet potatoes, peppers, kiwifruit, squash and grapes.

Astaxanthin, found in red or pink fish, crustaceans, fish eggs and red peppers.

Polyphenols, found in berries, Green tea and cocoa

Kale, leafy greens, cabbage, broccoli, spinach, legumes, pomegranates, walnuts, pecans, red and green chilli, red beets, purple cabbages, plums, pears, artichokes, elderberries.

Herbs and spices like cumin, star anise, coriander, oregano, thyme, rosemary, rosehips, turmeric, cloves, ginger, cinnamon, basil, mustard, curry, paprika.

Superfoods like Green tea, wheatgrass, barley grass, and phytoplankton.

SENESCENCE
– A Roadblock to Youth

'Senescence' is such a beautiful word – but unfortunately it isn't a beautiful process. Senescent cells are defiant cells that refuse to die as programmed and instead choose to live in a trance-like state beside healthy cells. They are dysfunctional cells, as they do not divide anymore, yet they cannot be regenerated back into healthy, dividing cells. These cells have no purpose. They wander around aimlessly in the blood creating toxicity and internal damage. They are caused by constant and prolonged exposure to stress and other forms of internal and external damage. They stop the body from absorbing nutrients; they promote fat gain and obesity, suppress immunity, disturb blood sugar balance, and harm the collagen turnover in the skin, accelerating ageing. In some people, senescent cells can make up 15% of their cells. These cells are very dangerous, as they love to promote inflammation and place a strain on the body's immune system. Luckily nature has some fantastic allies that can destroy these toxic, defiant cells.

SENESCENCE-FIGHTING FOODS AND NUTRIENTS

Vitamin E and mixed tocopherols, polyphenols like quercetin, catechins and resveratrol, rosmarinic acid, isothiocyanates, sulphides and carnosine all help to stop senescent cells.

Foods rich in these nutrients include:

Avocado, shellfish, Green tea, sweet potatoes, berries, garlic, ginger, beets, red peppers, dark grapes, pomegranates, turmeric, rosemary, broccoli, brussels sprouts, cauliflower, and collards.

Quercetin can result in a 50% reduction in senescent cells. The highest food sources of these include: elderberries, red onions, white onions, blackcurrants, coriander, cranberries, green chilli, kale, blueberries, red apples, romaine lettuces, pears, and spinach.

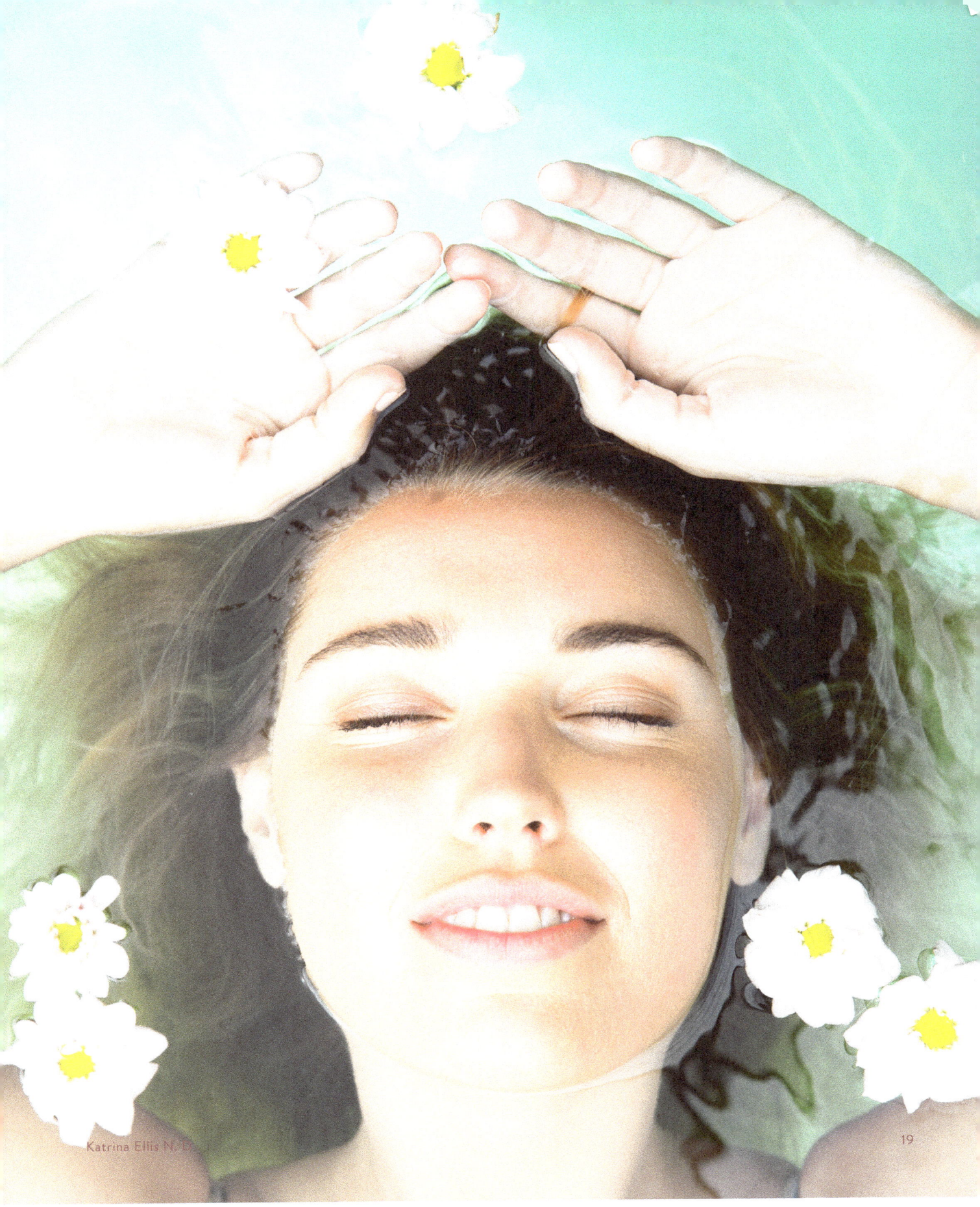

LONGER TELOMERES
= Longevity

At the end of each DNA strand is a telomere. These are like the protective plastic case or a cap at the end of the shoelace that protects it. As the cell replicates to replenish itself, the telomeres begin to shorten, yet the DNA stays intact. As the cell replicates over and over, the telomeres get too short to do their job and they fray. This can have a detrimental effect on the health of the DNA, leading to disease and ageing. Therefore, looking for ways to lengthen the telomeres can have a positive impact on wellness and beauty. Changes to your diet, stress management, the way we think and love, family support and other factors can result in longer telomeres. Feelings like anxiety, depression and loneliness can shorten telomeres, leading to advanced ageing. A study in Spain showed that positive practices like mindfulness meditation, when practiced daily, can promote healthy changes in telomeres and improve one's beauty and longevity.

Certain foods, lifestyle choices and emotions can have an impact on lengthening telomeres and improving your epigenetics. The next table highlights the best natural telomere troops to enhance natural beauty and anti-ageing.

"

A STUDY IN SPAIN SHOWED THAT POSITIVE PRACTICES LIKE MINDFULNESS MEDITATION, WHEN PRACTICED DAILY, CAN PROMOTE HEALTHY CHANGES IN TELOMERES AND IMPROVE ONE´S BEAUTY AND LONGEVITY.

TELOMERE TROOPS

Astaxanthin is a powerful antioxidant sixty times stronger than Vitamin C.
It can cross the blood-brain-barrier to work both inside and outside of a cell.
This is found in fish eggs and red salmon.

Fermented foods and **probiotics** – sauerkraut, kimchee, kefir, natto.

Selenium – found in blue corn, brazil nuts and bone broths.

Vitamin E – found in almonds, spinach, sweet potato.

Vitamin D3 – from safe sun exposure and found in oily fish.

Omega 3 fatty acids – found in flaxseeds, hemp seeds & oil, avocado, oily fish, blue-green algae.

Zinc – found in activated nuts and seeds, especially pumpkin seeds, seafood, fish, ginger.

Iron – spinach, pumpkin seeds, lentils.

Magnesium and Folate – found in green leafy vegetables, almonds, spinach, legumes.

Vitamin B12 – found in grass fed beef, fish, crustaceans, blue-green algae, prawns.

Vitamin C – found in peppers, kale, kiwifruit, limes, lemons.

Glutathione – made from sulphurous vegetables like artichokes, broccoli, brussels sprouts, cabbage, cauliflower, bok choy, watercress, radish, garlic, onions.

Manganese – found in melons, pecans, almonds, avocado, sweet potato, brown rice, pineapple.

Antioxidants like resveratrol, coenzyme Q10, grape seed, algae extracts and curcumin.

Polyphenols – found in cacao, Green tea and berries.

Deep sleep: eight hours + a night.

For women 3 ½ hours of vigorous **exercise weekly** can increase telomere length.

Intermittent fasting can dramatically enhance DNA repair and telomere length.

Stress and trauma shortens telomeres dramatically, so take a deep breath and RELAX!!!

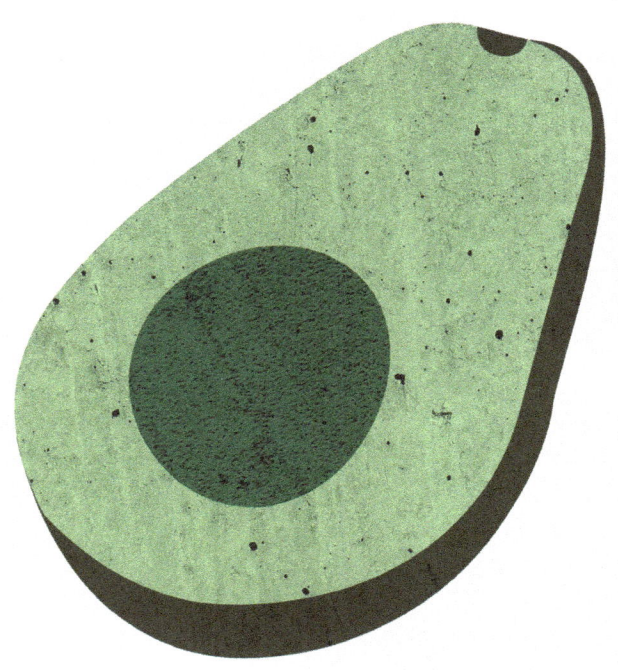

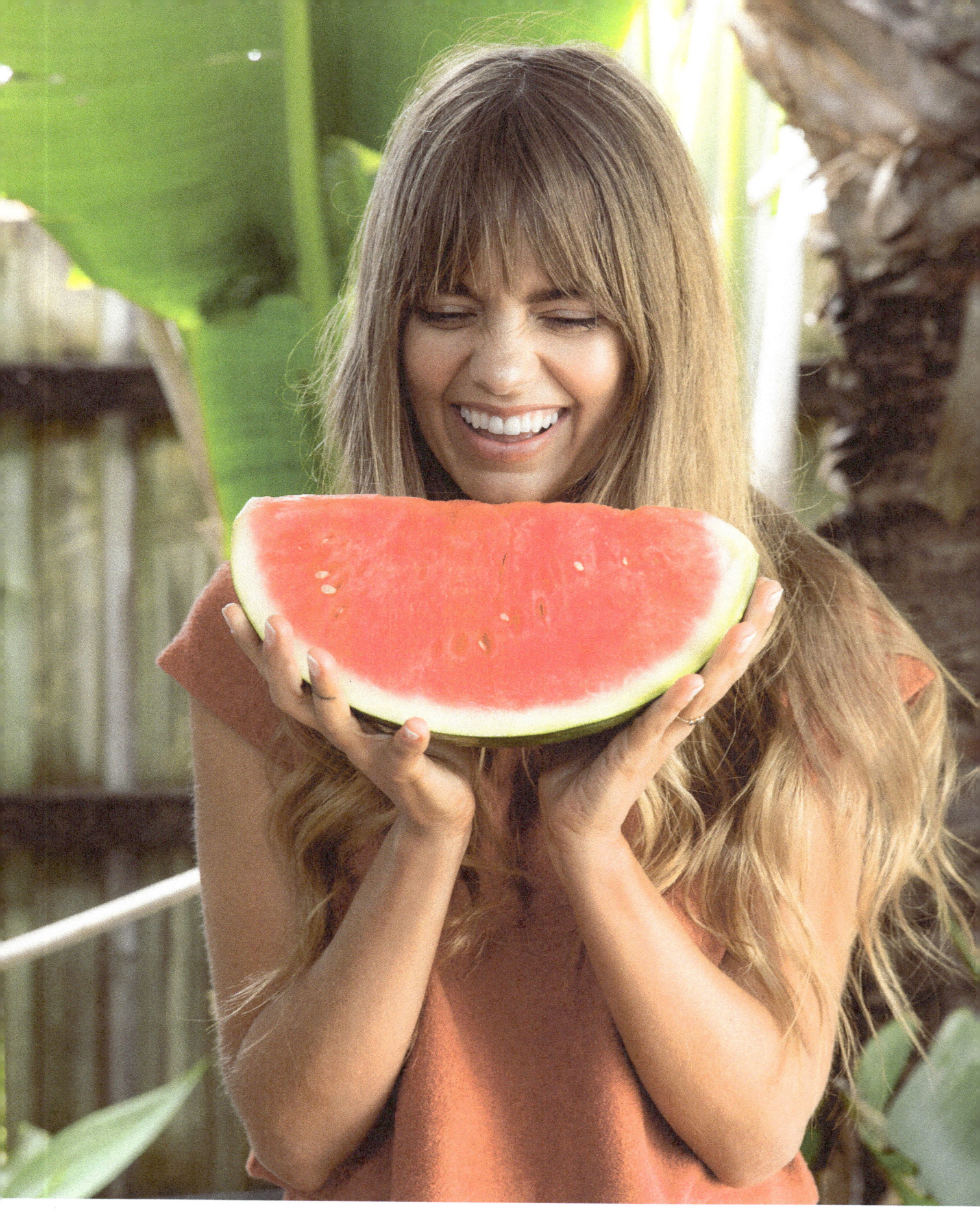

EXTERNAL AGEING THIEVES

There are many external factors that can contribute to reducing our beauty and health potential. Some of the worst of these include a lack of sleep and poor sleeping positions, low oxygen intake, obesity, stress, negative facial expressions (especially angry ones), a lack of exercise and a loss of fat between the skin and muscles.

BEAUTY FOOD THIEVES

Healing foods are without question one of the biggest keys to disease prevention, radiant beauty and happiness. The modern Western diet is lacking in youth-promoting nutrients and rich in toxic substances that advance ageing by encouraging a loss of skin tone and elasticity, leading to wrinkles, thin and brittle skin, age spots, cellulite and other signs of advanced ageing. Toxic processed foods strain the body's digestive system, use up valuable anti-ageing enzymes and put a strain on filtration organs. They also create free radical production. Foods that encourage this include an excess intake of animal products, too much caffeine and alcohol, preservatives, additives, table salt, GMO grains, saturated fats and sugars. Our beautiful collagen structures which help to prevent wrinkles require hydration and support from powerful antioxidants to protect against the damage of these 'beauty thieves'. Foods rich in Vitamin A, C, E, D, K2, indoles and polyphenols like lycopene, catechins and resveratrol kindly offer the protection needed to withstand the ravaging effects of these beauty-robbing monsters.

INTERESTING FACT

Did you know that there are communities in the world that remain beautiful, ageless and virtually disease free?

The top three include:

Okinawa in Japan – Okinawans owe their superb health to regular exercise, a nutritious diet high in seaweeds, fermented soy and ocean foods, alkaline water, beautiful social connections and abstaining from over-eating.

Sardinia in Italy – Although genetics play a big role, Sardinians follow a Mediterranean diet, as well as walking and exercising regularly, and having active and fun social lives.

Nicoya in Costa Rica – Nicoyans sleep eight hours every night, eat a nutrient rich diet and drink lots of alkaline water high in calcium and magnesium.

PROCESSED ANIMAL PRODUCTS

Most processed animal products like non-organic meats and dairy are wrinkle accelerators that promote arachidonic acid formation, an inflammatory substance which is formed when we eat too many foods containing Omega 6 fatty acids. Other foods rich in Omega 6 fatty acids include margarine and processed vegetable oils. Inflammation drives tissue damage and cell breakdown that causes the skin to lose its valuable moisture layer. Without this soothing moisture, the skin begins to wrinkle and sag. However, a small amount of grass fed, organic dairy and red meat can help to promote glutathione production in some constitutions. Glutathione is a powerful antioxidant that encourages heavy metal removal and guards against the ravaging effects of free radicals.

SUGAR
The Deceptive Thief

Sugar is a deceptive thief. It tastes so good and at first and tricks you into feeling great, but it ends up leaving you robbed of nutrition and loaded with poison. Eating lots of artificial, processed sugar is a perfect way to speed up ageing.

Sugar causes glycation in the body. This is a process where sugar attaches to a protein in the bloodstream and causes new molecules known as 'advanced glycation end products' or AGES to form. As AGES build up because of a high sugar intake, they damage collagen and elastin fibres, causing a loss of resilience and sagging skin. Even some grains, fruits and vegetables convert to glucose and feed this destructive glycation process.

Nearly all processed foods contain sugar, hidden cleverly behind names like barley malt, corn syrup, dextrose, fruit juice concentrate, maltose, molasses, rice syrup, fructose, high fructose corn syrup, mannitol and others. In fact, there are over sixty-one disguised names for sugar. To be safe, opt for organic fruits and healthier grains like quinoa, teff, brown and wild rice, amaranth and buckwheat and natural sweeteners like birch xylitol, stevia and monk fruit.

Artificial sweeteners are just as bad as sucrose. Aspartame, one artificial sweetener, excites neurons in the brain that encourage cell death, leading to dementia and even certain forms of cancer. Always avoid high fructose corn syrup. This is added to pastries, biscuits, lollies and soft drinks and labelled with many different names.

Even, so called 'natural sugars' like agave, stevia and xylitol can be toxic, if they are over-processed and exposed to high heats for long periods of time.

BAD FATS
cause Ageing Chaos

As I have constantly said in all of my books – 'not all fats are created equal'. There are many different types of fats found in foods. These include saturated, trans, monounsaturated and polyunsaturated fats. The modern age accelerators are 'trans and saturated fats'. Any oil which is heat-treated (causing it to change its original molecular structure) becomes a dangerous fat that can advance the ageing process.

Always choose cold-pressed, unrefined, organic oils in dark bottles that have not been exposed to heat or chemically altered. Be very careful with modern, processed oils like soybean, sunflower, corn, canola, cottonseed and safflower oils, as most of these are industrially made from genetically modified crops.

My favourite salad oils are hemp, macadamia, avocado, sacha inchi, olive, walnut, sesame, goji and black seed oils.

The best cooking oils are avocado (if kept below 500° F or 270°C), olive oil (if kept below 325° F or 160°C), organic macadamia and grass-fed ghee (for some constitutions). Ghee is rich in Vitamin A, D, E, K and CLA. I am fond of coconut oil as it has a high heating point, but I do not believe that it is the 'miracle oil' it is over-promoted to be. It definitely has some worthy anti-bacterial properties and works as a cooking oil, but it is high in saturated fats so for some European constitutions it should still be used in moderation.

I also like using water as the base of my cooking with lots of bone broth (and yes, there are vegan broths available made from miso, shiitake and algae – check out my recipe section).

PESTICIDE POISONS

Pesticides are used to increase crop production and to 'beautify' foods to ensure that more produce is sold for greater profits. However, these chemicals are extremely toxic as they are designed to kill agricultural pests – and in the end these toxins are consumed by you. Many wheat and grain crops undergo a number of sprays with Roundup to dry out their crops. This glyphosate-based pesticide is claimed to be 'harmless' by its developers Monsanto. How ridiculous!

After many years of scientific research, high levels of Roundup in food is being linked to health problems like ADHD, autism, birth defects, cancer, breast cancer, celiac disease, hypothyroidism, lymphoma, leaky gut and advanced ageing.

In animal farming, antibiotics and hormones are used to boost growth rates. Residues of these drugs are damaging and ageing to humans. They mimic the body's hormone levels adding to your hormone load. This can increase the risk of different types of cancer like breast, prostate, bowel, lymphoma, multiple myeloma and even brain tumours. For the health and wellbeing of your family, always opt for organic, local produce.

WATER
Liquid Gold

Drinking pure, alkaline, mineral-rich water has been a secret to perfect flawless skin and other beauty factors for many years. Our body is 80% water, so without the correct amount of water being consumed, the levels of acids, toxins and harmful substances begin to rise in the bloodstream.

Every organ of filtration requires mineral-rich water to function well. A long-term study performed by the World Health Organisation evaluated the reason why certain communities living in the world had a low incidence of disease and incredible longevity. One of the common factors amongst these communities was the quality of their WATER. The water was clean, rich in natural alkaline minerals and therefore highly oxygenated. Because of this, their blood pH was maintained in an alkaline state, free of toxins. Therefore, their organs were nourished and hydrated.

I drink mineral-rich water with a pH of around 9.5 that is rich in hydrogen. I also put my water into a VitaJuwel bottle with powerful crystals inside to restructure the water ions increasing its healing potential. I love clean, energized water!

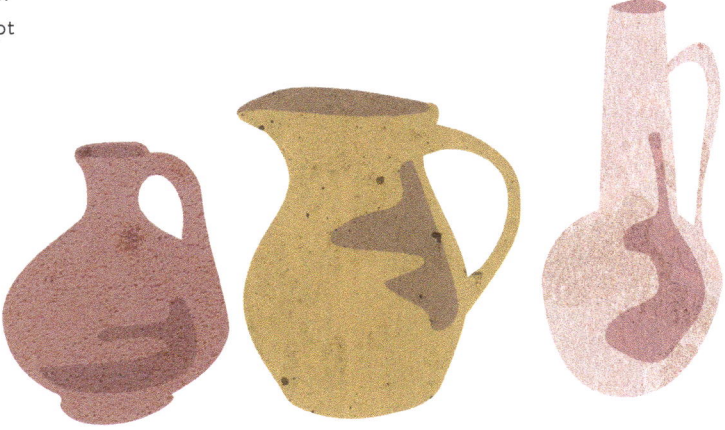

STRESS
The Beauty Robbing Mastermind

Every time we feel worried, depressed or stressed, our body's acid levels rise, increasing inflammation and shortening our body's telomeres. As these protective DNA caps shorten, their structure weakens, encouraging healthy cells to die faster. This leads to rapid ageing and an increased risk of diseases. Stress, anxiety and trauma can also drive a high adrenaline and cortisol release. Too much cortisol causes excess tummy fat, blood sugar problems, bone loss, fatigue, digestive upsets, lowered immunity and dry, wrinkled skin. On top of this, stress, anger and negative emotions, when regularly expressed, have the ability to paint permanent, unattractive lines on our faces, robbing us of our natural beauty.

To solve this, try laughing and smiling more often.

If you are feeling stressed practice yoga regularly and the powerful breathing exercises found in the spiritual beauty section to help you find your peace again.

SUN and RADIATION

Electromagnetic (EMR) frequencies from mobile phones, computers, 5G, flying, X-rays and dangerous UV radiation from the sun all generate free radicals which can damage a cell's DNA, leading to advanced ageing, skin damage and disease. Luckily nature has given us some effective natural sunscreens in the form of carotene, found in sweet potato, carrots, peaches and apricots, and lycopene, found in tomato products.

Mobile phones, computers and other electronic devices contain cadmium in the keys. Cadmium is a heavy metal that depletes zinc. Zinc helps to make powerful antioxidants to protect you against ageing and disease. Electromagnetic radiation from phones, computers and flying also depletes iodine stores. Iodine is a mineral that enhances metabolism, protects against cancer, beautifies the hair and boosts energy levels. To reduce the damage from harmful EMFs I use a Blushield in my home, office, in my car and on my body. Blushields radiate huge amounts of scalar waves to override the damaging and harmful effects of radioactive waves.

For more information on supplements and devices to protect against the danger of bad electromagnetic frequencies, please visit www.katrinaellis.com.au or www.wholistichouse.co

*Beautiful skin
is a reflection
of inner wellness*

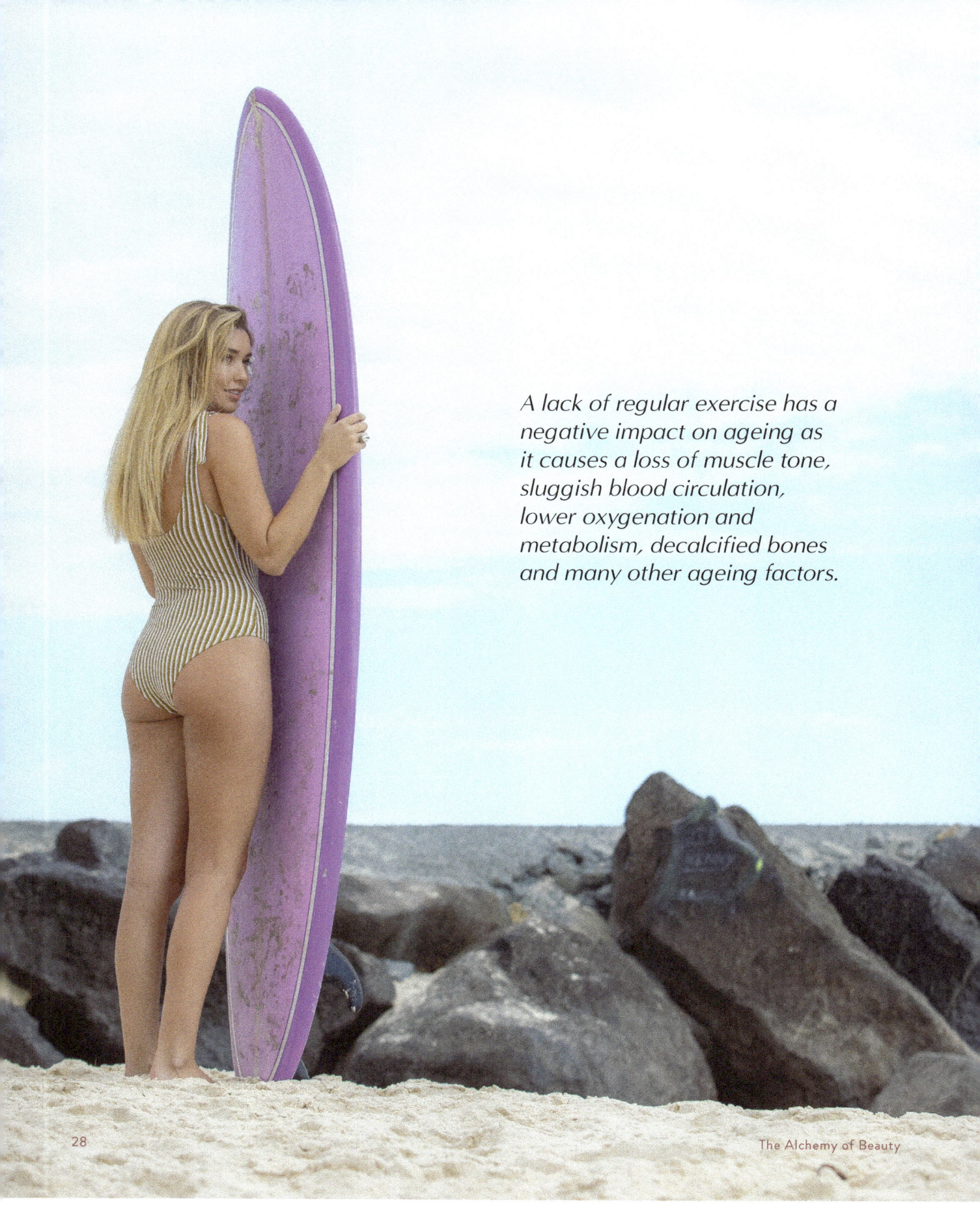

A lack of regular exercise has a negative impact on ageing as it causes a loss of muscle tone, sluggish blood circulation, lower oxygenation and metabolism, decalcified bones and many other ageing factors.

EXERCISE – The Right Movement

Exercise is a key factor to increasing happiness and for boosting blood, oxygen and nutrient flow to improve skin, hair, and nail quality. An elevated heart rate pushes blood through tiny capillaries in the skin, encouraging healthy new skin cells to rise to the surface. This promotes a healthy, radiant glow. Through sweating, the body is able to eliminate toxins and acid wastes, taking the pressure off the liver. Exercise lowers inflammation, balances hormones and reduces free radical damage. When you sweat, tiny capillaries in the skin open up, allowing more blood to reach the skin's surface to deliver nutrients to repair damage. This also speeds up the collagen-healing process reducing wrinkle formation. As we get older, fibroblasts in the skin (the cells that produce collagen) get sluggish, but luckily exercise can help pump them back up.

A lack of regular exercise has a negative impact on ageing as it causes a loss of muscle tone, sluggish blood circulation, lower oxygenation and metabolism, decalcified bones and many other ageing factors.

It is important to do at least thirty minutes of exercise daily to move your blood and nourish your cells.

Yoga is one of the best forms of movement as it reduces age-promoting stress hormones and transforms your body and mind through conscious movement, meditation and breathing. One of the best beauty exercises in the world is AERIAL YOGA. This allows more oxygen-rich blood to get to the brain helping to improve the glow to your skin and hair. By doing at least 30 minutes of cardiovascular exercise daily like fast walking, surfing, swimming, cycling and others and incorporating resistance exercises like pilates and yoga a few times weekly you will be surprised at how quickly you can transform your spiritual and physical beauty in a positive direction.

SLEEPING BEAUTY

Sleeping Beauty was onto it when she ate the apple and slept for many years. When she woke up, everyone around her was old and withered – yet Sleeping Beauty preserved her ageless beauty. She knew that good quality, deep sleep was the secret to healing and rejuvenating every cell and tissue in the human body. Skin produces the highest amount of collagen when we are in a deep sleep.

If you only get five hours of sleep per night, you will acquire twice as many wrinkles as someone who sleeps eight hours per night. Early in our nighttime sleep cycle, youth-promoting human growth hormone (or HGH) surges. HGH encourages the repair and rejuvenation of all tissues including our collagen matrix. Cell division peaks at two am, so if you go to bed too late or don't sleep at all, just imagine how quickly you will age.

Deep sleep also helps to counteract the effects of stress-driving cortisol. Sleep apnea invites quick ageing. When we breathe in more oxygen at night, the blood pH becomes more alkaline, collagen receives more oxygen for rejuvenation and all factors that contribute to disease decrease.

If you are having sleeping problems, taking a sleeping pill is not the answer. The body is giving you messages to tell you to fix something internally. Neurotransmitters like serotonin, melatonin and GABA help with peaceful sleep. If you suspect a neurotransmitter imbalance, ask your naturopath to order a urine neurotransmitter test and a saliva hormone profile. Hormone imbalances can have a big impact on sleeping problems. Always sleep in a dark room to boost your melatonin, and check for any deficiencies of zinc, magnesium, B6, tryptophan and calcium.

Age-Robbing Thieves and Youth Benefactors

AGE-ROBBING THIEVES	HOW DO THEY DO THIS?	YOUTH-PROMOTING BENEFACTORS
Sugar, artificial sugars: corn starch, corn syrup, dextrose, modified corn starch and other nasty sugars.	Sugar robs the body of B vitamins, zinc and other minerals. It creates glycation and destroys collagen.	**Natural sugars** like birch xylitol, stevia leaf, luo han guo or monk fruit (unheated and unprocessed).
Saturated fats, trans fats, processed vegetable oils that are heat-treated, and chemically-altered.	Refined, GMO vegetable oils increase inflammation, congest the liver and arteries and drive up all ageing and disease markers.	**Cold pressed oils** like flaxseed, olive, macadamia, sacha inchi, black seed, avocado and hemp oil – all oils should be organic and not exposed to heat or light.
Excess animal products: especially grain fed and antibiotic-filled.	Acid driving, age-promoting and time consuming on the digestive system to process.	Include **more plant-based options.** If you need to consume meat, only choose local, grass fed and eat it in small amounts.
Processed junk foods, artificial colours, flavours, additives etc.	Impedes filtration organs, drives acidity, devoid of any health benefit.	Choose predominantly **home-cooked, local produce free** from any nasties.
Stress and negative emotions like jealousy, anger, guilt, greed.	Creates high acidity, releases inflammatory hormones that cause collagen breakdown, depletes valuable youth nutrients, imprints ageing lines on the face.	**Happiness**, relaxation, meditation, feeling love, yoga, joy, freedom, stress relieving exercises.

AGE-ROBBING THIEVES	HOW DO THEY DO THIS?	YOUTH-PROMOTING BENEFACTORS
Acidic tap water filled with artificial fluoride and chemicals and reverse osmosis devoid of minerals.	Fluoride is a neurotoxin that damages the thyroid. Other toxins found in tap water are mercury, copper, aluminium, lead and chlorine. Aluminium depletes the silica needed for healthy collagen.	**Alkaline, mineral-rich water infused with hydrogen is pure healing water.** Clean mountain and river water. Vitajuwel crystal or vortex water energises and restructures the water for better hydration.
Lack of sleep.	Deep sleep is when most cellular rejuvenation occurs, body fat is burnt and DNA and RNA is repaired. It also promotes human growth hormone and collagen repair.	Plenty of **deep quality sleep before 10 pm.** It is important to sleep through and not have lots of waking periods. If you are waking often, there is a problem that needs repairing.
Too much caffeine, alcohol, nicotine, pharmaceutical drugs.	Congests the liver, digestive system and strips the body of valuable health promoting vitamins and minerals.	Replace excess caffeine with **green or herbal teas, bone broth**s, green smoothies and cold pressed juices.
Hormone imbalance: low oestrogen low progesterone, low testosterone.	Oestrogen helps to support the body's collagen network. Testosterone imbalances can cause acne, hair loss, oily skin and more.	Balance oestrogen, progesterone and testosterone with a **raw, plant-based diet** rich in cruciferous vegetables, nutrients and herbs
Toxins, heavy metals, environmental pollutants, pollution.	These toxins overload filtration organs ultimately driving dirty blood.	Regular **detoxification and fasting,** heavy metal chelation, near far infrared sauna therapy
Excess UV sunlight.	Advances skin ageing and pigmentation.	Use only **natural sunscreens.** Sunlight at the right time of day is important for healthy Vitamin D production.

CHAPTER TWO

NATURE'S SECRETS TO RADIANT BEAUTY

Alchemy of Beauty Diet

ALCHEMY of BEAUTY DIET

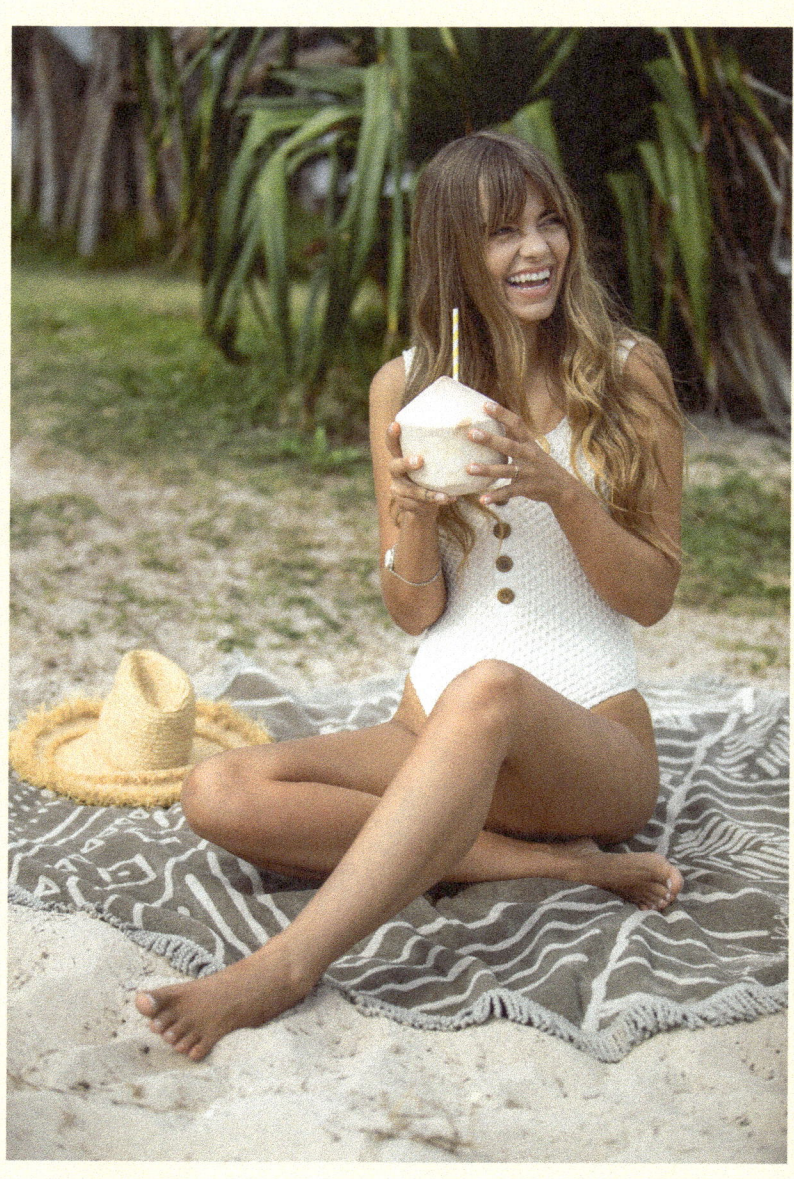

AS A KID I USED TO KEENLY WATCH SPACE AGE JETSON CARTOONS AND LAUGH WHEN I WOULD SEE THE PROCESSED, PACKAGED FOODS BEING CONSUMED AFTER PRESSING A BUTTON.

I thought this possible future was so far-fetched and hilarious! But now I know that the Jetsons were onto something, as the food we eat now is no different than the Jetsons' futuristic processed food. If you stroll through any commercial food market today, there are countless rows of food in boxes, cans, containers and jars. It is a wonderful assortment of modern processed foods, hidden sodium and sugars, toxic additives, adulterated fats and other age-promoting nasties – all perfect ingredients to promote premature wrinkles, thin and lifeless hair, tooth and bone decay, rapid mineral loss and of course, all of today's modern diseases.

The human body is not equipped to recognise foods that have been chemically altered, and to compensate, it tries to eliminate them as quickly as possible via its filtration organs. This causes purification systems like the liver, kidneys, lymphatics and digestion to become overloaded with unfamiliar wastes, which are not only beauty-robbing, but devoid of nutrition. If our body is overloaded with pollutants, it throws these dirty, unfamiliar toxins out via the largest organ of elimination, the SKIN. The skin then bubbles with anger, resulting in rashes, age spots, blemishes, dryness, wrinkles and other unwanted signs of premature ageing.

It is easy to shave years off your physical age just by choosing to eat a living, enzyme-rich diet. Our body is constantly under attack from external and internal age-promoting free radicals. The Alchemy of Beauty Diet provides you with the right tools to protect you against these beauty-robbing thieves. A predominantly raw, plant-based diet is beautifying in every way – physically, spiritually and ethically. Living foods add a sparkle to the eyes, a glow to the skin and a luscious body and shine to the hair.

One buzzword common in the beauty industry today is hyaluronic acid. This substance is naturally present in the skin. It helps to maintain hydration and a youthful, plump skin. As we age, levels of this deplete and so does the quality of our skin. One of the richest natural sources of this substance is found in RAW FOODS.

Proteins have anti-ageing qualities and can also repair skin damage. Everyone's skin is made of collagen, which is formed from the building blocks of protein. So, good amounts of absorbable protein in the diet, as well as Vitamin C, magnesium and silica are important for boosting collagen production for healthy and glowing skin.

FOODS WITH BEAUTIFYING QUALITIES INCLUDE THOSE WITH:

- Plenty of the minerals: sulphur, silica, iron, zinc, magnesium, manganese, potassium, iodine and copper.
- Foods high in vitamin A, C, E, D, K2, Carotenes, Folic Acid, B3, B5 and Biotin.
- Foods with anti-oxidants like polyphenols, flavonoids, resveratrol, lycopene and others.
- Foods containing fatty acids like Omega 3, 6, 9 and gamma-linolenic acid.
- Foods with a high hyaluronic acid content.
- Foods that are very alkaline in nature.
- Foods with anti-inflammatory actions.
- Foods with cleansing properties.
- Foods rich in 'living enzymes' like RAW, PLANT-BASED FOODS.
- Fermeted foods that enhance our living microbiome like kefir, kombucha, natto and sauerkraut.

TOP 15 BEAUTIFYING FOODS

1

Beautiful berries
*blueberry, aronia, maqui,
raspberry, etc.*

2 Avocado

3 Sweet potato

Ocean plants
*seaweeds, sea vegetables
and blue-green algae*

4

5 *Green leafy heroes*
*spinach, romaine lettuce,
kale and rocket.*

Soy
organic & fermented

6

Oily fish
*wild salmon (not farmed),
mackerel, herring, halibut etc.*

8

7 *Fermented foods*
sauerkraut, kefir, natto, kombucha.

9 *Omega oils*
*borage, hemp, buckthorn
and sacha inchi.*

Nuts and seeds
(activated), especially walnuts.

10

11 *Cacao and
dark chocolate.*

Green tea, organic
(matcha, sencha, etc.).

12

13 *Tomatoes and
bell peppers.*

Bone &
vegan broths.

14

15 *Cruciferous vegetables:*
*all cabbages, broccoli,
cauliflower, radishes, etc.*

RAW BEAUTY DIET LIST

FRUITS	VEGETABLES AND HERBS	ANIMAL KINGDOM	WHOLE GRAINS AND LEGUMES	NUTS AND SEEDS	OTHER
Açai berries	Basil	Organic eggs	Buckwheat	Almonds	Alkaline water
Apples	Broccoli	Oily fish like wild salmon, mackerel, mahi mahi, sardines	Millet	Chia seeds	Blue-green algae
Apricots	Cabbage		Amaranth	Flax seeds	Cacao
Aronia berries	Celery		Red kidney beans	Hazelnuts	Kombucha
Avocado	Chilli Peppers	Oysters	Quinoa	Hemp seeds	Kefir
Blueberries	Coriander	Scallops	Organic soy	Macadamia	Kimchi
Chokeberries	Cucumber	Grass-fed organic lamb and beef (in moderation)	Lentils	Pumpkin seeds	Miso
Coconut	Garlic		Teff	Pine nuts	Natto
Goji berries	Ginger			Walnuts	Sauerkraut
Grapefruit	Green leafy vegetables	Organic bone broths	(all of these are more beautifying when sprouted)	Sunflower seeds	Greek yoghurt
Honeydew	Horsetail herb			Sesame seeds	
Kiwi	Kale	Fish collagen broths		All of the cold-pressed oils from these seeds	
Lemons	Lettuce				
Limes	Mint			(always better when activated)	
Macqui berry	Nettles				
Mango	Onion				
Olives	Rocket				
Papaya	Romaine lettuce				
Pineapple	Spinach				
Pomegranate	Spring onions				
Strawberries	Sweet potato				
Tomatoes	Swiss chard				
Watermelon	Turmeric				
	Yarrow				
	Wheatgrass				

ALCHEMY
of BEAUTY

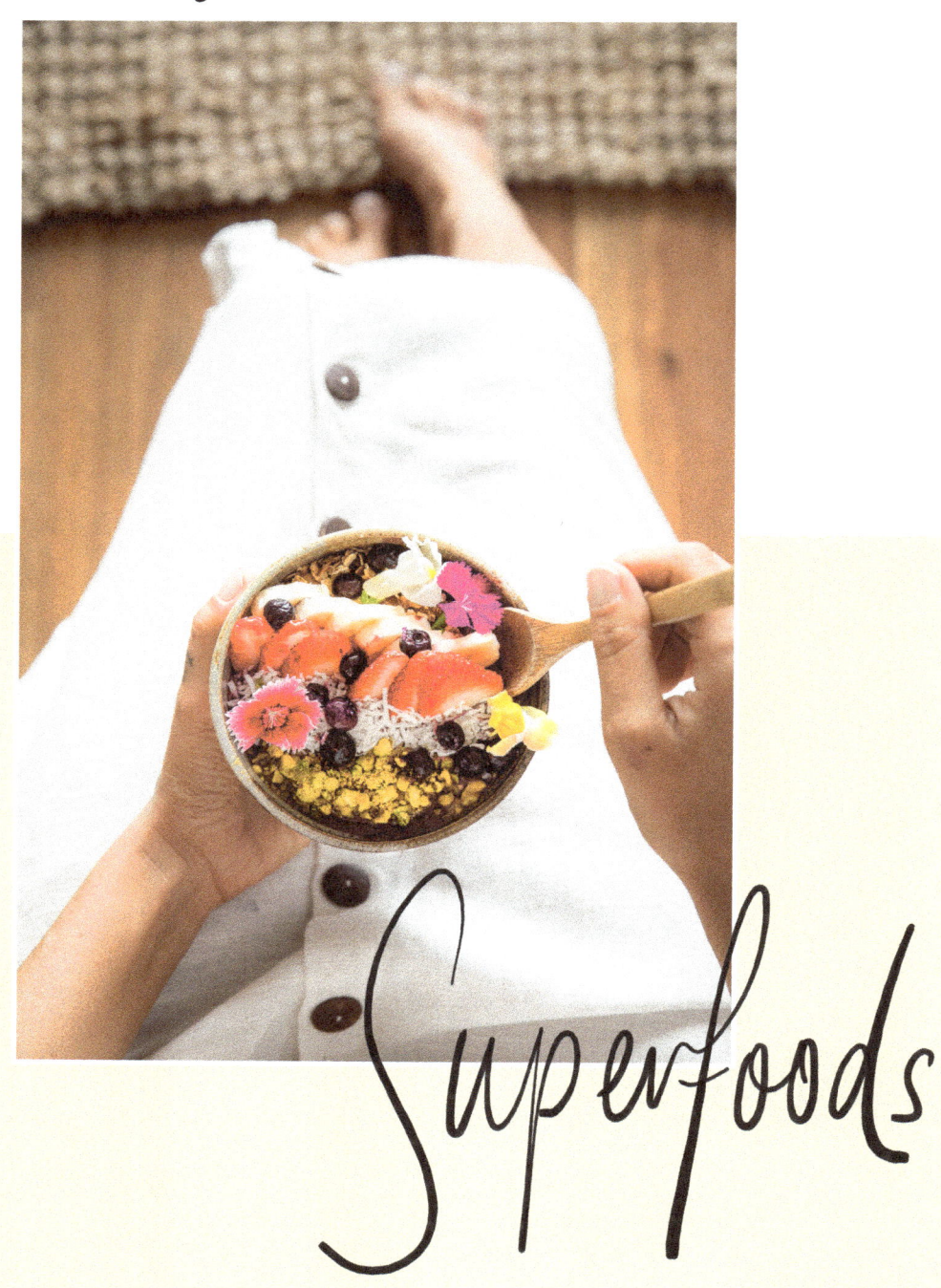

Superfoods

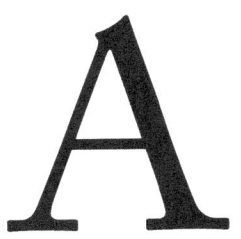

APPLES

Ever since I was a little girl I have loved the taste of apples. But apples are more than just a divine-tasting fruit that keeps the doctor away. They are a true beauty superstar! This little fruit is packed with the powerful anti-inflammatory flavonoid, quercetin. Quercetin shields against skin damaging UVB rays and cancer development. They also contain procyanidin B-2, a nutrient that encourages hair growth and thickness. On top of this they possess my favourite fibre, pectin. Pectin mops up heavy metals, viruses, yeast and toxins, keeping the bowels squeaky-clean and the skin glowing.

In summer, I love making an 'apple spritzer' with matcha green tea, Green apple juice, grated ginger, mint and lime! What a yummy way to beautify the skin and add a sparkle to the eyes!

ARUGULA OR ROCKET

Rocket would have to be one of my favourite salad vegetables. Just like broccoli, rocket is a superb source of indole-3-carbinol (I3C). This cleansing nutrient excretes harmful toxins and hormones that can cause breast, endometrial, colon and prostate cancer. It is also a great source of Vitamin K, a fat soluble vitamin that enhances cell renewal and collagen formation making your skin plump, youthful and smooth. Rocket also contains huge amounts of antioxidants like lutein, zeaxanthin, Vitamin C, folate, B vitamins and chlorophyll. Wow! No wonder I love rocket so much.

AVOCADO

Avocadoes are an incredible source of Vitamin A, D, E, lecithin, biotin, potassium and chlorophyll, which purifies the blood, strengthens nails and beautifies the skin. The luscious oils found in this fleshy fruit are a rich source of essential fatty acids. These nourish dry and sun-damaged skin and soothe eczema, dermatitis, psoriasis and early wrinkle formation.

AVOCADO REVIVE MASK

1 fresh avocado, mashed

1 egg white, beaten

¼ papaya, mashed

½ fresh lemon, squeezed

Mix all of the ingredients together until you have a paste. Apply to face and relax for twenty minutes. Wash off with warm water. Try this once a week to hydrate parched skin.

BEAUTIFUL BERRIES

Berries are the most nutritious fruit found on planet earth. Their vibrant colours, obtained from their proanthocyandins or OPC's, are not only visually appealing, but the source of their incredible healing properties. OPC's have the power to tone capillaries, veins and arteries and guard against free radical damage that causes wrinkles. Eating lots of berries prevents bruising and heals spider and varicose veins, hemorrhoids and broken capillaries.

They beautify the eyes, reverse sun damage, improve vision and are a true 'brain food'. Keep reading for some of my fav beauty berries.

Açai berries contain twice as many antioxidants as blueberries, as well as Vitamins A, E and flavonoids. These antioxidants coupled with Coenzyme Q10 help to guard against skin ageing caused by free radicals and pollutants. The rich Vitamin C, zinc and omega oils found in in açai boosts collagen, reduces pigmentation and increases skin, hair and nail radiance.

Blueberries have one of the highest ORAC values of any fruit on this planet. Just like their berry brothers, blueberries possess a very rich anthocyanin content coupled with huge amounts of Vitamin C. Vitamin C is needed to make collagen, remove dead skin cells and encourage two stages of hair growth resulting in hair that grows as fast as grass.

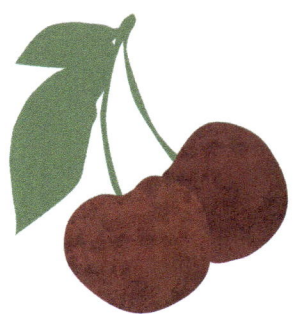

Cherries are the 'lullaby fruit' as they help to improve sleep. Anyone who sleeps at least eight hours of quality sleep per night is healthier, has a higher collagen repair time and therefore radiates more natural beauty.

Goji berries were eaten by Buddhist monks to promote a long and happy life. These berries are an incredible source of Vitamins A, C and E, calcium, potassium, iron, zinc and selenium. These nutrients fight off age-promoting free radicals thereby improving collagen and elastin production in the skin.

Macqui berries have the highest antioxidant potential of any berry on the planet. They contain more anthocyanins per weight than any other berry. When you add their Vitamin C, iron, calcium, magnesium and potassium content to this, you have a super powerful beauty berry that can reduce inflammation linked to arthritis, diabetes, ulcerative colitis, obesity, hair and skin damage and inflammatory bowel conditions.

Strawberries are a great fruit for keeping your skin looking amazing. Just one cup of strawberries supplies over 100 per cent of your daily Vitamin C needs. This vitamin acts as an important building block to collagen, the skin's support structure which prevents wrinkles and sagging skin. What a yummy way to get a natural Botox injection!

Raspberries are not as exotic sounding as a macqui berry, yet they still possess some incredible youth-promoting properties. They are a rich source of the cancer-fighting polyphenol, ellagic acid. Ellagic acid guards against many types of cancer including esophageal, bladder, breast, lung and skin cancer. The rich fibre, manganese and ketone content found in these red berries are brilliant for weight loss, fertility and digestive health. Raspberries can reduce pigmentation in the skin as they contain a ketone called tiliroside, that can balance out melanin production.

MY SECRET BLUEBERRY YOUTH MASK

2 cups of blueberries

3 tablespoons of yoghurt (sheep, cow's or coconut yoghurt)

1 tablespoon of raw, activated honey

Blend the blueberries, yoghurt and honey in a blender to make a paste. Leave on the skin for 20 minutes and you will be amazed at how beautifully your skin glows.

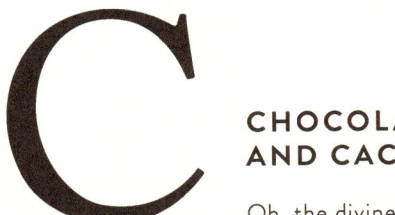

C

CHOCOLATE AND CACAO

Oh, the divine deliciousness of chocolate! Chocolate is definitely a girl's best friend! Chocolate is derived from cacao beans. Cacao is a rich source of polyphenol antioxidants, similar to those found in Green tea, raspberries and red wine. These polyphenols protect the skin against premature ageing. The magical cacao seed can increase blood flow, promote cellular healing and lower stress hormones making you feel happy.

Stress is one of the best ageing culprits so no wonder chocolate is such a superb youth-promoting food. One study in the Journal of Nutrition showed that people who drank cocoa for twelve weeks had smoother, more hydrated skin. Some of my favourite and healthiest chocolate brands are Alter Eco, Antidote (100% cacao), Raaka, Pana and Endangered Species. I am happily discovering more every day.

CABBAGE

As you can see from my recipes, cabbage is a regular addition to most of my beauty salads and soups. This leafy superstar contains waste-expelling nutrients like chlorophyll, chlorine, potassium and sulphur. Sulphur is nicknamed the 'beauty mineral' as it boosts the making of keratin, strengthening the hair, skin and nails. Cabbage is a great source of indole-3-carbinol (I3C), a powerful detoxifying substance that sweeps dangerous hormones and chemicals out of the body via the liver. On top of this its rich vitamin U content can heal stomach ulcers. Wow. What a true vegetable superstar!

CAPSICUM OR BELL PEPPERS – GREEN, RED, YELLOW, ORANGE

Bell peppers are loaded with huge amounts of Vitamin C. This enhances collagen production for healthier skin, hair and nails. Red peppers are a potent skin food because of their high content of Vitamins E, K, A, B6, folate and other powerful antioxidants. Research shows that women who eat green and yellow vegetables like capsicum have fewer wrinkles, especially around the eyes.

CHILLI PEPPERS – CHILLI, JALAPENO, PAPRIKA, CAYENNE

As you can see from my recipes, I add chilli to nearly everything. I acquired this love for chillies while living in Thailand. Living there was a great lesson in learning how to add food to dishes to speed up the metabolism. The active ingredient found in these hot little peppers, capsaicin, amps up the body's ability to burn fat. Capsaicin reduces the hunger driving hormone ghrelin and increases the appetite-suppressing hormone leptin. However, just like in the story of Cinderella, the effects are fleeting. Chillies need to be added to meals regularly to effect fat burning. On top of this, hot peppers are the perfect little skin protective vegetable. Nuclear transcription factors triggered by UV light cause skin ageing. The capsaicin in these peppers can block these transcription factors, thereby promoting beautiful, youthful skin. If you want some natural sunscreen, make yourself a guacamole and don't forget to spice it up with some paprika, jalapeño or cayenne. It will be the yummiest natural sunscreen that you have ever eaten.

CRAZY CRUSTACEANS

What a yummy way to eat yourself towards divine beauty! All crustaceans are super rich sources of the mineral zinc. Zinc is a 'beauty super star' as it is the key to healthy collagen and skin elasticity. A deficiency of zinc is a great way to lose your hair (and, God forbid – your eyelashes too). If your skin is dry or your scalp is flaky, a zinc deficiency is probably the cause. Just 100 grams of oysters can give you over 400% of your daily value of zinc – wow! Most of these ocean treats are also good sources of Vitamin D (the sunshine vitamin), B vitamins, protein and skin nourishing Omega 3 fatty acids. They help to boost immunity, act as a superb aphrodisiac, enhance blood circulation and even prevent osteoporosis. Some seafood can be high in mercury and other contaminants, so it is essential to always purchase from reliable, clean waters.

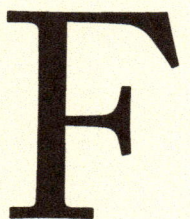

FERMENTED FOODS LIKE SAUERKRAUT, KEFIR, NATTO AND KOMBUCHA

The longest living cultures in the world include fermented foods as a staple in their diet. The Japanese have always known that fermented foods like miso, natto and tempeh contain some amazing isoflavones and Vitamin K2 to prevent skin ageing, cancer and heart disease. The Russians used fermented sauerkraut, the Koreans incorporated kimchee into their diets, and in fact, the fermenting of foods in the greatest living cultures dates back thousands of years.

One of my favourite authors and health promoters of all time, Donna Gates, pioneered the introduction of fermented foods and stevia into the modern western diet. Through her book, The Body Ecology Diet, she promoted the addition of fermented foods into a healthy diet to improve gut health, and, in the process, skin health, longevity and disease prevention. She coined the term the 'inner ecosystem'. She knew that fermented foods would heal the gut's 'living microbiome', maintaining ageless skin and a youthful mind.

Countless studies are now confirming the connection between the gut, the brain and skin health. Many of these have proven that people who regularly consume fermented foods in their diet have better skin hydration, less wrinkle formation and a brighter, more radiant skin tone.

FISH LIKE SALMON, TUNA, MACKEREL, SARDINES, HERRING, ETC.

Although this book is highly focused on raw fruits, vegetables, nuts and seeds and some legumes, food from the ocean earns a worthy place in the 'wellness and beauty' arena. Most oily fish are a wonderful source of protein, Vitamin D and Omega 3 fatty acids. These nutrients are not only needed for strong bones and teeth, but essential for producing collagen to prevent early wrinkle formation. Omega 3 fatty acids provide beautiful skin elasticity and encourage the growth of thick, resilient hair. They also help to reduce inflammation that can break down our collagen matrix and drive diseases like cancer, heart disease and Alzheimer's.

Salmon contains astaxanthin, a very powerful carotenoid that improves skin elasticity, tone and texture. Astaxanthin also guards vigilantly against heart disease and cancer. Farmed salmon has next to no astaxanthin content and it contains antibiotics and artificial colourings which can disrupt the body's happy microbiome. When choosing fish, only choose wild, oily, small catch fish from clean waters.

FLAXSEEDS

The healing properties of flaxseeds were known to the Greek physician Hippocrates, who recommended this seed for nearly every ailment. The oil derived from the seeds of this plant contain good amounts of fatty acids, particularly alpha-linolenic acid (ALA). ALA converts to Omega 3 fatty acids and then into DHA and EPA. These healthy fats help to beautify the skin, treating inflammation, dryness, eczema and psoriasis. In addition to ALA, flaxseeds contain a group of chemicals called lignans. Lignans provide protection against cancer, heart disease, constipation and hormonal problems. Flax seeds also contain the fat soluble-vitamins E and A and the 'sunshine vitamin', Vitamin D, in addition to Vitamins B1, B2, Vitamin C, soluble and insoluble fibre and every mineral known to humankind. Could you ever imagine that one little seed could contain so much healing magic?

Flaxseeds can reduce a high oil production in the skin, helping anyone with acne or blemishes. They nourish dull, lifeless hair and nails and stimulate their growth. Flaxseeds are easily prone to 'rancidity', so the oil has to be cold-pressed quickly in the right environment, then stored correctly. I personally love the brands Stoney Creek and Melrose.

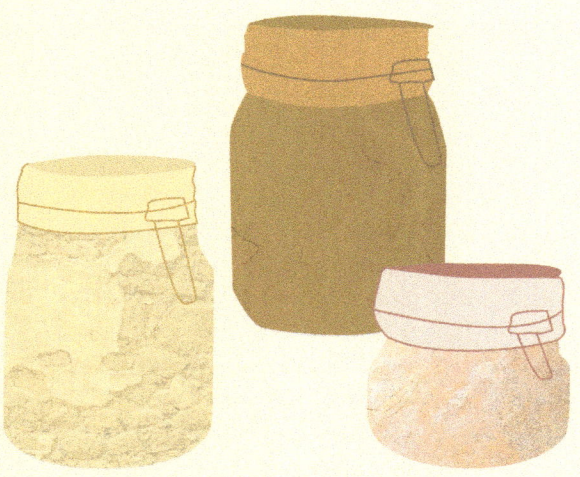

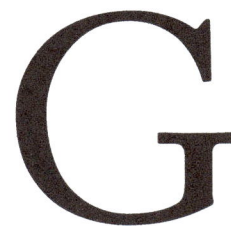

GREEN VEGGIES

Having beautiful, ageless skin into your eighties is not unachievable, especially if green leafy vegetables are the mainstay of your diet. Vegetables like spinach, broccoli, watercress and Swiss chard are a great source of Vitamin A, C and folic acid. These enhance the vibrancy and hydration of your skin, hair, nails and brain. These green powerhouses contain huge amounts of chlorophyll which detoxifies and oxygenates the blood. When the blood is clean and oxygenated the skin, hair and nails take on a beautiful glow.

GREEN TEA

Green tea is high on the list of skin-friendly drinks thanks to its impressive storehouse of antioxidant polyphenols like catechins. Catechins reduce inflammation and protect against free radical damage that causes skin breakdown and cancer. Studies have proven that Green tea can reduce the damage of sunburn and overexposure to ultraviolet light. It is especially rich in a compound known as EGCG, which may act as a 'fountain of youth' for dying skin cells to regenerate the skin faster. No wonder I love adding Japanese matcha powder to everything!

KALE

When I lived in Japan I used to pick kale from people's gardens to eat and the local people would look at me in horror. They had no idea that the ultimate source of longevity was growing abundantly in their own gardens. Kale is a very rich source of Vitamins C, E and K, beta-carotene, calcium, iron and phytochemicals including sulphoraphane and indoles. Indoles are respected for their ability to remove bad hormones that cause cancer. Like its other green leafy friends, kale contains chlorophyll, a potent blood cleanser. This leafy vegetable is a true beauty and youth-promoting superhero.

LEGUMES

Legumes and beans are a good protein source for vegetarians. Proteins speed the repair and regeneration of skin cells and collagen. Legumes are also a good source of fibre, which regulates blood sugar, cholesterol and positively affects weight loss. The only downside of legumes is that they contain anti-nutrients like phytic acid, lectins and saponins. These anti-nutrients can impair the absorption of minerals and damage the intestinal lining, resulting in leaky gut. However, 24 hour soaking, sprouting, fermenting and thoroughly cooking legumes can reduce their anti-nutrient content. My fav beauty legumes are black beans, kidney, lentils, adzuki, butter and soy beans.

ANTIOXIDANT TURMERIC AND CHICKPEA MASK

1 tablespoon of chickpea flour

2 teaspoons of almond oil

1 teaspoon of ground turmeric

2 teaspoons of raw, activated manuka honey

Mix all of the ingredients together. Apply to clean skin and leave on for twenty minutes. This antioxidant rich mask is brilliant for irritated, dull and inflamed skin.

LEMONS AND LIMES

Lemons and Limes are included in most of my juicing recipes, especially their skins. I love kick-starting my metabolism at the beginning of the day with a glass of alkaline water with a freshly-squeezed lemon or lime. These 'citrus beauties' are a terrific source of phosphorous (for strong bones, teeth, gums and nerves), sodium, (to purify the lymphatic system) and Vitamin C (to boost immunity and collagen). Many people think that lemons are acidic. This is true while they are in our fruit bowl, but as they enter your stomach they become alkaline. It is this quality that allows lemons to help maintain the correct pH in our body and also to act as a natural, internal antiseptic.

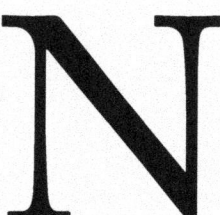

N

NUTS, SEEDS AND OILS

Almonds and almond oil

I have a secret love affair with almonds and it is no wonder, as they are one of the most nutritious nuts on this planet. Almonds were once worshipped by ancient people for their spiritual and healing qualities. King Tutankhamen took almonds to his grave and the Bible even designated almonds as being the symbol of birth, hope and values. Romans thought they were a fertility charm, which is interesting as almonds actually have a similar shape to ovaries, making them superb fertility tonics.

In fact, the beautifying nutrients in this nut are overwhelming. They contain protein, soluble and insoluble fibre, Omega 3 and 6 fatty acids, Vitamin E and most minerals including zinc, magnesium and calcium. They are also one of the best 'weight loss nuts' around, being packed with monounsaturated fats which boost the metabolism and curb cravings.

The high protein content found in almonds makes them the perfect building block for collagen, a substance that holds all tissues in place preventing sagging skin. Almonds are also a fantastic source of biotin. Biotin is a B vitamin which is essential for helping to heal eczema and dermatitis and for keeping the hair and nails healthy and strong.

Hemp seeds and oil

I love throwing hemp seeds into everything as they are super nutritious, containing all nine essential amino acids, every essential fatty acid and nearly all minerals, including iron. Hemp is rich in sulphur-building amino acids that help to build very strong hair, nails, muscles and connective tissues. They have the perfect balance of Omega 3, 6 and 9, including GLA to nourish the skin and regulate hormones. The lipids found in hemp oil are similar to those found in the skin making it one of the best natural moisturisers on planet earth.

If you want your hair to grow fast, add some hemp oil to your diet. The rich Omega fatty acid content combined with chlorophyll encourages rapid hair growth, while nourishing follicles for more beautiful hair.

Pumpkin seeds and oil

I add activated pumpkin seeds to nearly all of my salads as I know how rich this little seed is in zinc to help boost my immunity, enhance my collagen and give me some extra energy. If you want to feel happier and more relaxed, don't overlook this little seed – it contains all of the perfect ingredients to make the mood-uplifting serotonin and the anxiety-relieving GABA. Pumpkin seed oil is a rich source of key vitamins and fatty acids that can strengthen and hydrate hair follicles while blocking 5-alpha reductase to stop hair loss. No wonder I feed these hair-saving seeds to my hubby every day!

Sesame seeds and oil

Sesame seeds are one of the oldest crops on earth. The seeds can strengthen hair, improve nail, bone and tooth quality and add a beautiful, silky glow to the skin. Because of its anti-bacterial qualities, the oil can be used as a mouth gargle to kill plaque-driving bacteria.

I drizzle sesame oil onto all of my dishes, not only because it tastes beautiful but to ensure my skin, gums and hair stay strong and healthy.

Walnuts and oil

Everyone knows that when walnuts are broken in half, they look like a brain. So it is no surprise to learn that walnuts contain all the nutrients to nourish brain health. Their rich Omega 3 fatty acid content coupled with high levels of Vitamin E can improve skin elasticity and nourish hair and nail quality. The high copper content is brilliant for improving the formation of collagen and for preventing early greying of the hair. Only 7 walnuts contain 99% of the body's RDA of Omega 3 fatty acids – that's incredible. No wonder I love adding walnuts to salads!

OILS – COLD-PRESSED

My favourite skin, hair and nail beautifying oils are sacha inchi, hemp, pumpkin seed, sea buckthorn, borage, avocado, macadamia and sesame oil. For more info about these, refer to 'nuts and seeds'. Here's a peek at a couple of other beautifying contenders:

Borage oil

The borage plant produces a beautiful purple flower that is nicknamed 'starflower'. The seeds contain lots of essential fatty acids (EFAs). EFAs are fats that the body cannot make and so must be obtained from the diet. One of the most beautifying of these is gamma linolenic acid or GLA. Borage oil contains up to 25% GLA. GLA is needed to create prostaglandins, hormone-like substances that reduce inflammation and improve hydration, restoring suppleness to the skin. It is a great oil for skin dryness, eczema, psoriasis and PMS. Other oils that contain GLA, although in much smaller quantities are evening primrose and blackcurrant seed oil.

Sacha inchi (Plukenetia volubilis)

This native Peruvian plant is quickly climbing the ladder to superfood status, and it is no wonder, with its super rich natural oil content. The word 'sacha inchi' typically refers to the edible seeds of the plant, which are rich in essential fatty acids and have a nut-like flavour when roasted. Sacha inchi has a perfect balance of Omega 3 (in fact more than any other seed) and lots of Vitamin A and E to nourish the hair and skin with luscious oils while protecting it against advanced ageing.

Olives and olive oil

The olive tree is one of the oldest surviving trees on Earth. The oil is derived from the black and green fruits and the leaves are used medicinally to treat a wide range of health conditions. The olive leaf symbolises peace and prosperity and the fruit has been regarded as a culinary delight and as a precious oil for centuries. It is a rich source of monounsaturated fats which can prevent heart disease, inflammation, diabetes and dry skin. Olives contain antioxidants that offer incredible sun-protection against harmful UV rays. No wonder Mediterranean people never seem to burn.

ORANGE AND YELLOW VEGETABLES/FRUITS

All yellow and orange vegetables like apricots, pumpkins, carrots, mangoes and sweet potatoes are amazing sources of carotenes, including beta-carotene. Carotenes are powerful antioxidants that protect against collagen and elastin breakdown that cause advanced skin ageing. Studies around the world show that women who eat lots of these fruits and vegetables have more beautiful-looking skin, thicker hair and brighter eyes.

Sweet potatoes are one of the best natural beautifying vegetables on planet earth, which is why I include it in lots of my beauty recipes It is a great source of Vitamin A, E, C and magnesium, which aids in making hyaluronic acid. This substance gives our skin back the soft, squishy and hydrated look that we had when we were babies.

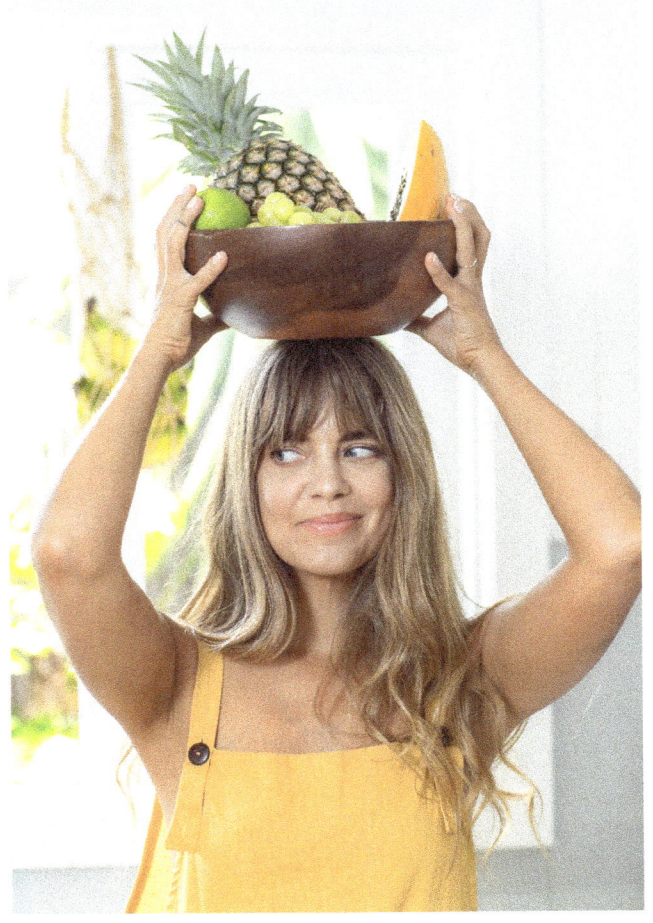

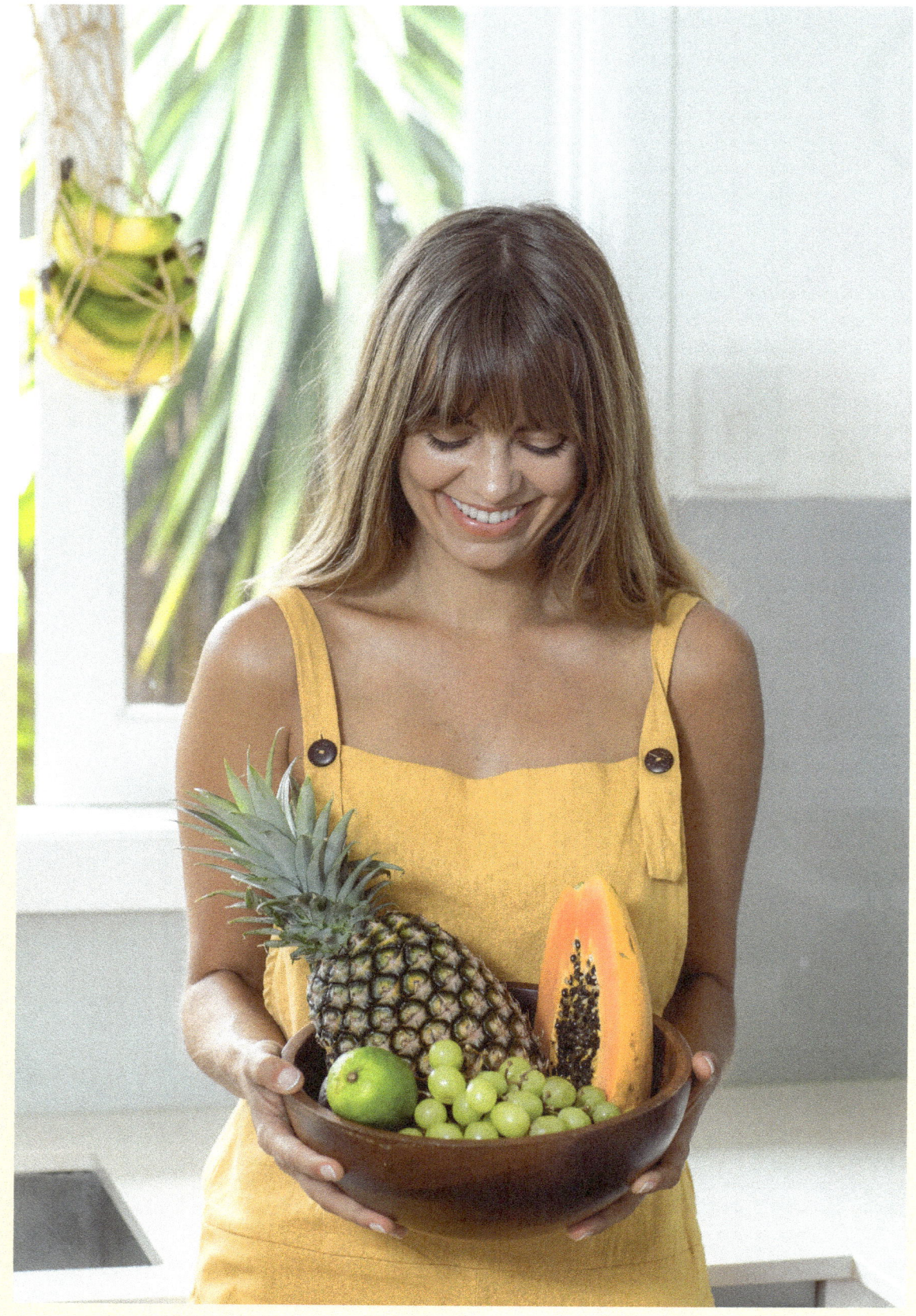

PINEAPPLE

I love using pineapple in my skin-preserving face scrubs and healing juices because of its high content of antioxidants, bromelain and alpha hydroxy acids. Pineapple is super rich in Vitamin C which reduces plaque, whitens the teeth and guards against gum disease. It also promotes the production of hyaluronic acid and collagen to add plumpness to the skin. It is one of the best natural remedies to help remove warts, moles, dark spots, freckles and wrinkles.

MAGIC SKIN PINEAPPLE SCRUB

¾ cup of Himalayan or Celtic sea salt or sugar

¼ cup of macadamia or jojoba oil

¼ pineapple

Place pineapple in a blender with salt or sugar. Remove and stir in the oil. Place this magical scrub in the fridge and apply to the skin a few times weekly. You will be surprised at how quickly your skin takes on a beautiful glow.

P

PAW PAW

Papaya or Paw Paw was a native fruit of Central America that was introduced to the world by Spanish and Portuguese explorers. Christopher Columbus nicknamed it 'the fruit of the angels' after tasting it for the first time. This beautiful fruit is an amazing source of Vitamin A, C, E, K, niacin and the minerals magnesium and potassium, which protect against skin damage and disease. I often use papaya as a skin mask to tone my skin and to lighten blemishes. Papaya contains a powerful anti-inflammatory known as papain, that assists with digestion and helps to reduce inflammation.

YUMMY PAPAYA BODY SCRUB

Sugar

Papaya

Honey

Olive or Macadamia Oil

Mix together until you get a scrub-like texture. Use as a daily body scrub to remove impurities leaving a soft and silky skin.

POMEGRANATE

When I was little we had a pomegranate tree and we would eat the seeds like lollies. No wonder we had such strong constitutions, considering all of the healing ingredients found in this magical fruit. This fruit is one of the best sources of cancer-fighting polyphenols, even higher than those found in Green tea. Polyphenols are antioxidants that fight free radical damage that causes skin ageing and disease.

They improve blood circulation to the skin, rallying youth-promoting nutrients, which improves the texture and quality of the skin. One cup of pomegranate juice supplies 40% of your RDA of folic acid, as well as huge amounts of Vitamins A, C and E. It is an amazing source of ellagic acid – a potent antioxidant that guards against carcinogenic changes to cells that drives cancer, particularly skin cancer. It also contains punicic acid, an Omega 5 fatty acid which helps with cell regeneration and skin hydration.

Q

QUINOA

Quinoa is an ancient food that dates back 3000 years to when the Incas ate it as a staple food source. It is a rich source of fatty acids, minerals, protein and vitamins, making it a superb food for brightening the skin, reducing wrinkles and melanin-clustering skin pigmentation. It blocks the activity of matrix metalloproteinases (MMPs), substances that destroy collagen and advance sun spots. It is also a good source of magnesium for healthy skin, teeth and bones, and manganese, a mineral that helps to make a powerful age-fighting antioxidant known as 'superoxide dismutase' or SOD. Quinoa is a protein superstar as it contains nine amino acids that can strengthen the hair and nails, preventing breakage. One of these amino acids, known as tyrosine, helps to maintain hair colour and stops the loss of melanin. No wonder the Incas had such flawless skin and shiny hair.

RADISH

Radishes contain huge amounts of antioxidants which enhance skin cell renewal and repair and plenty of minerals to boost oxygen, strengthen nails, bones and teeth and improve skin hydration. Just like Green tea and berries, radishes contain plenty of healthy cancer-fighting catechins and nutrients to guard against sun damage, age spots and pigmentation.

SEAWEEDS LIKE WAKAME, ARAME, DULSE, HIJIKE, KOMBU

Seaweed is an ancient superfood revered in many cultures for its ability to enhance longevity, beauty and health. These ocean plants are a girl's best friend. They can make your hair grow like grass, shrink your waistline, strengthen weak nails and bones, remove aches and pains, strip you of cellulite and kick wrinkles to the kerb. Seaweeds not only absorb minerals from the ocean, but they also harness the power of the sun.

Iodine is deficient in the Earth's soils, and because of this, diseases like cancer, fibrocystic breast disease and thyroid problems are on the rise. Seaweeds are the best natural source of absorbable iodine. Iodine nourishes the thyroid gland to boost the metabolism, strip away unhealthy fat, protect against radiation and beautifies the skin and hair. A lack of iodine is a major cause of hair loss. My favourite sea vegetables are wakame, hijike, arame, kelp, kombu, and dulse and I also love blue-green algae from the Klamath Lake in Oregon.

SOYBEANS

Soybeans are a healthy food that has received a bad rap in the media. Don't get me wrong – there are some bad forms of soy, particularly if they are genetically modified and made via a poor extraction process. But if your soybeans are organic and fermented naturally you will surprised at how they can improve health and wellbeing. The minerals and proteins found in soybeans can reduce skin pigmentation, wrinkles and beautify the skin. The best forms of soy are organic fermented edamame, natto, tempeh, tamari and miso.

Collagen, the fibrous protein that keeps skin firm, youthful-looking and wrinkle-free, begins to decline in your mid-twenties! Eating edamame and other soy foods rich in isoflavones may help to preserve skin-firming collagen. In a study published in the Journal of the American College of Nutrition, mice fed isoflavones that were exposed to ultraviolet radiation had fewer wrinkles and smoother skin than mice that were exposed to UV light but didn't eat isoflavones. The researchers believe that soy-rich isoflavones help prevent collagen breakdown. In another study on women that were given 40 mg of soy-rich isoflavones they were found to have fewer crow's feet, their skin had better elasticity and less wrinkles were likely to form. Wow! What a delicious way to beautify your skin.

The Alchemy of Beauty

S SPINACH

Spinach was made famous by Popeye, who in times of emergency ate cans of this green superfood to power himself into action. Popeye was on the right track. Spinach is a potent nutrient mix that is a rich source of powerful minerals and antioxidants like lutein, quercetin, Vitamin K and E, folic acid and Vitamin C. It is an excellent blood-boosting and detoxifying vegetable that cleanses impurities from the body. The iron, beta carotene and folate in spinach helps to keep hair follicles nourished and healthy.

T TOMATOES

Tomatoes are rich in cancer-fighting and heart-protective carotenoids like lycopene. Lycopene guards against free radical attacks that break down the supporting structures in hair, skin and nails. It is also an incredible sun warrior. A German study found that lycopene-rich tomato paste helped prevent sunburn when combined with olive oil. No wonder Mediterranean people never seem to burn, when cooked tomatoes are a main part of their diet. Removing the seeds and skin and cooking tomatoes increases their lycopene content. Keep in mind that these are nightshades, so if you are prone to arthritis you may need to remove them from your diet.

TURMERIC

In India, turmeric is nicknamed the 'King of Spices', but it should really be called the 'King of Anti-Inflammatories'. The curcuminoids found in turmeric are responsible for its amazing antioxidant, anti-ageing and anti-inflammatory properties. Curcumin protects the collagen-producing fibroblast cells from damage. It has also been demonstrated that turmeric provides superb protection against UV related sun damage that causes skin-ageing. It can stimulate cell regeneration and turnover, making it ideal for adding a youthful, vibrant glow to the skin.

Y YOGHURT (ESPECIALLY GREEK)

Greek yoghurt is a beauty-promoting food. It is packed with calcium and protein to beautify and whiten the teeth and bones. Yoghurt also contains natural live active cultures or 'good' bacteria that aid digestion, leading to a flat and 'happy' belly! The live bacteria in yoghurt can help to boost gut immunity, thereby benefiting the body's entire immune system. If you are dairy-intolerant, opt for camel, sheep, nut or coconut yoghurt.

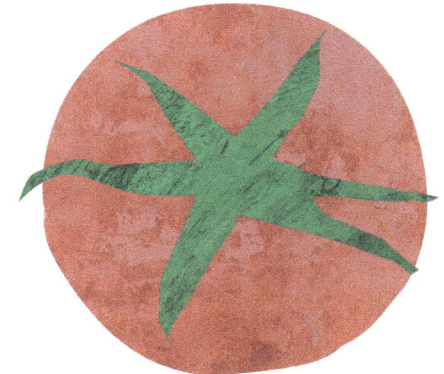

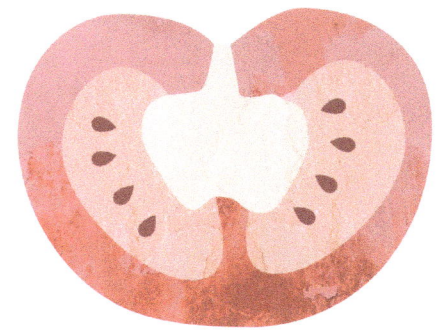

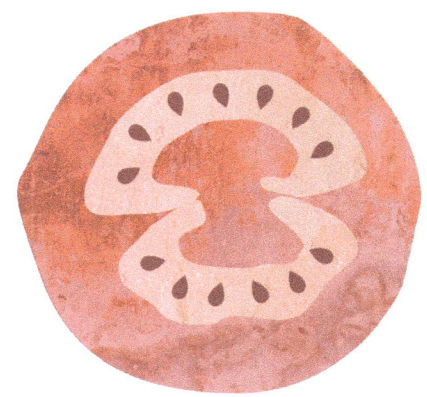

CHAPTER THREE

NATURE'S SECRETS TO RADIANT BEAUTY

Alchemy of Beauty Nutrients

ALCHEMY of
BEAUTY NUTRIENTS

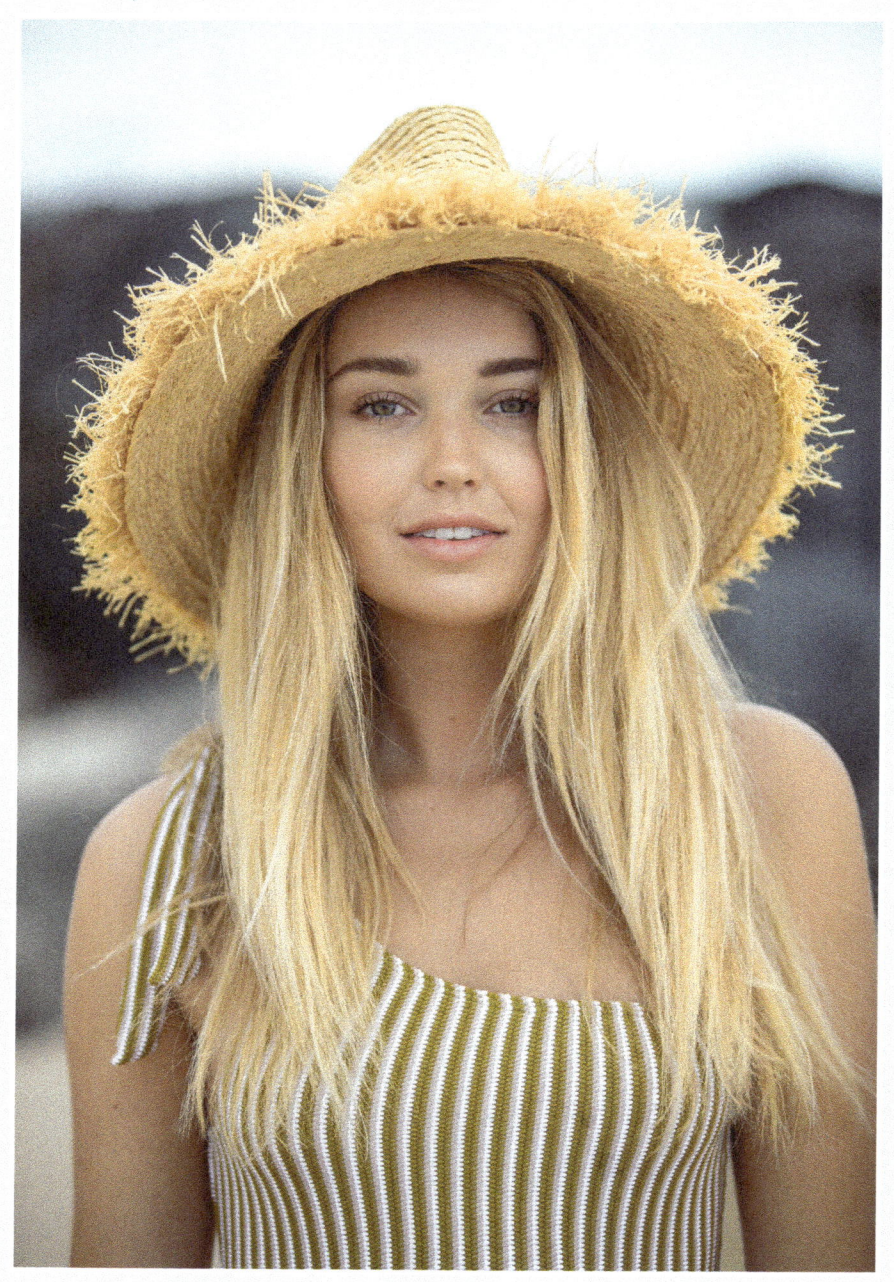

NATURE IS FILLED WITH AN ABUNDANT SOURCE OF PROTECTIVE AND BEAUTIFYING NUTRIENTS. ATTAINING AGELESS BEAUTY AND VIBRANT HEALTH IS HIGHLY DEPENDENT ON THE TYPE OF FOODS THAT WE CHOOSE TO EAT, AS EACH DIFFERENT TYPE OF FOOD CONTAINS A UNIQUE ARRAY OF PHYTOCHEMICALS THAT CAN GUARD AGAINST SKIN DAMAGE AND CELL BREAKDOWN. EATING WHOLESOME, ORGANIC AND NUTRIENT-RICH FOODS IS A MAJOR KEY TO ATTAINING BEAUTIFUL SKIN, LUSCIOUS HAIR, STRONG NAILS AND EVEN TO BALANCING YOUR EMOTIONS.

PROTEIN – THE COLLAGEN BUILDER

Proteins are molecules that contain a range of different amino acids. A complete protein has all twenty-two amino acids. Incomplete proteins have different combinations of these, but not the whole range. Proteins are the building blocks of life. They help with growth, repair, development and structure. The skin is made up of collagen, which is formed from these amino acids. Collagen is the cement that holds our bodily structures together, so without it our skin begins to sag and droop. Healthy protein foods are one of the best ways to enhance collagen production. Amino acids are also a key to making serotonin, GABA and dopamine, chemicals that make you feel happy, focused, calm and motivated.

Complete proteins are found in animal foods and incomplete proteins are found in plant foods, nuts, seeds, seaweeds and legumes. Eating too much of the wrong animal protein is a great way to speed up ageing, especially if a person's digestive system is poor. Good forms of digestible animal protein are organic eggs, oily fish, small catch seafood like oysters, mussels and prawns, and organic grass fed-meats in moderation.

If you are a vegetarian, beans, legumes and whole grains are probably your protein go-to. But it is important to remember they contain substances like phytic acid that can inhibit absorption of minerals. To help break down the 'anti-nutrients' in these foods, soak, sprout or dehydrate them.

As unique beings, we are not all the same. Because of this, some constitutions need a little bit of organic, grass-fed red meat in their diet, but it is still important to eat in moderation and to make living, plant foods the mainstay of your diet.

Signs of protein deficiency: Brittle or slow-growing nails, thin and lifeless hair, poor muscle tone, white horizontal bands on nails, cellulite, skin pigmentation, fatigue, scaly or thin skin, full moon shaped face, low blood pressure, muscle weakness, constipation.

SOME OF MY FAV BEAUTY PROTEIN FOODS
AMOUNT OF PROTEIN IN GRAMS PER SERVING SIZE

Almonds, walnuts, macadamia, pumpkin and sunflower seeds
(best when soaked and activated) – average 5 grams to 8 grams per cup

Avocado (1 medium size) – 4 grams

Bee pollen (per 100 grams) – 24 grams

Black beans, kidney beans (per cup) – 15 grams

Blue-green algae like Klamath Lake and Spirulina (per 100 grams) – around 55 grams
of protein plus 18 amino acids (harvesting time changes protein levels)

Brewer's yeast (per 2 tablespoons) – 16 grams of protein with 8 amino acids

Buckwheat (per cup) – 24 grams

Chia seeds (per 2 tablespoons) – 4 grams

Green vegetables (peas, kale, spinach, brussels sprouts collard, broccoli, parsley, asparagus,
rocket, artichoke, watercress) – average is 4 to 5 grams per cup

Hemp seeds (per 3 tablespoons) – 10 grams and hemp protein (3 tablespoons) – 18 grams

Lentils, chickpeas (per cup) – around 18 grams

Marine phytoplankton (per 2 tablespoons) – 14 grams

Mature grasses like barley and wheatgrass (per 100 grams) – around 25 grams

Oily fish like sardines, mackerel, herring, halibut, salmon, tuna (wild caught, small catch)
– ranges from 30 to 35 grams per 100 grams of fish

Oysters (1 oyster) – 5 grams

Quinoa, teff and seitan (per 85 grams) – around 30 grams

Scallops (1 scallop) – 3 grams

Tempeh and tofu (organic) – 40 grams per cup

Wild and brown rice (especially sprouted) – 7 grams per cup

SUPER FATS FOR HYDRATION

Essential fatty acids (EFAs) are called 'essential' as the body is unable to make them on its own. They need to be sourced from a healthy diet. They are one of the KEYS to optimal health, beautiful hair and skin, longevity and wellbeing. There are two important families of EFAs: Omega 3 and Omega 6. The Omega 3 family is made up of alpha-linolenic acid (ALA) and eicosapentaenoic acid (EPA) and docosahexaenoic acid (DHA). These are found in oily fish, flaxseeds, pumpkin seeds, walnuts, soybeans (tofu, tempeh), dark green vegetables (kale, chard, parsley etc.), blue-green algae, and cereal grasses like wheatgrass. The Omega 6 family is made up of linoleic acid (LA), gamma-linolenic acid (GLA), and arachidonic acid (AA). Omega 6 fatty acids are found in meat, nuts, seeds, legumes, grains and dairy.

The beautifying and healing benefits of EFAs are diverse. They are needed for:

- Healthy cell membranes

- Healthy thyroid and adrenal function

- Fertility and hormone balance

- Regulation of blood pressure, liver health, immune and inflammatory responses

- The transport and breakdown of cholesterol

- Healthy skin, hair and nails, and much more...

By improving the structure and function of every cell membrane, they can build a strong and flexible skin barrier. This results in less water loss, leaving the skin hydrated, glowing and protected. Their ability to lower inflammation creates more collagen and protection against dangerous UV rays.

The metabolism of these in the body is complicated. The Omega 3 pathway is a healthy one as it converts ALA to EPA to reduce inflammation, increase oxygen and improve blood flow. The Omega 6 pathway converts Linoleic Acid (LA) to GLA (Gamma-linolenic Acid) and then to DGLA or Arachidonic Acid (AA). Arachidonic acid, which is mainly found in animal products, can be dangerous as it increases inflammation, allergies and platelet stickiness whereas DGLA has the opposite effect. Oils high in GLA like borage and evening primrose oil can reduce AA, thereby beautifying the skin and in doing so, reverse psoriasis, dermatitis and dry skin problems.

For beautiful, glowing, dewy skin, I include lots of healthy Omega 3 EFAs and GLA in my diet. I drizzle hemp, pumpkin seed, udos or another balanced Omega oil onto my salads, along with lots of avocado. I also add super green powders rich in phytoplankton and blue-green algae to my cold-pressed juices. Without enough healing oils in the diet, skin and hair can become dry, dehydrated and lifeless.

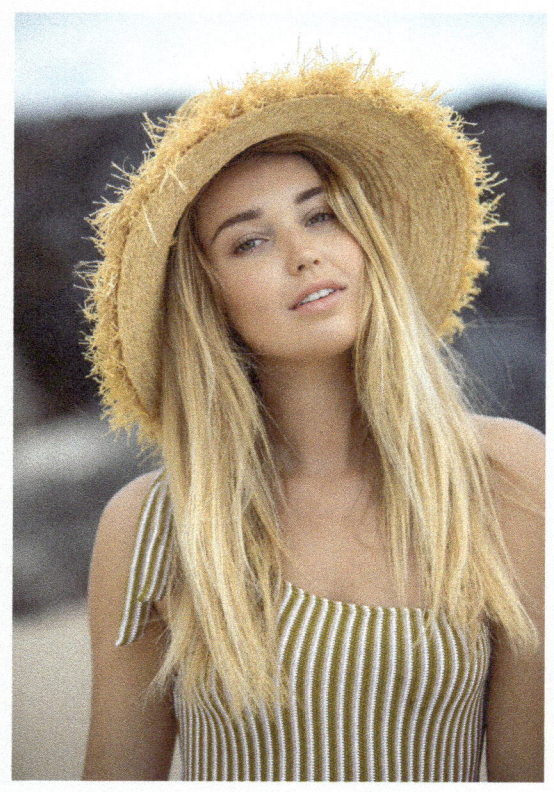

HYALURONIC ACID FOR YOUTH

Hyaluronic acid is the 'it' word in the beauty industry at the moment. And it does have some fantastic anti-ageing properties. It is a naturally occurring polysaccharide (glycosaminoglycan) found in the skin, hair, eyes, joints and other tissues. It holds water and forms a gel-like substance to lubricate and hydrate these areas and in doing so improves the moisture, plumpness and firmness of the skin. Even tissues around our nerves and joints contain hyaluronic acid, which acts as a cushion.

Babies are born with huge amounts of hyaluronic acid, which is why their skin is soft, dewy and squishy. Unfortunately, our reserves of this yummy, anti-ageing substance depletes with age, especially after the age of forty, and skin then starts to lose its plumpness. But never fear, there are some fantastic natural foods, nutrients and herbs that can boost hyaluronic acid production.

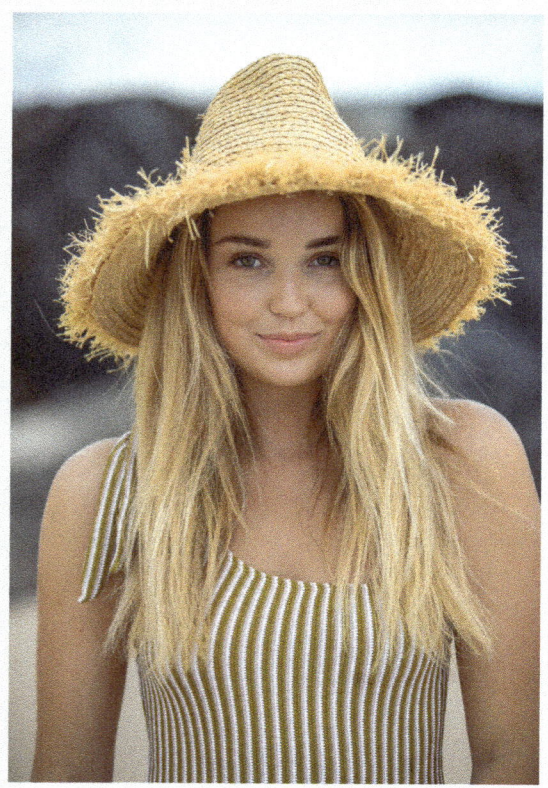

HYALURONIC ACID SUPER FOODS

Root vegetables – taro, sweet potatoes, yams

Vitamin C – bell peppers, strawberries, kiwifruit, kale, citrus

Magnesium – green leafy vegetables, asparagus, avocado, broccoli, lettuce, cauliflower, sweet potatoes, carrots, root vegetables, soybeans, apple, green beans

Fermented organic soy like natto, miso, tempeh, tofu

Bone and algae broths

Protein foods – organic eggs, Greek yoghurt, lean white meat, oily fish, legumes, seafood

Herbs – parsley, coriander, chilli

Grape seed extract or dark grapes can boost production (a glass of organic red wine)

A HAPPY MICROBIOME MEANS *HAPPY* SKIN.

The skin-gut connection has been studied since the 1930s and we still do not know all the names and roles of each bacteria that lives within our gastrointestinal tract. There are millions of different organisms, some friendly and some not so friendly, that co-exist within our gut, mouth, and other body parts. Everyday we discover more. We do know that the gut microbiome can influence inflammation, oxidative stress, blood sugar, allergies and sensitivities and in many people play a role in the health of skin conditions like eczema, psoriasis, acne and rosacea.

An easy way to start positively balancing your microbiome is by adding fermented foods like kefir, natto, tempeh, sauerkraut, kimchi and yoghurt into your diet. If you feel this doesn't work for you, you may have small intestinal bacterial overgrowth also known as SIBO. A large percentage of people with skin problems suffer from SIBO. This can be tested with a simple hydrogen breath test. SIBO is an overgrowth of micro-organisms that produce a substance called D-lactic acid.

Unfortunately, many probiotics contain strains like lactobacillus acidophilus that produce D-lactic acid and this can make the condition worse. Soil based organisms do not produce a lot of this and are a much better choice. Restoring your microbiome is a vital key to glowing skin and graceful ageing.

MAGNETIC MINERALS FOR BEAUTY

As you can probably tell, I love to rave on about minerals. It is no wonder as minerals are the prime beauty elements. They are involved in an incredible 95 per cent of our body's activities including hydration, filtration, hair and nail growth and alkalinity. I have an amazing German device that I use in my naturopathic practice that can accurately pick up on mineral deficiencies. After testing thousands of clients, I have found that over 90 per cent of people are mineral deficient, with the most common deficiencies being magnesium, silica, iodine and zinc. This doesn't surprise me, as our environment and food supplies are overloaded with huge amounts of heavy metals and chemicals and minerals act as the buffer to help protect us against these.

So how do you get enough minerals from food sources to satisfy the body's needs when the earth's soils are so depleted? Even if we eat 100 per cent organic all of the time and primarily raw it is still easy to experience mineral deficiencies, as stress, poor digestion and absorption, heavy metals, drinking too much caffeine, soft drinks and alcohol and even medications can deplete and disrupt our stores.

Green plants are definitely the number one 'beauty food' as they contain most of the minerals we need to enhance every factor that contributes to natural beauty and wellness, including the replication of collagen and elastin. To get a higher mineral content, it is always best to eat most greens raw, although some greens like broccoli, broccolini and bok choy suit being steamed to unlock some of their beautifying nutrients. Eating 80 per cent raw foods in the diet is a great way to boost your mineral levels and to enhance all beauty and wellness factors. If you activate or sprout your nuts, seeds and pulses you can boost your mineral absorption even more.

THE BEST MINERAL RICH GREENS

Seaweeds and sea vegetables	Spinach	Swiss chard
Broccoli and broccolini	Bok choy	Kale
	Celery	Mustard greens
Rocket	Dandelion greens	Wheatgrass

For an added beauty boost, eat organic greens, because minerals enter the plant from the soil and organic soil has a higher mineral content than traditionally farmed soil.

CALCIUM – THE BONE STRENGTHENER

Everyone knows that calcium builds healthy teeth and bones, but many people do not realise its unique skin beautifying qualities. Calcium exists abundantly in the epidermis and here it regulates cell turnover by replacing old cells with new ones. If you do not have enough calcium in the skin, cell regeneration slows down, causing thin, aged and tired looking skin. Calcium, along with magnesium, silica and Vitamin D are essential to the integrity of all bones in the human body. If calcium levels are low, bones in the face begin to deteriorate, causing a loss of symmetry and sagging skin.

This handy little mineral is 'alkaline' in nature, so along with its friends, magnesium, potassium and sodium, it helps to keep the blood pH balanced and oxygenated. Calcium is a great natural fat burner – if more calcium is in the cells, fat is burnt more efficiently.

Signs to look out for with a calcium deficiency include soft nails, coarse hair, muscle cramps or weakness, fatigue, brittle teeth and cavities, psoriasis, dry and thin skin, headaches, acidity, poor sleep and irritated nerves.

CALCIUM SUPER HEROES

Beans, nuts (almonds, pistachio), sardines, leafy greens, Greek yoghurt, raw milk, spinach, broccoli, sesame seeds, tahini, organic tofu, bone broths

Too much soft drink, alcohol, red meat, coffee and stress can deplete calcium stores

COPPER – THE ELASTIN BOOSTER

Copper is the third most abundant mineral found in our body. It cannot be made, so we need to absorb this by eating the right foods. Along with zinc it encourages the production of collagen and elastin which gives skin its beautiful strength and elasticity. Copper works in harmony with selenium to help protect the skin against damage from harmful UV rays.

Warning signs of copper deficiency include early hair greying, fatigue, low body temperature, anemia, irregular heartbeat, bone fractures, skin pigmentation, paleness, thinning hair, bruising, frequent illness and brittle bones

COPPER SUPER HEROES

Sunflower seeds, mushrooms, soybeans, cashews, oysters, oily fish, black pepper, purple onions, dark green leafy vegetables, kale and Shiitake.

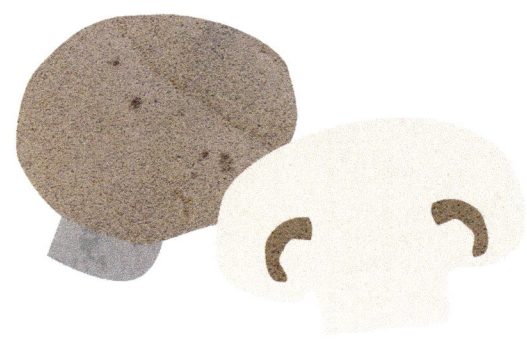

MAGNESIUM – THE HAPPY NUTRIENT

Magnesium is the most underestimated beauty mineral in the world. It is involved in three hundred biochemical reactions in the body, with one of these being the absorption of calcium to strengthen bones and teeth and to enhance fat burning. It is one of the main ingredients in making serotonin and melatonin – two important sleep chemicals. If you do not get your beauty sleep regularly, your skin can age very quickly. It boosts hyaluronic acid to plump the skin and helps to stop the shortening of telomeres, extending their lifespan.

Warning signs of a magnesium deficiency include leg or menstrual cramps, muscle tension or tremors, headaches, fatigue, shaking tongue, nausea, dizziness, poor memory, confusion, high blood pressure, anxiety, weakness, arrhythmias, sleep problems, depression, anxiety and moodiness.

MAGNESIUM SUPER HEROES

Spinach, Swiss chard, kale, asparagus, artichokes, avocado and collard greens, seaweed, oily fish, soybeans, root vegetables, black-eyed beans, chickpeas, lentils, brown rice, quinoa, millet, buckwheat, cacao, sesame seeds, cashews, pine nuts, pecans, brazil nuts, pumpkin seeds and dried apricots.

People are often surprised when they learn they have a magnesium deficiency, especially when they eat so well. So many factors cause a depletion of magnesium from the body, like drinking too much coffee, alcohol, tap water, soft drinks or tea, high stress, over-exercising, sweating, diarrhea, heavy metals like mercury, sugar, antibiotics, asthma medications, birth control pills, diuretics, pyrrole disorder, ComT gene issues and so much more. Understanding this, it is no wonder that 80% of people have a magnesium deficiency in today's world.

SILICA – COLLAGEN'S BEST FRIEND

Silica is the most common deficiency I see in clients of every age. This is not surprising, as silica helps to remove aluminium from the body and with our water supplies, foods and environment being flooded with this heavy metal it is understandable why most people's silica stores are being used up. Silica is found in the bones, cartilage, tendons, nails and connective tissues, where it provides strength and stability for collagen, the cement that holds everything together. When we are babies, our silica stores are very high, but once we get into our twenties they start to decline rapidly.

Along with its friends Vitamin C and compounds known as glycosaminoglycans or GAG's, silica enhances moisture in the tissues and improves the firmness, elasticity and strength of your skin, hair and nails.

Warning signs of a silica deficiency include brittle and ridged nails, slow hair growth and breakage, premature wrinkles, osteoporosis, poor muscle tone, cellulite, stretch marks following pregnancy, dental caries, acne, eczema, boils, scarring, kidney stones, gallstones, and brittle teeth.

SILICA SUPER HEROES

Apples, oranges, cherries, raisins, banana, mango, cabbage, onions, endive, carrots, eggplant, pumpkin, celery, beets, cucumber (the skin), bamboo shoots, alfalfa, artichoke, radish, romaine lettuce, spinach, asparagus, watercress, green beans, tomatoes (the skin), brown rice, barley, millet and oats.

Herb sources include horsetail, nettles, comfrey, chickweed and burdock root.

SELENIUM – THE AGEING GLADIATOR

Sadly, skin damage and most diseases are often a result of free radical driven 'oxidation' or ROS. External free radicals come from cigarette smoke, drugs, pollution, alcohol, heavy metals, toxins and harmful UV rays. Internal free radicals are created from poor digestion, stress and a diet high in saturated fats, sugar and processed foods. Selenium, along with its best friend, Vitamin E, can mop up some of the age-promoting damage of these destructive free radicals and in the process improve skin elasticity, sun protection, and minimise age spots. Selenium is a powerful cancer fighter that protects against many forms of cancer, including skin, prostate, breast, lung and liver cancer.

Warning signs of a selenium deficiency include mood swings, fatigue, garlic smelling breath, hair loss, diarrhea, indented nails, muscle pain, hypothyroidism and mental fatigue.

SELENIUM SUPERHEROES

Tuna, crab, oysters, prawns, turkey, wheat germ, chicken breast, mushrooms, eggs. Only 3 to 4 Brazil nuts daily can help you get your RDA of selenium.

SULPHUR – THE DETOXIFYING KING

Sulphur is part of the chemical structure of three different amino acids, cystine, cysteine and methionine. Sulphur is found abundantly in keratin, a protein that strengthens the hair, skin and nails. It is often referred to as 'nature's beauty mineral,' as it helps to make elastin, a protein that helps keep skin flexible and young.

It is a naturally-occurring mineral that is found near hot springs and volcanic craters. It has a delightful 'rotten egg' smell (just kidding) that is caused by sulphur dioxide gas escaping into the air. Its two prime supplement forms, dimethyl sulfoxide (DMSO) and methylsulfonylmethane (MSM) are both effective remedies for inflammation and skin health.

SULPHUR SUPER HEROES

Broccoli sprouts, cruciferous vegetables (broccoli, cauliflower, brussels sprouts, cabbage), egg yolks, berries (raspberries, blueberries, strawberries), brazil nuts, fish, GARLIC, onions, leeks, chives, spinach, fennel, asparagus.

ZINC – THE IMMUNE GUARDIAN

Zinc is the 'immunity guardian' that protects against viruses, infections and other nasties. It is involved in over 120 enzyme functions daily, including appetite regulation, stress protection, healthy sleep, taste and smell, libido and healing. Zinc protects the body's cells against age-promoting free radicals that result from ultraviolet light, radiation, nicotine, and air pollution.

Zinc is very important for anyone who suffers from acne as it balances hormones, controlling the production of oil in the skin. It is excreted in large amounts in people who have 'pyrrole disorder'. This is quite a common, genetic condition that causes large amounts of zinc, biotin, B6 and magnesium to be excreted from the body when a person is stressed or going through hormone changes.

Warning signs of a deficiency include a poor appetite, taste or smell, stunted growth, poor wound healing, skin abnormalities (such as acne, atopic dermatitis and psoriasis), hair loss, warts, herpes, delayed sexual maturation, white spots on the nails, depression, anxiety, poor sleep, irritability, cold sores, dry skin and cracks in the heels.

ZINC SUPER HEROES

Oysters, crab, fish, crustaceans, chicken, turkey, pumpkin seeds, almonds, sesame seeds, hazelnuts, mushrooms, ginger, grass-fed meats.

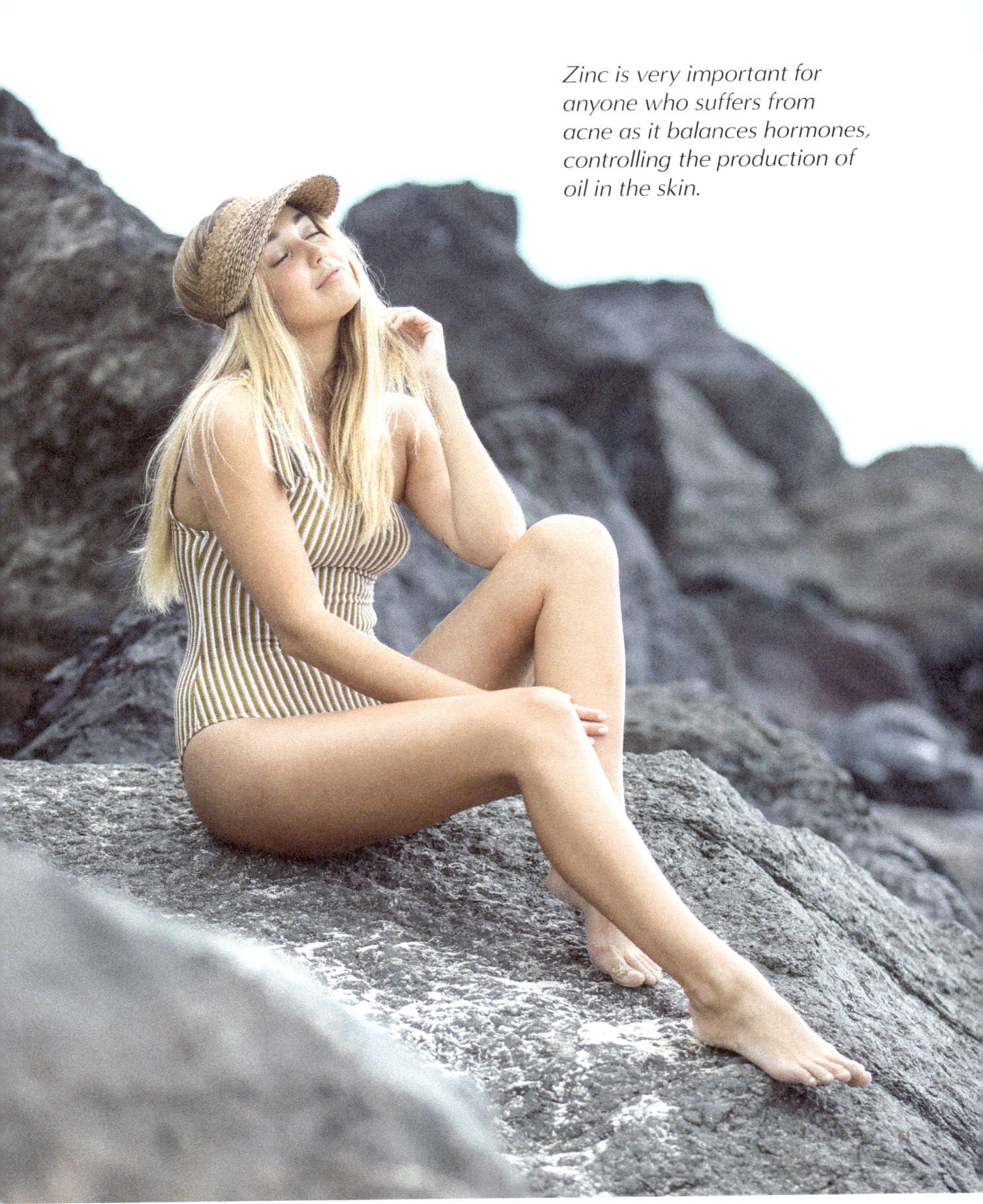

Zinc is very important for anyone who suffers from acne as it balances hormones, controlling the production of oil in the skin.

Natural Beauty Vitamins

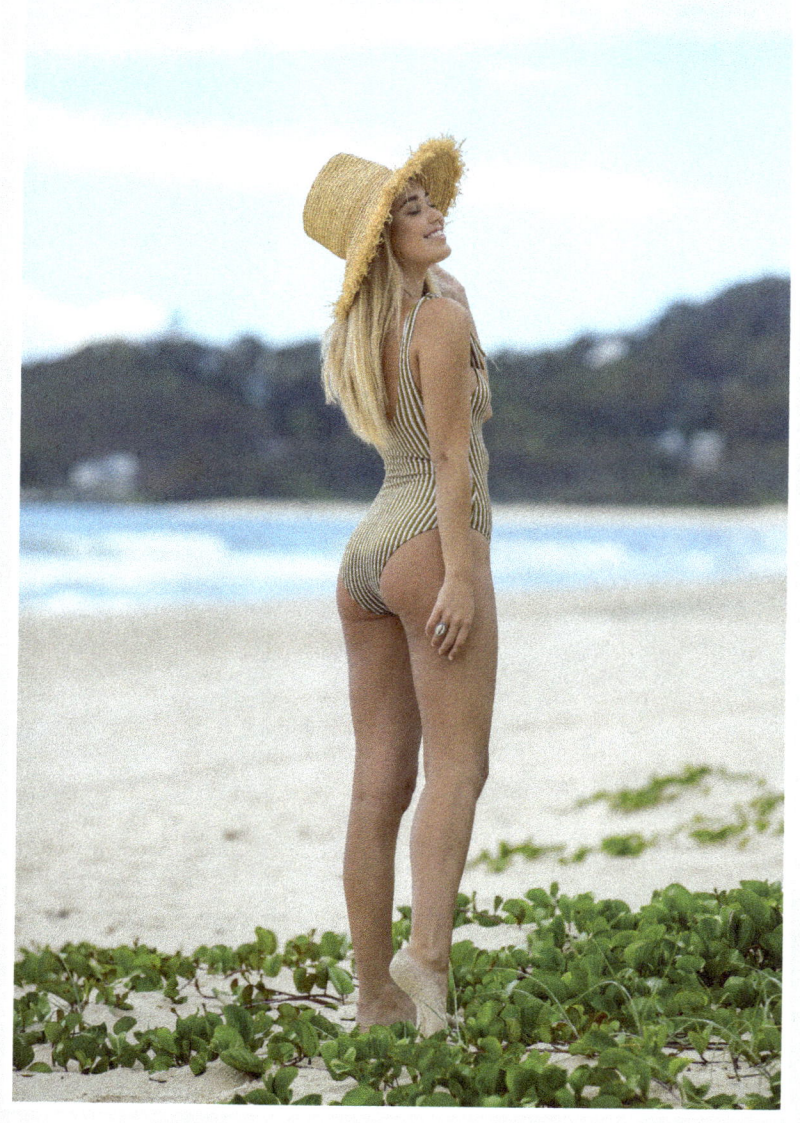

VITAMIN A – THE PEEP PROTECTOR

Vitamin A is a powerful antioxidant that puts a roadblock on skin-destroying free radicals, reducing their ability to advance wrinkles, age spots and stretch marks. It is a true skin warrior that provides amazing protection against sun damage and plays a big role in protecting against all forms of skin cancer. If your skin is oily or pimply, Vitamin A will stop an over-production of sebum. And don't forget, if you want incredible vision, add some Vitamin A rich foods into your diet as this is the best nutrient for improving the health of your peeps.

Warning signs of a deficiency include night blindness, poor immunity, inflammatory bowel problems like Crohn's and Ulcerative Colitis, stretch marks, acne and skin pigmentation.

VITAMIN A SUPER HEROES

Animal Vitamin A sources; grass fed butter, dairy products, eggs, liver, ghee.

The carotene containing vegetables which help to produce Vitamin A are apricots, cantaloupe, carrots, red or orange bell peppers, mango, pumpkin, sweet potato, kale and spinach.

VITAMIN C – THE ALL-ROUNDER

Vitamin C is another big player in the war against advanced skin ageing and disease. Collagen cannot be made without Vitamin C. Without collagen our skin begins to sag and wrinkle. It fights an admirable battle in the protection against free radicals that advance ageing and cause disease. Vitamin C is one of the cofactors in producing hyaluronic acid, a cushioning substance that makes skin plump and hydrated. As vitamin C is water-soluble it needs to be replaced daily through food.

Warning signs of a deficiency include frequent colds and flus, fatigue, paleness, sunken eyes, bleeding & tender gums, poor wound healing, scars, easy bruising, dry and splitting hair, nosebleeds, rough/dry/scaly skin, weight gain, leaky gut and poor immunity.

VITAMIN C SUPERHEROES

Guava, blackcurrants, berries, bell peppers (all colours, although red contains the highest amount), broccoli, cantaloupe, melons, kale, mango, citrus (lemon, lime, grapefruit, orange), pineapple, snow peas, tomatoes, kiwifruit, papaya and cauliflower.

VITAMIN D – THE SUN WARRIOR

Did you know that Vitamin D not only protects against cancer, immune diseases and strengthens the bones and teeth, but it also acts as a superb weight loss nutrient? This sun warrior is essential for the absorption of calcium, and low calcium can make fatty acids turn calories into fat. No wonder it is easy to lose weight when you spend holidays in hot, tropical climates. Vitamin D is needed for skin renewal, so it plays a vital role in reducing the flakiness linked to eczema and psoriasis. Skin colour is produced by the formation of melanin in the skin and this requires Vitamin D.

Sunlight encourages the body to make Vitamin D. People with very dark skin need 20 times more sunlight to absorb Vitamin D and using sunscreen all over your body can block its absorption. Unfortunately, many people carry genes that are unable to convert Vitamin D from sunlight into its active form, so in these cases you may need to supplement. Inflammatory bowel diseases, low levels of essential fatty acids, magnesium or zinc deficiency and many other reasons can inhibit its absorption.

THE BEST VITAMIN D SUPER HEROES ARE:

Sunlight

Fatty and oily fishes like salmon, cod, herring, halibut, sardines, tuna, mackerel, trout

Portobello and shitake mushrooms (organic)

Egg yolk (one contains around 40 IU of Vitamin D)

Organic tofu (firmer tofu contains more)

Raw cow's milk (not pasteurised)

Lots of fortified sources like grains and dairy products (although these aren't the healthiest option)

VITAMIN E – THE AGEING GUARDIAN

Vitamin E is one of the body's greatest skin guardians. It is a fat-soluble vitamin that protects the skin against free radicals generated from harmful UV rays. Nearly every cell in the human body contains Vitamin E. It works alongside Vitamin C to provide anti-ageing skin protection. It also helps to regulate sebum production in the skin, helping to stop irritation, inflammation and skin dryness. It is one of the best natural remedies to help heal burns and scars.

Warning signs of a deficiency include hair loss, muscle weakness, anaemia, balance and coordination problems, very dry skin and vision problems.

VITAMIN E SUPERHEROES

Wheatgerm, nuts and seeds, olive oil, swiss chard, spinach, leafy greens, sweet potato.

VITAMIN B3 OR NIACIN – THE BLOOD FLUSHER

There are so many B vitamins all with their special roles to play in the human body. This vitamin affects how your body draws energy from fats, so it plays a big role in making you feel energized. Nicotinamide, an activated form of Vitamin B3, has received rave reviews for its ability to reduce the formation of squamous and basal cell skin cancers by over 25% when taken regularly. If you want a perkier pout, don't forget to add some niacin to your program, as this vitamin can increase blood flow to your lips. Coffee is rich in niacin, so drinking a cup of organic coffee daily is a great way to reduce skin cancer risk and to add some extra plump to your lips.

Signs of a deficiency include poor concentration, fatigue, anxiety, restlessness, apathy, depression, cold hands and feet, high cholesterol and skin cancers.

VITAMIN B3 SUPERHEROES

Shiitake, salmon, wild rice, organic chicken, turkey, avocado, Portobello mushrooms, sunflower seeds, tuna, broccoli, asparagus and coffee.

VITAMIN K – THE ANTI-WRINKLE QUEEN.

Japanese women are considered to have flawless, wrinkle-free skin, even when they reach a prime age. One of the reasons for this is the high amount of Vitamin K in their diets. This is found in fermented foods like natto, miso and tempeh. Vitamin K prevents calcification in the elastin of the skin. Elastin is the protein that gives the skin its flexibility to bounce back, thus helping to reduce wrinkling. Vitamin K is essential for carrying calcium into bones, so without this, bones begin to weaken, leading to osteoporosis and a lack of symmetry. If you want beautiful strong teeth, don't forget Vitamin K. This vitamin helps to produce dentin, which carries calcium into the teeth.

Vitamin K also helps to maintain the integrity of all the blood vessels and capillaries that feed the skin. A lack of this nutrient can cause a loss of tone in the veins, leading to varicose veins. Because Vitamin K helps with skin elasticity, a deficiency is a major driver towards those dreaded stretch marks too.

Signs of a deficiency include easy bruising, dark circles under eyes, stretch marks, heavy periods, osteoporosis, bleeding problems, varicose veins and nosebleeds.

VITAMIN K SUPERHEROES

Vitamin K1 is found in green leafy vegetables like spinach, kale, brussels sprouts, cabbage, broccoli, collards, spring onions and asparagus. The conversion of K1 into K2 is very limited at a 10:1 ratio.

Vitamin K2, which is considered more easily absorbable, is found in sauerkraut, kefir, swiss cheese, hard cheeses, fermented foods like tempeh and natto, grass-fed meat, butter and egg yolks.

BIOTIN – AS HARD AS NAILS

Biotin is often overlooked in the world of beauty, but since the discovery that biotin plays a role in skin, hair and nail health it has taken on celebrity status! Biotin helps to metabolise carbohydrates, fats and protein into energy. It is needed for the formation of our genetic material, our DNA and RNA. It is a natural nail, hair and skin reinforcer that reduces eczema, dermatitis, greying hair, cradle cap and other dry skin conditions.

Signs of a deficiency include hair loss, scaly dermatitis, depression, pale skin, high blood sugar, nausea, sore tongue, dry and flaky skin, high cholesterol, sensitivity to touch, inflamed eyes, weight gain and cradle cap in children.

BIOTIN SUPERHEROES

Swiss chard, carrots, almonds, walnuts, goat's milk, eggs (but not raw eggs), halibut, strawberries, raspberries, salmon, sardines, tuna, buttermilk, cauliflower, lettuce, cucumber, spinach, avocado, banana, goji berries and beer, wine and coffee (can you believe it?).

OTHER NUTRIENT SUPERHEROES

Polyphenols are powerful phytochemicals that develop in plants to guard them against damage from environmental predators. When a human ingests these substances they also receive this vital protection. Some of the most well known polyphenols are curcumin (found in turmeric), quercetin (found in onions), resveratrol (found in grape skins), catechins (found in green, oolong and white tea) and lycopene (found in tomatoes).

Resveratrol is a polyphenol that is found in high amounts in red wine, cocoa, grape skins, grape seed extract, blueberries and cranberries. Just like its other polyphenol brothers, it vigilantly guards against cancer, cardiovascular disease, skin damage and premature ageing.

Anthocyanins are a type of polyphenol that belongs to the bioflavonoid family. They are antioxidants that paint plants and berries with their magnificent blue, red and purple colours. These powerful substances SHIELD against the free radical damage that causes ageing and skin breakdown, as well as against other diseases. Good sources of these are found in purple carrots and all blue or purple berries.

Ellagic acid is an influential antioxidant polyphenol that protects the skin from sun damage and hinders the formation of an enzyme that breaks down elastin and collagen in the skin. When you combine ellagic acid with anthocyanins you have the perfect wrinkle-destroying team. The best sources of this are found in green tea, blackberries, cranberries, raspberries, and strawberries.

Glucosamine is an amino acid that most people take for inflammation and joint damage. However, it is so much more than that. It is a true beauty warrior as it can plump up the hyaluronic acid stores in the skin, reducing the formation of wrinkles. Glucosamine or GAGS are found abundantly in bone broths.

Coenzyme Q10 is not often talked about in the beauty world, but now that its cell rejuvenating effects are coming to light it is making a welcome appearance. We all make coenzyme Q10 in the body, but unfortunately as we start to age, production of it slows. It plays a vital role in cellular ATP or energy production, so without it our cells' energy cycle begins to slow down. This leaves us more vulnerable to free radical destruction, which can cause a great deal of skin ageing. Foods rich in coenzyme Q10 include fatty, cold water fish like salmon, tuna and herring, grass-fed meats, broccoli, cauliflower, peanuts, sesame seeds, pistachio nuts and strawberries.

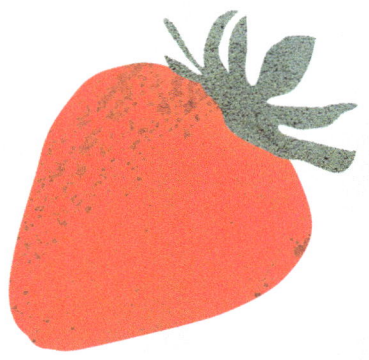

CHAPTER FOUR

NATURE'S SECRETS TO RADIANT BEAUTY

Seeds of Beauty: digestion

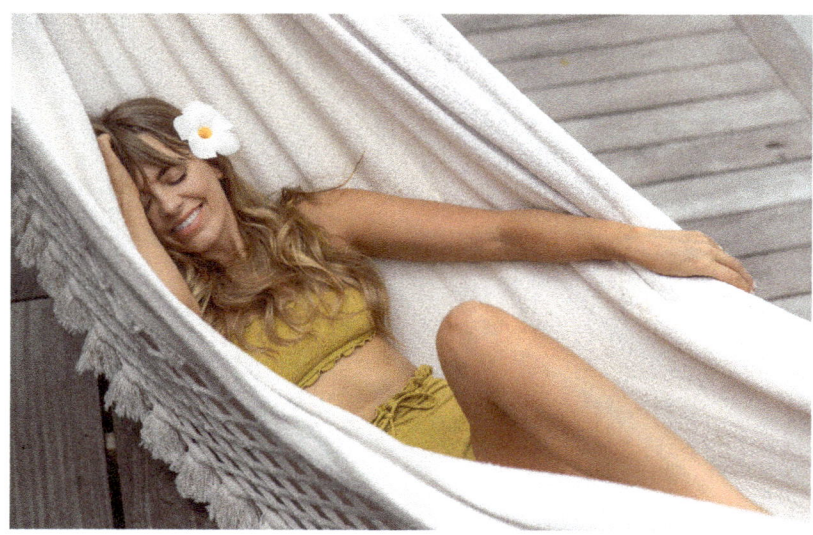

SEEDS OF BEAUTY: DIGESTION

THE DIGESTIVE SYSTEM'S ROLE IN ENHANCING BEAUTY AND OPTIMAL HEALTH IS NOW BEING EXPLORED MORE THAN OTHER 'BEAUTY OR WELLNESS FACTOR'.

A resilient and healthy digestive system begins the moment of conception. If our mum dined on a cocktail of sugar, soft drinks and processed foods before and during pregnancy, this poor nutrition can affect the quality of our microbiome and our intestinal lining, as well as our ability to absorb nutrients to create strong teeth, bones and gums. If we were lucky enough to have been fed nutrient-rich mother's milk, weaned on living, enzyme rich foods and not given antibiotics, then our digestive systems have had the best start in life.

Sadly, this is not the case for many. Some children are introduced to man-made formula milk at birth, given antibiotics, fed refined sugar products and exposed to artificial additives, preservatives and other nutritionally devoid foods that can wipe out a thriving digestive system. So why is a healthy diet from conception so important? When a beautiful seed blossoms into a strong plant it requires nutritionally rich soil to grow healthy and strong, enabling it to withstand any environmental dangers.

The body's intestinal ecology is not unlike a plant. If its microbial environment is rich in the right flora, it can withstand any disease and enhance the absorption of life-giving and beauty-enhancing minerals to renew every cell in the human body.

This living bacterial ecosystem, consisting of over 100 trillion organisms, is not only found in our digestive system, but in our gums, our noses and on our skin. We call this living, breathing orchestra our 'microbiome'.

Some of these organisms are 'friendly' and some are not so 'friendly', but as long as they coexist in balance they remain harmonious.

The majority of these bacteria take up residence within the gut, and because of their intelligence, they are now nicknamed our 'second brain'.

Here these clever organisms can regulate our physical and emotional health via their own neural network, known as the enteric nervous system. This system is quite complex as it contains 100 million nerves found in the gut lining. These nerves, along with the smart microbiome, are uniquely connected via a complex symphony of hormones, neurotransmitters and electrical impulses. This allows the upper brain, the nervous system, the immune and the digestive systems to communicate in order to keep a harmonious balance, just like a brilliantly composed symphony.

SO HOW DOES DIGESTION WORK?

As soon as we catch a whiff of that yummy chocolate our mouth begins to salivate with anticipation. This enzyme-rich saliva softens the food so it can easily slide down the oesophageal slippery slide into the stomach. Glutamic acid, pepsin and betaine are released into the stomach (and with the help of zinc creates a hydrochloric acid like mix) and a swirling motion breaks the big food particles into smaller ones.

This is the beginning of how proteins and minerals are drawn from foods. Food can stay here for forty-five minutes or three hours depending on what was eaten and how healthy your digestive system is. Just like in a concrete mixer, the food is swirled into a liquid called 'chyme'. When the mixture is ready, it is passed into a 20-foot-long tunnel

known as the small intestine. Chyme puts its breaks on and takes a leisurely stroll through here passing through the duodenum to absorb minerals, into the jejunum to absorb water-soluble vitamins, carbohydrates and protein and then into the ileum to absorb fat soluble vitamins, cholesterol and bile. The small intestine secretes lots of digestive and protective substances with the help of its friends the pancreas, liver and gallbladder. A majority of the bacteria that make up the 'microbiome' live within the small intestines, helping with absorption, elimination and neurotransmitter production.

After most of the good stuff is extracted from the food, the leftovers pass into the large intestines where more water and electrolytes are absorbed. Microbial fermentation of fibre, starch and undigested carbohydrates occurs here, and short chain fatty acids like butyrate, propionate and acetate come to life. These clever little hydrogen-bonded molecules balance the microbiome here, helping to lower inflammation, create energy and boost immunity. After extracting what it needs the large intestines (or colon) escorts the toxic waste from the party area, kicking it out.

The digestive system's friends, the pancreas, gallbladder and liver, don't like to be left out, so they offer their assistance too. The pancreas makes enzymes to break down fats, starches and proteins. This balances glucose creating energy and prevents food intolerances. The gallbladder holds bile produced in the liver in order to absorb fats and fat-soluble vitamins and to soften stools.

When the body's digestive system is healthy, the skin takes on a beautiful glow. However, many lifestyle and dietary factors can affect its performance. The intestinal walls can easily become damaged from eating processed foods, alcohol, stimulants, drugs or medications, from chemotherapy or radiation, constipation, parasite and bacterial overgrowth and long-term stress. Stress is the biggest culprit in disabling the health of the digestive system.

As naturopaths, we are told over and over 'fix the gut and you will repair everything'. And now I'm happy that this 'health mantra' was drummed into me, as this saying is turning out to be 100% true, especially when it comes to rejuvenating beauty, spiritual wellness and enhancing longevity.

The Healthy Colon Test

How healthy is your colon? Rate the occurrence of each question then calculate your total score.

Rating Scale: 0 = Never | **1** = Rarely | **2** = Occasionally | **3** = Often | **4** = Occasionally with severe symptoms | **5** = Always

Acne	0	1	2	3	4	5
Appendicitis	0	1	2	3	4	5
Bad breath	0	1	2	3	4	5
Bloating straight after meals	0	1	2	3	4	5
Bloating at any time	0	1	2	3	4	5
Boils	0	1	2	3	4	5
Bowel movements less than once daily	0	1	2	3	4	5
Coated tongue	0	1	2	3	4	5
Colon cancer or polyps	0	1	2	3	4	5
Constipation	0	1	2	3	4	5
Diarrhoea	0	1	2	3	4	5
Diverticulitis	0	1	2	3	4	5
Dry stools	0	1	2	3	4	5
Eczema, dermatitis, rashes	0	1	2	3	4	5
Dairy intake more than 5 times week	0	1	2	3	4	5
Red meat intake more than 5 times week	0	1	2	3	4	5
Sugar in diet more than 5 times week	0	1	2	3	4	5
Fatigue	0	1	2	3	4	5
Food allergies or intolerances	0	1	2	3	4	5
Gas or flatulence	0	1	2	3	4	5

Headaches or migraines	0	1	2	3	4	5
Heartburn	0	1	2	3	4	5
Haemorrhoids	0	1	2	3	4	5
Hernia	0	1	2	3	4	5
Inability to break down fats	0	1	2	3	4	5
Indigestion	0	1	2	3	4	5
Lower back pain	0	1	2	3	4	5
Nausea	0	1	2	3	4	5
Need for laxatives (natural or pharmaceutical)	0	1	2	3	4	5
Stomach pains	0	1	2	3	4	5
Ulcers	0	1	2	3	4	5
Varicose veins	0	1	2	3	4	5
Weight gain around the middle	0	1	2	3	4	5

If you scored 1 to 13 you have a mild digestive problem

If you scored from 14 – 25 you have some moderate digestive issues

If you scored from 26 – 40 this indicates a severe digestive imbalance

If you scored from 41 + this indicates a very bad problem that needs to be fixed quickly.

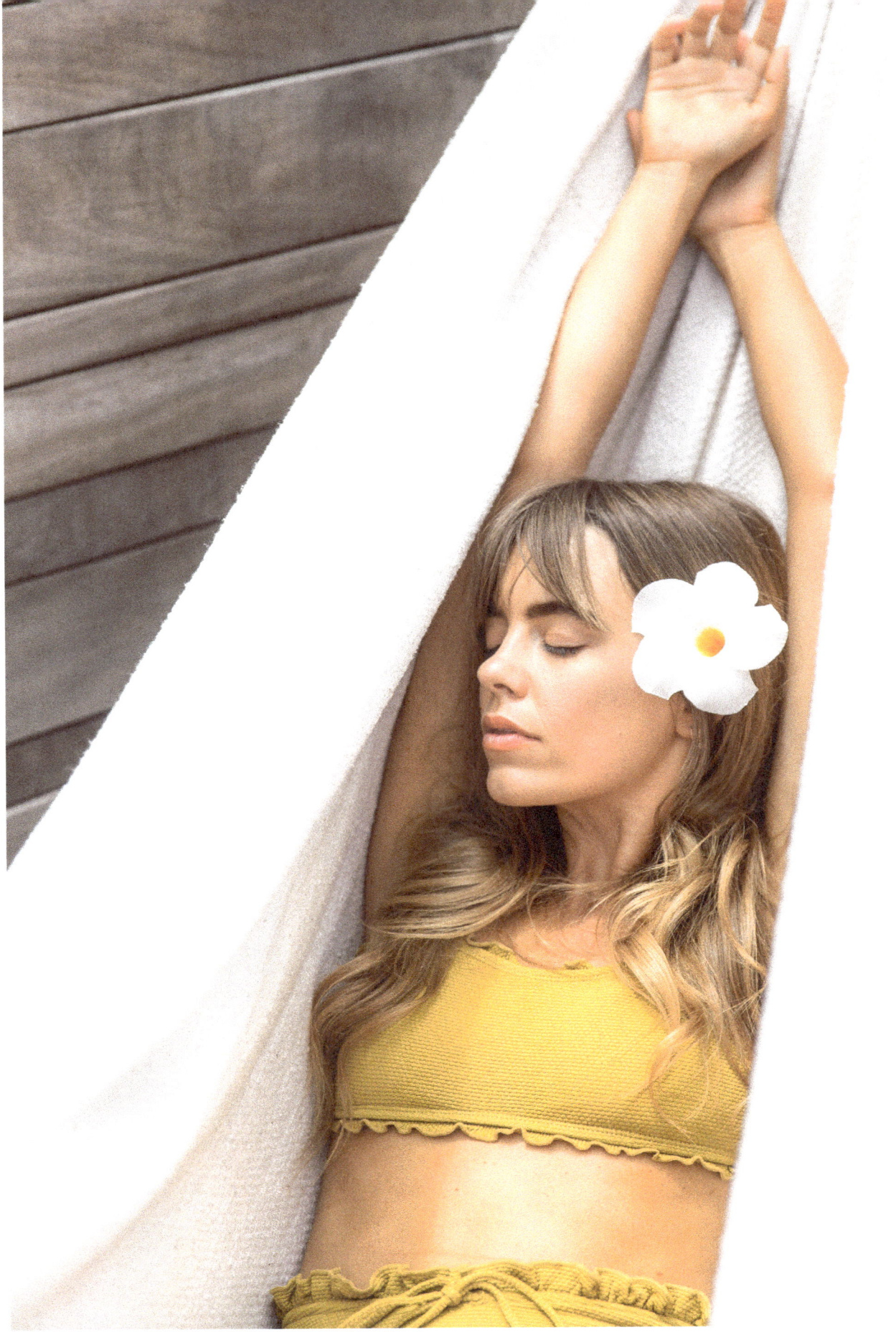

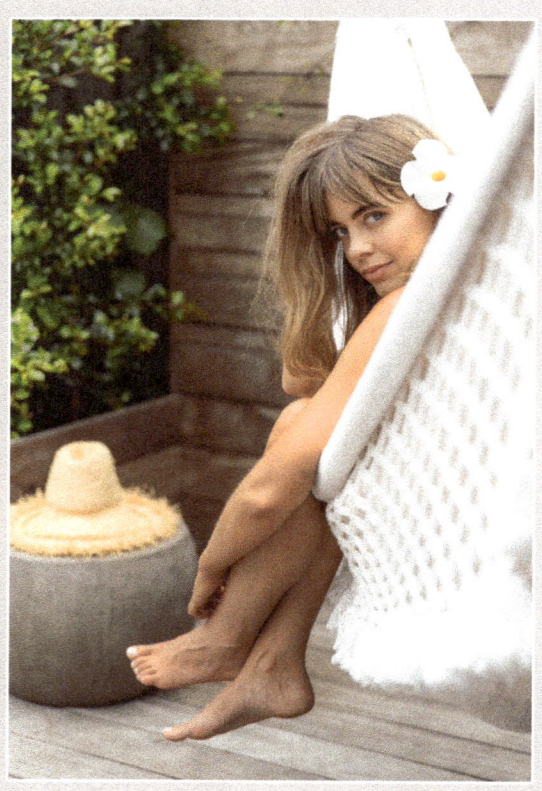

THE BODY'S DIGESTIVE FIRE – HYDROCHLORIC ACID

Hydrochloric acid (HCL) is the main gastric acid secreted by the stomach. It helps to break large food particles into smaller ones, preventing food intolerances and symptoms linked to this. When gastric acid is released, it also triggers the release of alkaline bicarbonate into the blood, helping to regulate blood PH.

HCL coordinates signals to the nervous system to open and close the gate from the stomach to the esophagus, known as the esophageal sphincter. Proper opening and closing of this muscle prevents acid reflux, GORD and Barrett's. If the food decides to get lazy and sits in the stomach because HCL levels are too low, the natural reaction of the body is to push it up through the gate into the esophagus to get it out. This can cause heartburn, indigestion and discomfort.

HCL is also the body's first barrier against parasites, microbes, viruses and bad bacteria including the ulcer driving bacteria H Pylori. HCL denatures proteins, basically melting them apart, and activates a substance called pepsin via its conversion from pepsinogen. Pepsin is essential for protein digestion and proteins are needed for healthy collagen, elastin, hair, skin, nails, enzymes, muscles, and neurotransmitters. It is also essential for the absorption of minerals like calcium, zinc and magnesium. Without these alkaline minerals the body becomes very acidic, resulting in advanced ageing, skin and bone breakdown and disease. Zinc is needed to help convert pepsin into pepsinogen for healthy digestion.

SYMPTOMS AND SIGNS OF LOW GASTRIC ACIDITY

- Abnormal bowel flora
- Adrenal fatigue (poor protein digestion raises cortisol and in turn raises blood glucose causing adrenal fatigue)
- Anemia or iron deficiency
- Bad breath
- Bloating, belching, burning or gas after meals
- Body odour
- Brittle, split or cracked nails
- Butterfly rash on face
- Candida and yeast overgrowth
- Diarrhoea or constipation
- Difficulty digesting foods
- Dilated capillaries on the cheeks
- Dry skin
- Fatigue
- Food allergies/intolerances
- Gallstones
- H Pylori infection
- Hair loss, especially in women
- Itchy anus/rectum
- Leaky gut
- Loss of appetite for high protein foods
- Low B12 levels
- Mineral deficiencies of calcium, magnesium, iron, zinc, copper, chromium, manganese, molybdenum, selenium
- Nausea after taking supplements
- Parasites
- Post adolescent acne
- Protruding stomach
- Red rash with pimples
- Stools – pale, greasy or floating
- Tooth problems and periodontal disease
- Undigested food in stools
- Vitiligo (loss of skin pigmentation)
- White spots on nails
- Worms

Certain health conditions are thought to be linked to low HCL levels including acne, asthma, alcoholism, hives, dermatitis/eczema, rheumatoid arthritis, Helicobacter, Addison's disease, autoimmunity, diabetes, hepatitis, hypothyroidism, lupus and osteoporosis.

CAUSES OF 'LOW STOMACH ACID'

- B vitamin and/or zinc deficiency
- Iodine deficiency – iodine is used by parietal cells to concentrate chloride – a component of HCL
- A high sugar, protein, grain or processed food intake
- Antacid or proton pump inhibitor use
- Overuse of anti-inflammatory drugs and antibiotics
- Stress and worry
- Drinking too much caffeine, alcohol or stimulants
- Age-related HCL depletion
- Eating too quickly or on the go

How to FIX your 'DIGESTIVE FIRE'

Diet is an essential tool in rebuilding the 'chemical balance' of HCL in your tummy. It is important to remove sugar, processed foods, excess caffeine, alcohol and saturated fats. Never eat when you are upset or in a hurry and don't drink icy cold drinks while eating.

OTHER IMPORTANT KEYS INCLUDE:

BETAINE HCL supplements are the fastest way to help boost HCL production. These contain the essential tools of hydrogen and chloride. Take 1 capsule ten minutes before meals and when you begin to feel a warm sensation in your tummy after taking for a while, stop.

FERMENTED FOODS like sauerkraut, kefir, kimchee, natto, tempeh, miso and similar can help.

RAW APPLE CIDER VINEGAR is also helpful. Dilute one teaspoon into a little water and drink ten minutes before eating.

CELERY juice contains natural sodium salts to help stimulate digestion. Begin the day with a glass of cold pressed celery juice and don't forget to add a bitter like lemon skin or ginger.

BITTER FOODS like radicchio, chicory, dandelion, rocket or endive are helpful.

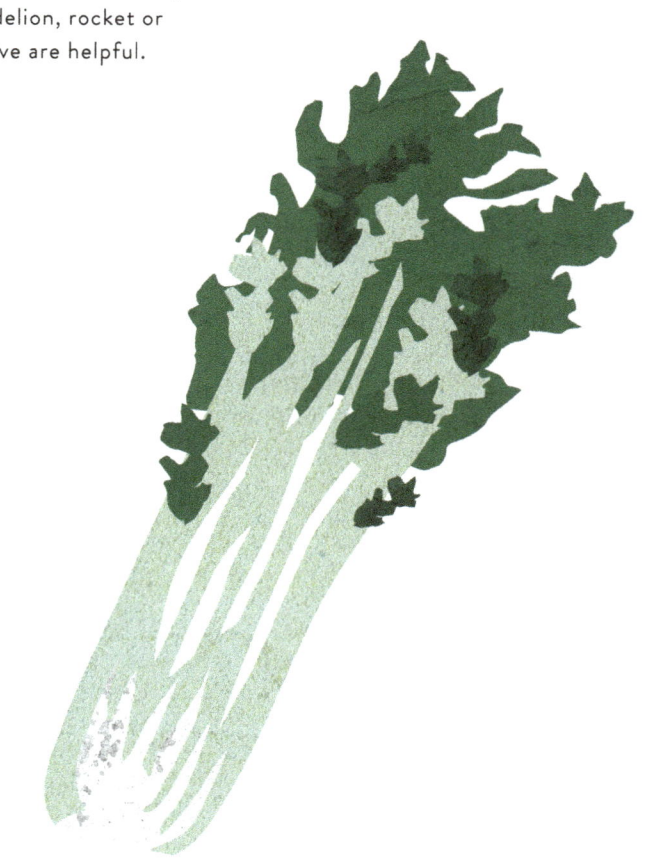

DIGESTIVE BITTERS – I love creating herbal 'bitter' tonics to improve stomach acid. My fav herbs for this are gentian, meadowsweet, agrimony, dandelion root & milk thistle.

ZINC is a cofactor in HCL production. Foods rich in this include activated pumpkin seeds, ginger, mushrooms, shellfish, oily fish, cacao...

ACTIVATED B VITAMINS are essential for stomach health.

Ginger, cumin, orange peel, galangal, kale, spinach, wheat grass, barley grass and black olives can really help stimulate HCL.

BONE or VEGAN BROTHS are fantastic healing remedies too

ANTACIDS ARE DANGEROUS BEAUTY ROBBERS

In my twenty-five years of practice, I now see that at least 30% of people have been prescribed antacids or proton pump inhibitors by their practitioners. Antacids are natural beauty robbers as they reduce protein and mineral absorption needed for healthy collagen and elastin production in the skin. They also affect adrenal, pancreas and liver health. HCL in the stomach is the body's first line of defense against harmful bacteria, microbes and parasites. Long-term use of these medications can destroy your microbiome and leave you vulnerable to different forms of parasites, bacteria and even cancer. Many of my clients are put on these for reflux or heartburn. Wouldn't it be smarter to actually fix the cause of problem rather than placing a person on a pharmaceutical that causes multiple nutrient deficiencies, leading to worse problems in the future?

RAW FOODS ARE ENZYME REJUVENATORS

The food that you choose to eat shapes your skin health, cell rejuvenation, spiritual state and ability to manifest at a higher level. Raw, plant-based foods are living sources of antioxidants, minerals, vitamins, fibre, hyaluronic acid, water and enzymes. When you consume raw, living food, hair becomes luscious, the eyes sparkle with vitality and the skin glows with vibrance. This is largely due to the fact that plant-based foods are brimming with living enzymes. Enzymes are the spark plugs to millions of biochemical reactions in the human body. They are the catalysts to creating beauty and wellness on both a physical and spiritual level. Rejuvenating enzymes become depleted when we consume lots of processed and over-cooked foods.

Within our bodies we have thousands of enzymes that are activated by certain minerals. Minerals are abundant in living plant foods and with the help of enzymes they activate cell and tissue repair and create harmony on a deep level. Many raw food enthusiasts claim that you can only achieve beauty by eating a 100% raw, plant-based diet. I definitely believe that a raw foods diet is beautifying in every way, however I believe there are some situations in life and certain genetic constitutions that require a small amount of heated foods to achieve this balance.

ENZYMES – THE SECRET TO NATURAL BEAUTY

1. Enzymes control the release of adenosine triphosphate (ATP) to increase vitality.

2. Enzymes mop up toxic sludge and wastes that dull the complexion.

3. Enzymes are the catalysts for mineral absorption.

4. They are 'living proteins' that put energy into all internal metabolic processes.

5. They help to repair our DNA/RNA.

6. They help to make hormones.

7. They balance immunity and reduce inflammation.

8. They reduce blood viscosity, preventing clots and strokes.

9. They enhance tumour breakdown.

PARASITES – BEAUTY SCAVENGERS

It's very funny when my clients visit a practitioner and they are told 'don't worry about getting rid of parasites. They won't affect your health'. I hear this statement often from clients who are suffering from fatigue, inflammation, irritable bowel and similar digestive problems. All parasites are opportunistic organisms that rob the body of vital nutrients needed for optimal health, immunity and beauty. They often reside in the intestines where they steal nutrients, destroy the microbiome, weaken the intestinal lining and reduce immunoglobulins, setting up a multitude of modern day diseases.

Common symptoms of parasite overgrowth includes fatigue, itching anus, abdominal pain, weight loss or gain, diarrhea or constipation, gas and bloating, irritable bowel symptoms, tooth grinding, granulomas (lungs, liver, kidneys), anemia, skin rashes, anxiety, food intolerances, waking around 2 to 3 am, nose picking in kids, floaters or dark spots in eyes, craving for sugar or starch, toe fungus, sores on mouth or lips and recurrent vaginal or urinary tract infections.

A diet rich in starches, carbohydrates, SUGAR, saturated fats and processed foods is a perfect food supply for these nutrient-sucking scavengers. If your diet is full of enzyme-rich, anti-parasitical living foods like pumpkin seeds, pomegranate, raw garlic, beets, onion juice, coconut oil, papaya seeds, cloves, oregano, thyme, cinnamon, bitter melon and green onions, parasites will not be welcome in your digestive space.

If you need some extra herbal support to kill these nutrient sucking scavengers consider herbal killers like sweet wormwood, epazote, male fern, black walnut, berberine, goldenseal, neem and tea tree. Parasites are becoming more resistant to medication. If this is the case for you I would suggest using a biofilm dissolver, large doses of liposomal Vitamin C to flush your colon and rife frequency devices.

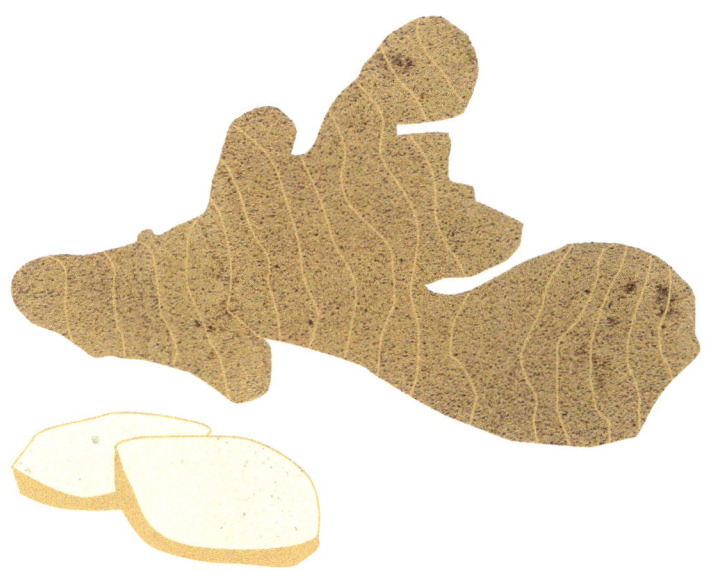

LOVE your
microbiome Diet

AM BEAUTY TONIC

¼ to ½ cup of purified, alkaline water

1 to 2 teaspoons of apple cider vinegar (made from 'mother')

½ lemon or lime

1 knob of ginger, finely grated or juiced

2 celery stalks, juiced

1 tbsp of aloe vera juice (100% pure from leaf – no sodium benzonate)

1 teaspoon of liquid colostrum (optional)

If you have a cold pressed juicer, put celery, lemon or lime and ginger through this. Stir in the apple cider vinegar and aloe vera juice. If you do not have a juicer, simply mix all of the ingredients and leave the celery out, adding more water if needed. This 'tummy tonic' boosts stomach acids, nourishes the microbiome and heals a damaged intestinal lining. Drink at the start of every day to improve your absorption and digestion.

LOVE your microbiome Diet

Begin the day with a glass of lukewarm, **alkaline water with a squeeze of fresh lemon** or lime OR drink one glass of the **AM BEAUTY TONIC** (recipe on previous page 77)

Two days a week it can be helpful to do intermittent fasting in the morning. Simply have your last meal at 6 or 7 pm the night before and try not to eat until 11 am the next day.

Aim for as many **vegan or bone broths** as you like throughout the day. These healing soups contain lots of minerals, amino acids and GAGS which boost stomach acids and help nourish the intestinal lining. There are some delicious recipes in this book.

Include at least **one serve of fermented foods** in your diet daily. My fav's are kimchee, sauerkraut, miso, natto and organic tempeh. I also love coconut kefir, kombucha and other fermented super drinks.

Eat plenty of **prebiotic foods** to help build up your natural gut bacteria in the large intestines. Prebiotic fibre, found in certain foods like beets, flaxseeds, apples, citrus, asparagus, garlic, carrots, chicory root, onions, Jerusalem artichokes, radish, jicama, dandelion greens and chia seeds, can help to produce short chain fatty acids like butyrate to inhibit bad bacteria in the gut while improving the production of the youth-promoting substance glutathione.

If you have a cold pressed juicer, don't forget the magic of **fresh wheatgrass juice**. Wheatgrass is packed full of chlorophyll to oxygenate the colon clearing impurities. I also love **cabbage, celery, ginger and lemon juice.**

While following this digestive healing diet, **avoid sugar, saturated fats, vegetable oils, processed foods, gluten, dairy products** (unless specified in the table), **non-organic meats** and other artificial foods.

Drink 6 to 8 glasses of alkaline, mineral rich water daily to help flush impurities through the colon.

Follow the **food list below** to help build a healthy microbiome and in doing so improve all factors towards wellness, beauty and spiritual happiness.

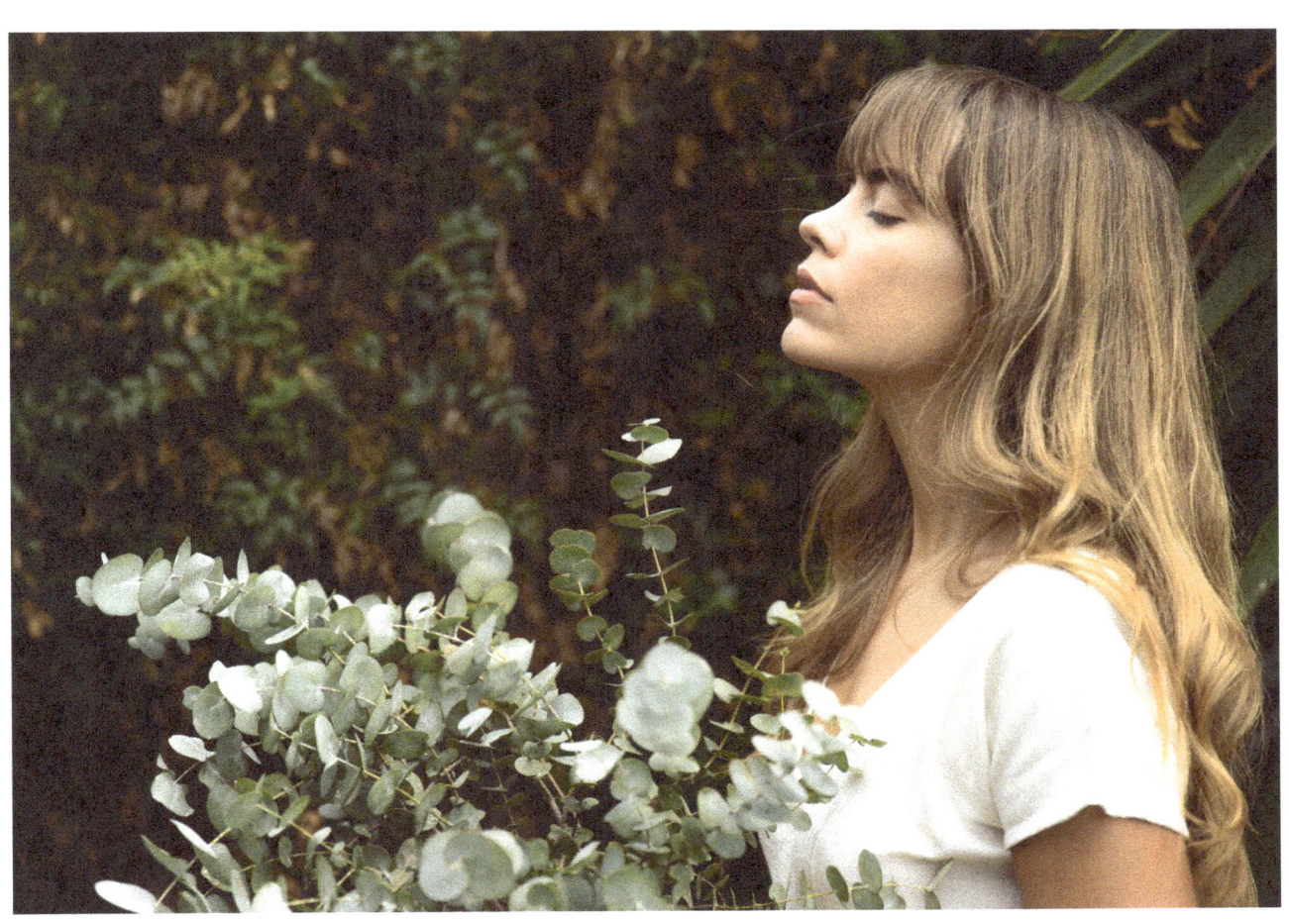

LOVE YOUR MICROBIOME FOOD LIST

OILS First cold pressed, organic, in dark bottles	NUTS & SEEDS ¼ cup day max – organic, soaked & activated	HERBS & SEASONING
Avocado oil – cook, raw	Almonds	Aniseed
Coconut oil – cook & raw	Brazil nuts	Basil
Ghee – cook	Chia seeds	Cayenne
Hemp seed oil – raw	Sesame	Celtic salt
Macadamia oil – cook	Flaxseeds	Chili
MCT oil – raw	Hazelnuts	Cinnamon
Olive oil – cook low heat	Hemp seeds	Cloves
Perilla oil – raw	Macadamia	Coriander
Pumpkin seed oil – raw	Pecans	Dill
Red palm oil – raw	Pine nuts	Fennel
Sacha inchi oil – raw	Pumpkin seeds	Ginger
Sesame oil – raw	Walnuts	Himalayan salt
Udo's oil – raw		Mint
Walnut oil – raw		Paprika

VINEGAR Make sure its raw, from the mother

	Parsley
Apple cider vinegar (raw)	Turmeric

SWEETENERS

Birch xylitol	Monk fruit
Erythritol	Stevia – leaf powder
Inulin	Yacon syrup
Luo han guo	

Rice vinegar
Coconut vinegar

FERMENTED FOODS Aim for 1 to 2 serves/day

BEANS, GRAINS
Organic, pre-soaked for 24 hours – eat in moderation, higher in carbs, if following keto, reduce or avoid

Kefir
Kimchee
Kombucha
Miso

COCONUT PRODUCTS

Adzuki	Millet
Amaranth	Quinoa
Black beans	Teff
Buckwheat	Rice – brown and wild

Natto
Sauerkraut

Coconut kefir
Coconut milk
Coconut flour
Coconut yoghurt (sugar-free)

VEGETABLES

Artichokes	Collards
Asparagus	Cruciferous vegetables
Beets	Cucumber
Bok choy	Daikon radish
Broccoli	Garlic
Brussels sprouts	Leeks
Carrots	Mushrooms – Shitake
Celery	Onions
Chicory root	Radish
Chives	Swiss chard

GREEN LEAFIES
Aim for 3 cups of salad veggies daily

Butter lettuce	Mustard greens
Cabbage – all types	Radicchio
Dandelion Greens	Rocket
Endive	Romaine lettuce
Kale	Spinach
Mesculin lettuce	Watercress
Mizuna	

ROOT VEGETABLES

Sweet potato	Yams
Taro	

DAIRY PRODUCTS

Avoid most dairy products. If you can tolerate, choose small amounts of:

Grass-fed butter	Goats' cheese
Parmesan and/or mozzarella cheese	Goats yoghurt
	Greek yoghurt

FRUITS

Apples	Lime
Avocado	Nectarines
Berries (all kinds)	Papaya
Grapefruit	Peaches
Kiwifruit	Pineapple
Lemon	Pomegranate

DRINKS

Activated nut milks

Alkaline water – PH 8 +

Ceremonial grade cacao

Beautiful vortex water

Green tea – matcha, sencha or genmai

Hemp milk

Hydrogen infused water

Herbal tea – chamomile, ginger, fennel, tulsi, mint, marshmallow

OTHER

Algae extracts

Aloe Vera Juice (100 % - inner leaf)

BONE BROTHS – organic, grass fed bones – concentrated is best

Braggs amino acids

Dark chocolate - cacao

Nutritional yeast

Seaweeds

Slippery elm powder

PLANT-BASED PROTEIN

Organic tempeh
– soy, chickpea or other

Legumes
– only if soaked & preferably sprouted

ANIMAL PROTEIN

Some people need animal protein in their diet to thrive. If this is you, choose organic, grass fed meats no more than twice weekly.

Organic, uncaged eggs not fed grain or corn are fine

Organic chicken/turkey

SEAFOOD
Aim for 2 to serves weekly if you are not vegetarian

Oily fish – mackerel, salmon (unfarmed – sockeye), sardines, herring, halibut

Oysters

Crustaceans – in moderation

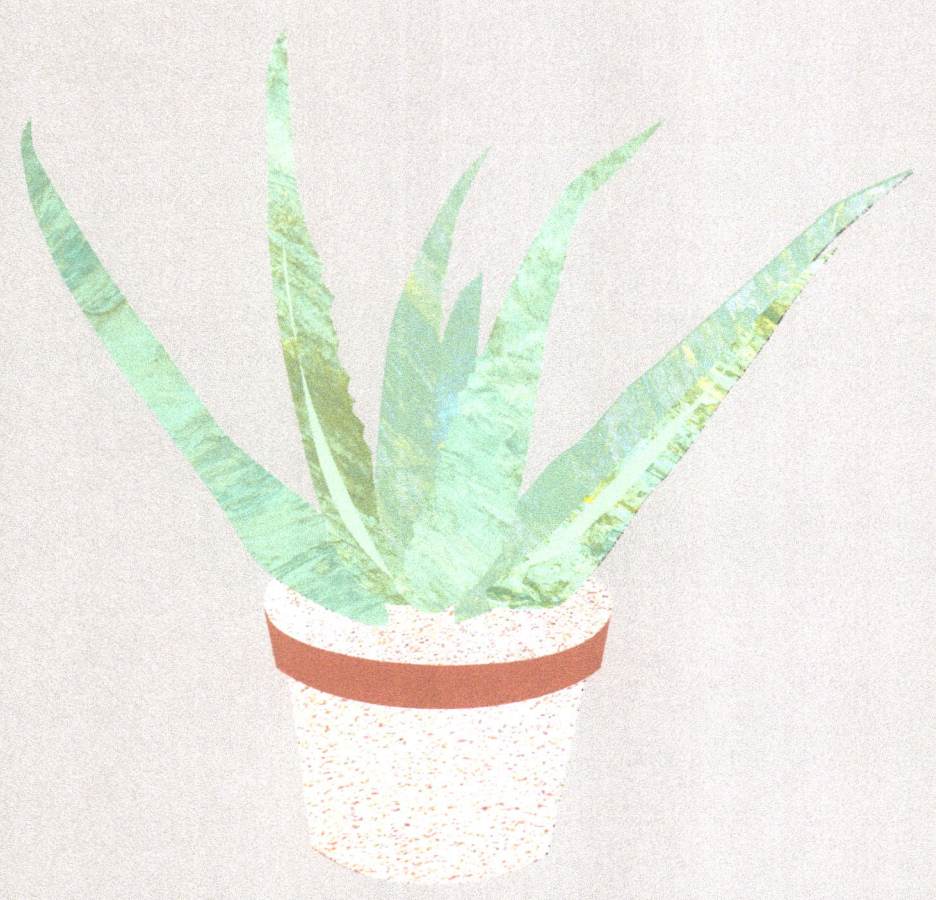

BOWEL BROOM

This drink is great for anyone prone to constipation or if you need to do a deep cleanse. This drink leaves your insides clean and your skin glowing with health.

1 teaspoon of partially hydrolyzed guar gum (PHGG)

1 tablespoon of 100% organic aloe vera juice

1 teaspoon of pre-soaked flaxseeds or golden flaxseed meal

½ cup of freshly squeezed pear or apple juice (optional)

2 cm chunk of ginger (optional)

½ to 1 glass of alkaline or purified water

If you have a juicer, juice apple or pear and ginger and then add the rest of the ingredients. If you do not have a cold pressed juicer, simply leave ginger and apple or pear out and add more water. If you cannot find PHGG, add psyllium husks instead.

DIGESTIVE HEALING FRIENDS

PROBIOTICS

Nature provides the body with trillions of bacteria, both good and bad. These microbes make up our body's diverse and unique microbiome. Although bad bacteria can overgrow because of a number of dietary and lifestyle reasons, if we keep our good bacteria plentiful, our digestion will thrive. Probiotics are the fertilizers that can flourish the body's microbiome, however they will not flourish in balance unless prebiotics foods or supplements are used in combination. The most well-known probotic species are lactobacillus and bididobacteria.

LACTOBACILLUS

Lactobacillus is the working bee – it is the most abundant and friendly bacteria in the small intestines. This diligent microbe produces lactic acid to protect against the entrance and growth of 'bad' organisms that cause disease. It has many sub-species which include:

STRAIN	SPECIAL ROLE
L. Rhamosus	Digestive Support, Eczema, Food Poisoning, Diarrhea from antibiotics, urinary tract infections
L.Aciophilus	Vaginal health, urinary health, diarrhea, acne
L.Casei	Immunity, brain function – anxiety, depression, diarrhea
L. Plantarum	Inflammation, bloating, IBS symptoms, gut lining health, makes L-lysine to boost immunity, calcium absorption
L. Gasseri	Supports healthy weight, balanced blood sugar, digestion
L. Lactis	Guards against 'leaky gut', digestion,
L. Paracasei	Fatigue, cavities, environmental sensitivities
L. Johnsonii	Skin health, protects against UV damage

BIFIDOBACTERIUM

Bifidobacterium are also lactic acid producing bacteria that produce vitamins, antibacterial chemicals and antibiotic type substances. The key difference between lactobacillus and bifido is that this super hardy microbe also makes acetic acid to reduce the growth of yeasts and moulds. This makes it a handy probiotic to guard against problems in the vaginal and urogenital tracts. Some of its unique species include:

STRAINS	SPECIAL ROLE
B. Lactis	Immunity, digestive support, wheat digestion
B. Longum	Constipation, memory, brain support
B. Bifidum	Keeps pathogens at bay, supports inflammatory bowel conditions, immunity, allergies
B. Breve	Anti-ageing, protection against UV damage, glowing skin, chronic constipation in kids
B. Subtilis	Protects against moulds and aflatoxins, enzyme production, beautiful digestion and skin
L. Johnsonii	Skin health, protects against UV damage

Streptococcus thermophilus is a youth-promoting probiotic. It helps to increase ceramides in the skin barrier to improve skin hydration.

Saccharomyces boulardii can withstand the low pH in the stomach and travel to the intestines where it is resistant to antibiotics. It prevents antibiotic-induced diarrhoea as well as traveller's diarrhoea, irritable bowel and bowel inflammation. So, if you are considering partaking in Asian street food, do not forget to take a bottle of SB probiotic with you.

Fructooligosaccharides (FOS) is a natural prebiotic that can promote the growth and activity of friendly bacteria within the gut.

There are billions of bacteria each with different roles that are being discovered every day.

NATURE TIP – SOIL-BASED PROBIOTICS

What? Did I just suggest eating probiotics straight from the soil?

Not quite, but as the name suggests soil-based probiotics emerge from the soil. Now I don't mean that you should go out and eat a handful of dirt (although I'm sure if it was fertile, you could get plenty of nutrients from it). These probiotics are not taken from the soil, but are grown from soil microbiome. The soil requires its own clever bacteria to increase the nutrient content within the soil so it can produce a healthy plant. When humans consume these organisms, they can travel to exactly where they need to go to deposit their healthy 'mini bacteria' for ideal gut health. The bonus is these bacteria are resistant and hardy to any breakdown from corrosive digestive juices, so they always travel exactly where they need to go to deposit their goodness. Wow! How clever is nature?

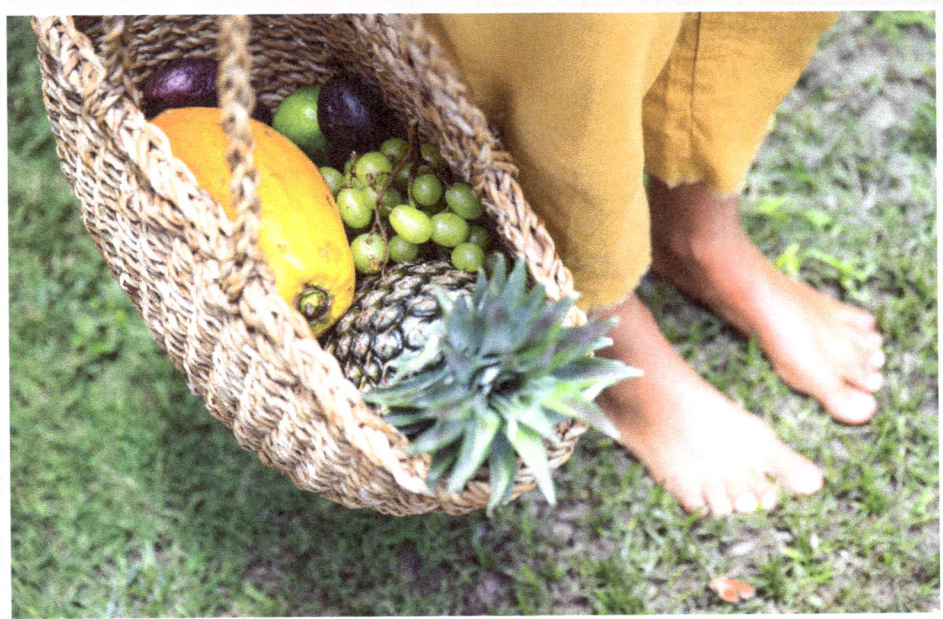

ENZYMES – PROTEASE, AMYLASE, LIPASE, LACTASE, BROMELAIN ETC.

Broad spectrum digestive enzymes reduce digestive problems like heartburn, indigestion and bloating by helping to break down undigested food into smaller particles for better absorption. When taken during a meal, enzymes can improve the absorption of proteins, thereby stopping them from leaking across the intestinal wall where they cause food allergies, intolerances and inflammation that can drive disease and ageing.

FIBRE

Soluble fibre attracts water and forms a gel in the digestive tract. This slows digestion and lowers sugar and starch absorption, which in turn, reduces cholesterol, inflammation and enhances weight loss via satiety. Psyllium husk, pectin, konjac root, glucomannon and the soft parts of fruits and dried beans are good examples of soluble fibre.

Insoluble fibre is the portion of plant cells that gives the wall its structural integrity. Insoluble fibre can be found in the peel of fruits, such as apples and grapes. It acts as a natural laxative by giving stool its shape and helps to move it quickly through the gastrointestinal tract aiding constipation, diarrhea and diverticulosis. It also offers protection against colon cancer.

B COMPLEX

B vitamins nourish the digestive system by boosting microflora production. The muscular tone of the bowel that helps us go to the toilet is affected by B vitamins. Most B vitamins are urinated out of the body (in fluorescent yellow wee), so it is important to take liposomal or activated B vitamins.

VITAMIN C

Vitamin C helps to flush heavy metals and toxins out of the colon, preventing constipation and guarding against many digestive type cancers. To get the best absorption of Vitamin C try a liposomal Vitamin C as it has a 90% absorption rate. Always look for GMO free phospholipids without any PEG's I have created my own special brand 'LIPO SUPER C' that is powerful and free of nasties.

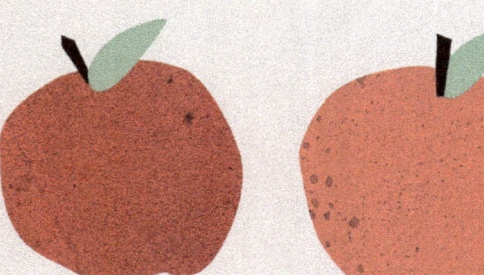
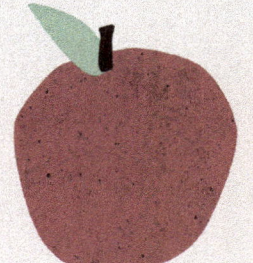
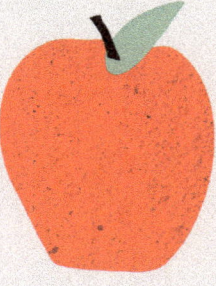

MAGNESIUM

Magnesium is a natural 'bowel relaxant' that flushes toxins through the colon. If you are deficient in magnesium, bowels can become sluggish and bacteria begins to breed in the large intestines overloading the liver.

GREEN GIFTS OF NATURE

Chlorophyll is the substance that gives plants their beautiful green colour and is responsible for photosynthesis (the conversion of sunlight into carbohydrates in plants). Chlorophyll resembles haemoglobin, the oxygen-carrying molecule found in red blood cells. The key difference between haemoglobin and chlorophyll is that the metallic atom in the middle of the human haemoglobin is iron and the metallic atom in the middle of chlorophyll is magnesium. Chlorophyll increases alkalinity, removes heavy metals and improves oxygenation to the body's microbiome and intestinal lining. The best natural sources of this include wheat grass, barley grass, spirulina and blue-green algae.

L-GLUTAMINE

L-Glutamine is an amino acid that fuels the mucosal linings in the gastrointestinal tract. It preserves the health of the mucosa and the microvilli in the intestinal wall. Because of this it helps with diarrhea, food sensitivities, ulcers and inflammatory bowel diseases like ulcerative colitis and Crohn's disease.

My other fav digestive friends are aloe vera, prebiotics like inulin and larch arabinogalactans, lactoferrin, colostrum, slippery elm, collagen and glyconutrients.

EXERCISE FOR BEAUTIFUL DIGESTION

Regular exercise boosts blood supply to the digestive system and stimulates natural peristalsis, leading to superb bowel motions. The bowel is a muscle and it requires exercise just like any muscle in the body, otherwise it gets very lazy. The end result can be a toxic bowel.

Try exercising for thirty minutes daily. It is important to increase your heart rate to pump blood through your capillaries oxygenating tissues, organs and cells. Beach or mountain walking floods the body with the oxygen-rich air needed for healthy digestion. Yoga, Tai Chi, Pilates and stretching keep the body supple. Special postures like the cat pose, the triangle and breathing exercises are all good for digestives health.

BOWEL MOVER – APANASANA

Lie on your back, relax, inhale and place your hands on your knees. Exhale and hug your knees to your chest. Rock your knees from side to side for five to ten breaths and then release your knees. Relax and repeat two to three times.

This is a great exercise to remove bloating, gas and to encourage bowel motions.

CHAPTER FIVE

NATURE'S SECRETS TO RADIANT BEAUTY

Inner Beauty Purification & Fasting

INNER BEAUTY
PURIFICATION
& FASTING

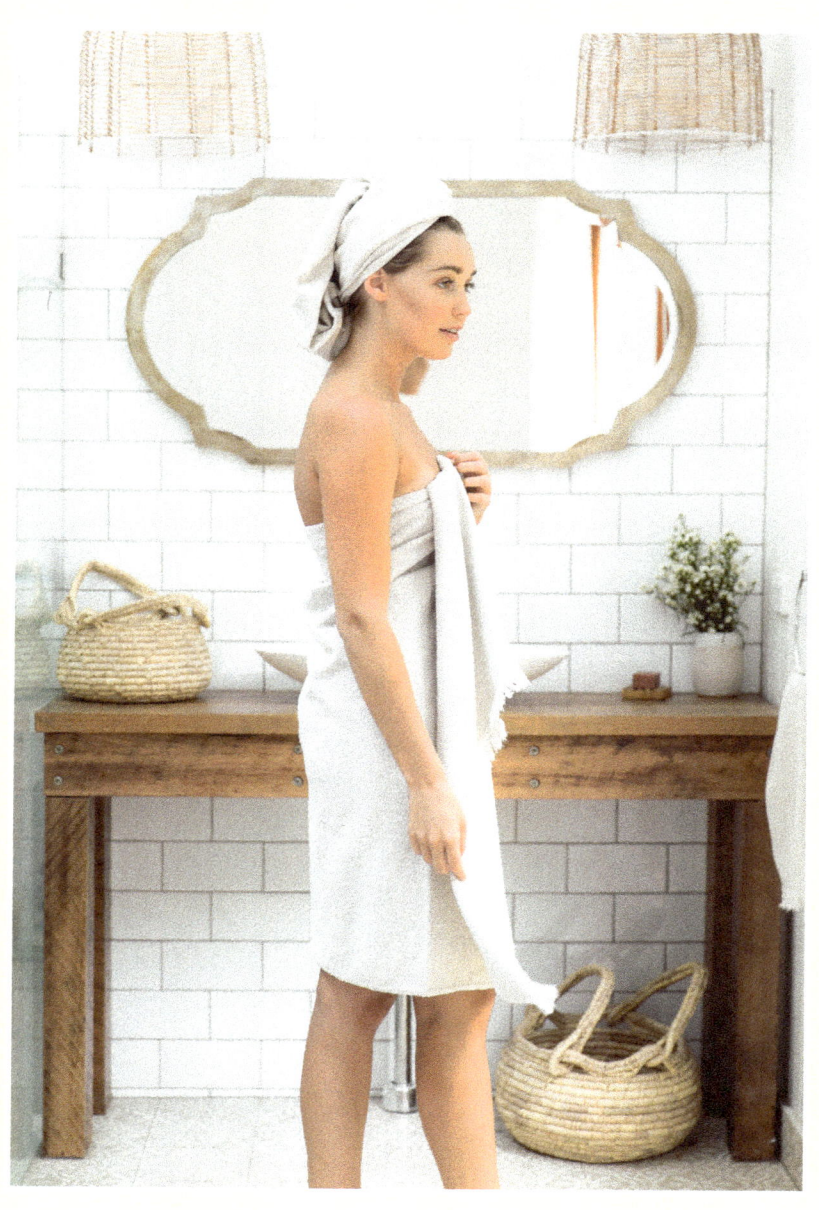

In the past century over 84000 chemicals have been created and have found themselves in our environment, our food and in the products we use daily. Most of these chemicals are fat soluble, which means they find a safe place living within your body's fat cells. Some of the most common nasties we now face include:

- **MOULD TOXINS** are very difficult to eliminate and to visually see. They are linked to problems like sinusitis, chronic fatigue, immune suppression, cancer and other health ailments. They are found in the environment and on foods like grains, nuts and seeds that are stored in silos for long periods of time.

- **HEAVY METALS**, such as cadmium (electronics, computers, mobile phones), lead (gasoline, water pipes, paint, food, cheap glass), mercury (dental amalgams, plastics), arsenic (fertilisers, non-organic wine, rice), copper (pipes, chlorinated water etc.) and aluminium (fluoridated water, make-up, tins, cookware) are found everywhere.

- **PESTICIDES AND HERBICIDE**s are abundant in our environment, with glycophosphates (round up) being the worst culprit as it is used at a rate of 5 billion pounds per year. These dangerous poisons do not break down in the environment and accumulate in our fat stores. They mimick hormones driving diseases like cancer.

- **BISPHENOL A (BPA) AND PHTHALATES** are chemicals used to make plastics and resins. These do not break down in the environment and like pesticides mimic our hormones driving cell breakdown and disease.

- **POPS OR PERSISTENT ORGANIC POLLUTANTS** are fat soluble toxins. They often come from agricultural and industrial chemicals like pesticides, fertilizers, polychlorinated biphenyls (PCB's), dioxins, plastics and flame retardants found in non-stick cookware, upholstery and cabinets. POPS accumulate in the environment and our foods and increase reactive oxygen species (ROS) leading to inflammation, insulin resistance, obesity, diabetes, cardiovascular disease, advanced ageing and even cancer.

- **HETEROCYLIC AMINES** are chemicals that form when foods are cooked at high temperatures, like when boiling, frying or grilling.

- **DANGEROUS EMF FREQUENCIES** are pervasive as they are everywhere in the form of wifi use, computers and mobile phones.

- **GENETICALLY MODIFIED FOODS** are modern day disease predators. Foods that have undergone genetic modification disrupt the body's metabolism, create insulin resistance, infertility and advanced ageing. When animals eat genetically modified crops, many of them die in weeks from their stomachs splitting open, so you can only imagine the effect on humans. In Australia, nearly all corn and canola crops are GM, but there are many more coming into the country.

The chemical exposure to the average human being in the last forty years has now become disastrous. If we wish to survive in a healthy state it is important for every individual to contribute by learning smart ways to reduce our ecological footprint on the planet. Easy ways to begin doing this is by purchasing as much organic as possible, preparing lots of plant-based meals, saying NO to plastics, choosing chemical-free make-up, skincare and cleaning products and by ensuring these practices become a daily habit.

Our body forgives us time and time again for overindulging in unhealthy foods and practices. However, if we continuously fall victim to this emotional pattern, the body will begin to show cracks in the form of niggling pains, dull eyes, lifeless hair and skin blemishes. If you do not correct these poor eating and living patterns, signs of discord will worsen into more serious symptoms like joint deterioration, injuries, extreme fatigue and even premature ageing. Our body is our friend and it wants to repair anything that could cause us harm. Eating restorative, healing foods and taking the strain off the body's eliminative organs forces the body to spend its precious time mopping up free radicals, inflammation and disease-promoting agents. One of the easiest ways to do this is by returning to ancient methods of healing in the form of cleansing or fasting.

THE POWER of FASTING

Fasting is an ancient healing practice that has been used by many cultures, religions and healers for thousands of years as a spiritual and health restorative tool. In Greek, Indian, Catholic and Egyptian scriptures fasting was regularly used to help bring one closer to god and to heal a myriad of mysterious diseases. Hippocrates, 'the father of medicine' understood the healing principles behind fasting. He stated 'If the body is cleared, the more you feed it the more you will harm it. When the body is fed too richly, the disease is fed as well...excess is against all nature'.

Modern research has backed up this ancient practice by proving that fasting has many proven regenerative benefits. As a naturopathic healer I was always taught to encourage detoxification through different methods depending on a person's individual needs, toxic load and genetic make-up. Because of this, there are many different types of fasting methods being used today that suit different situations and constitutions. Some of these include:

- **Water fasting** – complete abstinence from food and drinking only water for a number of days. This can be dangerous and should only be done under medical supervision. This can cause a huge amount of toxins to be released and if the body's detox organs are not balanced the body will simply reabsorb these toxins creating more problems.

- **Juice fasting** – drinking only cold-pressed juices for a number of days – a fantastic way to cleanse the body of toxins and impurities

- **Raw fruits and vegetables** – eating only raw fruits and vegetables for a number of days – this can take the strain off the body's digestive organs.

- **Keto fasting** – reducing your calorie intake to around 600 calories of nutrient-dense foods. This is normally done 1 or 2 times weekly following an intermittent fast.

- **Intermittent fasting** – this involves fasting for 14 to 16 hours daily and eating all of your meals in 6 to 8 consecutive hours. For example, eating the first meal of the day at 11 am and the last meal at 6 to 7 pm giving the body a 17 hour window of healing.

Fasting has many proven benefits including weight loss, reducing insulin resistance and detoxification of harmful chemicals. Most dangerous toxins found in the environment today are fat soluble and because of this they learn to store in our body's fat cells. Fasting enhances weight loss and as the body loses weight it also releases stored toxins from the fat cells into the bloodstream. When your body converts from burning carbohydrates for energy to burning fats for energy, it releases not only stored energy but all of the toxins that are stored in there. This is one of the reasons why a 'ketogenic' or 'paleo' type diet is so beneficial to health.

Fasting can also boost autophagy and mitophagy. These are the body's natural cleansing functions that help to remove diseased tissues, senescent cells and age-promoting body materials. It can also trigger the replication of stem cells and of new mitochondria.

INCREASED PHYSICAL
& EMOTIONAL
AWARENESS OF FOOD
AND ENVIRONMENT

IMPROVING SKIN HEALTH
AND RADIANCE

PREVENTING
DISEASE

REDUCING
OXIDATIVE STRESS

VITALITY IS
BOOSTED

LOWERING INSULIN
RESISTANCE

DETOXIFICATION

Benefits of fasting include

INCREASING
OXYGENATION

APPETITE REGULATION
AND WEIGHT LOSS

BOOSTING IMMUNITY

LYMPHATICS, DIGESTION,
KIDNEYS AND LUNGS ARE
REVITALISED

EYES BECOME BRIGHT
AND SPARKLY

PROMOTING
YOUTH-PROMOTING
HUMAN GROWTH
HORMONE (HGH)

Intermittent fasting is my favourite curative and youth-promoting remedy that I use in both my naturopathic practice and personal life daily. At least two days per week I stop eating the night before at 6 pm and I do not eat until 11 am the next day. On this day I only consume two nutritious meals and lots of bone or vegan broths, cold-pressed juices, keto or paleo based recipes and alkaline water. This gives my body around 17 hours of reprieve from digestion allowing it to put all of its vital energies into healing.

If you're not ready to commit to intermittent fasting, but you still want to detoxify, try switching to a raw food diet for 14 to 28 days. My plant based recipe book Raw Addiction focuses on showing people how to convert to a raw food diet to improve healing and rejuvenation on all levels and in the process raise your healing and beauty vibration.

For more information on this book, go to katrinaellis.com.au or wholistichouse.co

THE QUEEN of FILTRATION – the LIVER

Most detoxification diets or fasting methods improve the performance and function of the body's detox organs. The body uses the lungs, skin, kidneys, lymphatics and the liver to remove harmful toxins, with the liver being the 'Queen' of filtration organs. The liver can filter three pints of blood per minute and clear nearly all toxins, heavy metals, bacteria and other nasties before they re-enter the blood circulation. If the liver is overloaded or functioning poorly, many of these toxins re-enter the blood, creating cell breakdown, advanced ageing and disease.

Unhappy Liver Test

If you have more than three of these symptoms, your liver needs a clean.

- [ ] Abdominal fat
- [ ] Abdominal bloating or discomfort
- [ ] Acne rosacea
- [ ] Allergies
- [ ] Bad Breath
- [ ] Body odour
- [ ] Cellulite (excess)
- [ ] Chemical sensitivity
- [ ] Darkness around the eyes
- [ ] Digestive problems
- [ ] Depression
- [ ] Easy bruising
- [ ] Easy to anger
- [ ] Eczema
- [ ] Excess sweating
- [ ] Fatigue – severe
- [ ] Gallstones
- [ ] Headaches
- [ ] Heartburn, reflux
- [ ] High cholesterol and triglycerides
- [ ] Hormone imbalances like hot flushes or PMS
- [ ] Hot or overheated body
- [ ] Hot and burning soles of feet
- [ ] Inability to lose weight even when dieting
- [ ] Intolerances to fatty foods
- [ ] Itchy skin
- [ ] Joint aches and pains
- [ ] Liver spots on body or hands
- [ ] Nausea
- [ ] Pain under ribcage
- [ ] Psoriasis
- [ ] Red swollen eyes
- [ ] Rashes or skin breakouts
- [ ] Recurrent infections
- [ ] Tongue coating
- [ ] Yellowing in the eyes
- [ ] Vertical lines in between eyes

The liver can filter three pints of blood per minute and clear nearly all toxins, heavy metals, bacteria and other nasties before they re-enter the blood circulation. If the liver is overloaded or functioning poorly, many of these toxins re-enter the blood, creating cell breakdown, advanced ageing and disease."

The liver can make toxins harmless by chemically changing them, either by an oxidation reaction known as phase one or by a conjugation reaction known as phase two. Phase one detoxification neutralises all kinds of toxins by using a group of enzymes known as cytochrome P450 enzymes. These enzymes can alter a toxin by making it water soluble, so the body can wee it out. Foods that help with this phase include indoles found in cruciferous vegetables like broccoli, cauliflower, brussels sprouts and kale, protein found in oily fish, eggs and grass-fed meat and citrus (but not grapefruit), berries and Green tea.

The second method of detoxification works by a number of different pathways. It allows the liver from phase one to convert the toxin into a more active form for the phase two metabolites to break this down. This intermediate process can create high amounts of free radicals and tissue damage if accessory nutrients like B vitamins, zinc, magnesium, selenium and others are low. Some foods that can assist phase two detoxification pathways include asparagus, avocados, cabbage, broccoli, Brussels sprouts, kale, bok choy, watercress, mustard, horseradish, turnips, citrus peel, papaya, beets, blue-green algae, onions, garlic and shallots.

Once the liver has processed these toxins, the wastes are delivered to the bile and secreted into the intestines to be excreted out through the bowel.

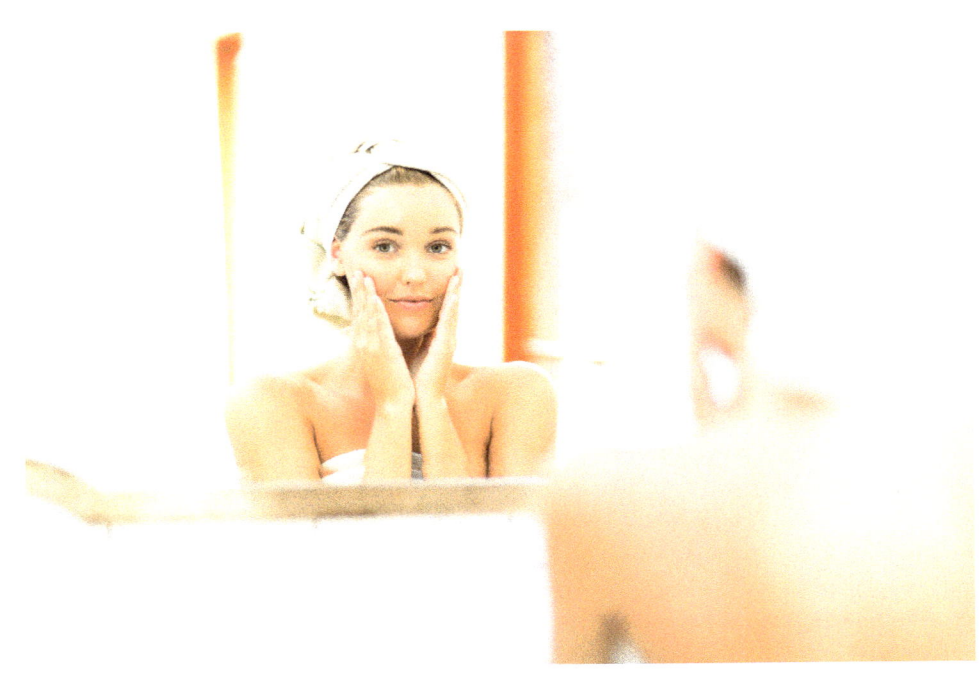

BEAUTY PURIFICATION DIET

This seven-day 'Beauty Purification' was created to help you remove dirty toxins that impede your liver, lymphatics, kidneys, skin and brain. If you follow this cleanse well, you will notice a dramatic increase in energy, more beautiful skin, hair and nails, a boost in your happiness and the ability to shift some unwanted kilos in the process too.

HOW TO START

If you haven't regularly cleansed for some time, you may experience some 'detox' symptoms like headaches, nausea, insomnia, body odour, skin flare-ups or changes in bowel motions in the first forty-eight hours, but this should disappear quickly if you sleep well, drink plenty of water and use near far infrared sauna or mineral baths. Consider adding fresh lemon juice, organic bi-carb of soda or chlorophyll to your water to reduce die-off or detox symptoms.

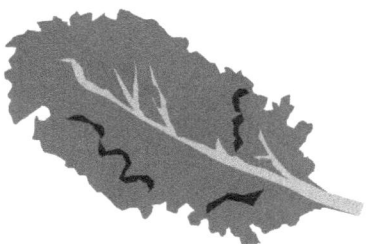

TIPS FOR THE BEAUTY PURIFICATION DIET

Before cleansing, make sure your bowels are clean. Use a small amount of magnesium oxide or BOWEL BROOM (my brand) a day before you start the cleanse. If you normally have sluggish bowels, continue this every night while doing the cleanse to ensure your colon stays toxin free. It doesn't hurt to incorporate some coffee enemas into any cleansing protocol.

If you are wanting to do an intermittent fast two days a week or even on alternate days, simply swap breakfast selections below and place into lunch at 11 am. Finish eating at 7 pm the next night and allow at least 3 hours before going to sleep. The longer the window where you abstain from food the greater period of repair and restoration.

NO

THE JUST SAY NO TO DETOX FOODS

- Dairy products –ALL
- SUGAR – including soft drinks, cordials, energy drinks
- Alcohol
- Coffee and tea
- Dried fruit
- Red meats

- Grains including wheat, rice, corn, rye, barley, oats
- Canned products
- Packaged foods or sauces from a jar
- Pasta or bread
- Fried foods of any kind

YES

THE JUST SAY YES TO DETOX FOODS

- **Fruit** – any fresh, organic and in season – include dark berries, honeydew melon, red papaya, apples, pears, citrus, watermelon, avocado.
- **Vegetables** – any fresh, organic and in season – aim for a rainbow of five to eight different vegetables daily – include sweet potato, beetroot, taro, yams, carrots, celery, capsicum, broccoli, asparagus, cauliflower, spring onions, broccolini, radish, kohlrabi, green beans, cucumber, tomatoes, mushroom, peppers, turnips, onion, garlic, brussels sprouts and artichokes.
- **Salad vegetables** – aim for at least 3 cups daily to include kale, spinach, swiss chard, lettuce, endive, mesculin, romaine lettuce, microgreens, rocket, bok choy, dandelion, watercress and sprouts.
- **Organic tempeh, miso** and **natto** are great protein sources for vegetarians
- **Cold pressed, omega oils** like avocado, olive, hemp, walnut, pumpkin seed and flaxseed oil. Use on all foods including salads, smoothies and steamed vegetables. Aim for at least 3 to 5 tablespoons of oil per day
- For cooking – use only **ghee, olive oil** (low heat), **avocado oil** or water.
- **Smoothies and cold pressed juices** – for a great selection refer to the recipe section in this book.
- **Collagen beauty broth** (See page 102) or organic bone or vegan broths. Drink as many as you like throughout the day.
- **Activated seeds** – pumpkin, sesame and sunflower.
- **Activated nuts** – almonds, walnuts, hazelnuts, pecans and brazil.
- Use lots of **herbs and spices** like turmeric, ginger, basil, cardamom, star anise, coriander, parsley, cinnamon, oregano, cumin, fenugreek and mustard seeds.
- Use a little **Celtic/Himalayan sea salt** and **black pepper.**
- Drink **herbal teas** like lemongrass, burdock root, yellowdock, dandelion leaf, red clover or matcha green tea or my PURIFY brand tea as often as you like.
- For extra cleansing feel free to add **organic wheatgrass, barley grass, seaweeds, spirulina, blue-green algae, zeolites, aloe vera juice** and other cleansing friends

AFTER 7 DAYS SLOWLY ADD IN:

- Pre-soaked beans like red beans, haricot beans, kidney beans and butter beans
- Oily, small catch fish like salmon, tuna, herring, halibut, snapper, sea bass – make sure they are sourced from small catch, clean waters

EVERY DAY ON RISING:

- Drink one glass of fresh purified water with ½ fresh lemon or lime. This is an old remedy – but still a beauty. If you have hydrogen water, feel free to use too.

CLEANSING SOUPS

The Collagen Beauty Broth (see page 102) can be drunk any time you feel peckish. To give your thyroid a helping hand, add a few dulse or wakame flakes with a little Bragg's amino acid seasoning for extra iodine.

RAW FOODS

Reduce cooking during this cleanse and switch to home-made, mostly raw foods. Raw foods are packed with nutrients and living enzymes which rejuvenate cells, tissues and organ function. When making a salad, add fresh sprouts like broccoli, snow pea or alfalfa sprouts. Make a detox dressing for your salad from raw Apple Cider Vinegar or lemon juice, coriander and hemp seed oil or use the beautiful, cleansing recipes throughout this book. If you have severe digestive problems, you may need to heat up some of your foods or slow cook your meals.

CLEANSE YOUR MIND

A detox is a perfect time to clear your mind of negative emotions. Try doing at least fifteen minutes of meditation daily. Alternatively, use the deep breathing and oxygenation exercises found in Spiritual Beauty. This is a perfect way to expel toxins out through the lungs, leaving a clear, uplifted and happy mind.

PURE WATER

Pure water is the key to detoxification. Aim for two litres of alkaline water daily in addition to your cold-pressed juices and soups. This flushes toxins through the kidney, liver and lymphatics.

Hydrotherapy and Body Brushing is a great way to increase detoxification through the skin. Use a dry, natural bristle brush in long strokes towards the heart. Always finish your shower with a burst of cold water to stimulate blood circulation.

NEAR FAR INFRARED SAUNAS

Near Far Infrared Saunas are a fantastic way to drive toxins from your fat cells out through your skin. Aim for at least two sessions weekly while cleansing. Near Far Infrared treatments stimulate collagen and elastin production to beautify your skin, while encouraging heavy metal removal. There is a difference between Far Infared sauna therapy and Near Far Infrared therapy. The main difference is the frequency of the light – Near Infared is just beyond the spectrum of visible red light, going from 700 nanometres to 1400 nanometres, and Far Infared is 3000 to 100000 nanometres. Near far IR can penetrate into your body up to 3.9 inches while far IR only penetrates a few millimetres. Sunlight contains 40% more UVB in the near IR spectrum so exposing the body to near far IR is the most effective way to enhance detoxification on a deep level. Near far IR can also activate your mitochondria improving the function of every cell in the human body. For more information on Near Far Infrared Saunas in Australia please refer to my website www.wholistichouse.co

SLEEP

Sleep is one of the most important ways to rejuvenate the body. When we are in deep sleep, the body repairs its cells, tissues and organs. It is also a fantastic way to burn fat naturally. When we rest well, the next day we tend to eat less calories and make less ghrelin and leptin. These hormones help with appetite, fullness and fat burning.

BEAUTY IN A BOTTLE

2 green apples (skin on)

A handful of fresh wheatgrass

2 cm of ginger

1 garlic clove

½ fresh lemon or lime (use some skin)

1 tablespoon of bentonite or zeolite liquid or powder

1 tablespoon of chlorophyll liquid

If you have a cold pressed juicer, juice apples, ginger and garlic. If you can find fresh wheatgrass, throw a handful of this in too. Stir in chlorophyll, bentonite or zeolite liquid or powder and add some purified, alkaline water. If you do not have a juicer, mince garlic and ginger and squeeze lemon in (leaving the apples and wheatgrass out). Add the chlorophyll and bentonite or zeolite powder at the end. If you want extra cleansing, feel free to add any organic wheatgrass, barley grass or blue-green algae powder. This is the ultimate beauty enhancing and detoxification drink.

A SAMPLE DAY

If you are going to do an intermittent fast, simply swap the breakfast choices for lunch (around 11 am) and choose from Lunch and Dinner choices for dinner. Leave out mid-morning and mid-afternoon snacks.

AM

BREAKFAST

One of the following fruits:

Red papaya, grapefruit or pomegranate with a few berries like blueberries/raspberries/strawberries AND if still hungry a 'glowing green smoothie' (see page 140) with one cup of collagen beauty broth or bone or collagen broth with wakame (see page 102) OR

Smoothies or juices in the back of this book.

MID-MORN

Cold pressed vegetable juice like:

- Carrot/apple/lemon/ginger OR
- Celery/apple/kale/ginger OR
- Pineapple/mint/apple/ginger OR
- Pineapple/coriander/apple/lemon with skin OR
- Carrot/beetroot/celery with tops/kale/garlic OR
- Carrot/celery/turmeric/lemon/apple/ginger OR
- A handful of activated pumpkin seeds and almonds.

PM

LUNCH

A rainbow beauty salad made with different coloured
vegetables like spinach, romaine lettuce, kale, cabbage,
capsicum, sweet potato, red onion, coriander, mint, basil,
watercress, beet, cucumber and sprouts. Use flaxseed,
avocado or hemp oil with pure Apple Cider Vinegar or
lemon juice and chopped garlic or ginger as the dressing or
use one of the beauty dressings found in this book. If you
need extra protein, grill some tempeh and sprinkle with
activated seeds.

MID-ARVO

Fresh celery, cucumber or bell pepper sticks with the
turmeric lovgevity dip (see page 163) OR two cups of
collagen beauty broth (see page 102) or chicken or vegan
broth with wakame or dulse flakes.

DINNER

A rainbow plate of steamed vegetables and as much
collagen beauty broth or bone broth as you like or
choose from one of the beauty salads (see page 222)
or mains in the recipe section (see page 238).

COLLAGEN BEAUTY BROTH

2 carrots, unpeeled

2 sticks of celery, with tops

2 beets with tops, chopped in quarters

1 medium potato, brush the skin

A hand full of parsley, chopped

A handful of spinach, chopped

1 brown or white onion, peeled
and chopped up

1 medium sized zucchini, with skin

1 medium sized parsnip

4 to 6 shitake mushrooms

1 litre of purified water

1 teaspoon of Celtic salt

1 teaspoon of cumin powder

2 tablespoons of tamari or
braggs amino acid seasoning

2 tablespoons of apple cider vinegar

Seaweed (added at the end)

Place all of the ingredients into a saucepan, bring to the boil and simmer on the lowest heat for 4 hours. Add Bragg's or tamari, Apple Cider Vinegar and seaweed at the end. Strain the vegetables. Store in the fridge and drink as often as you like while cleansing.

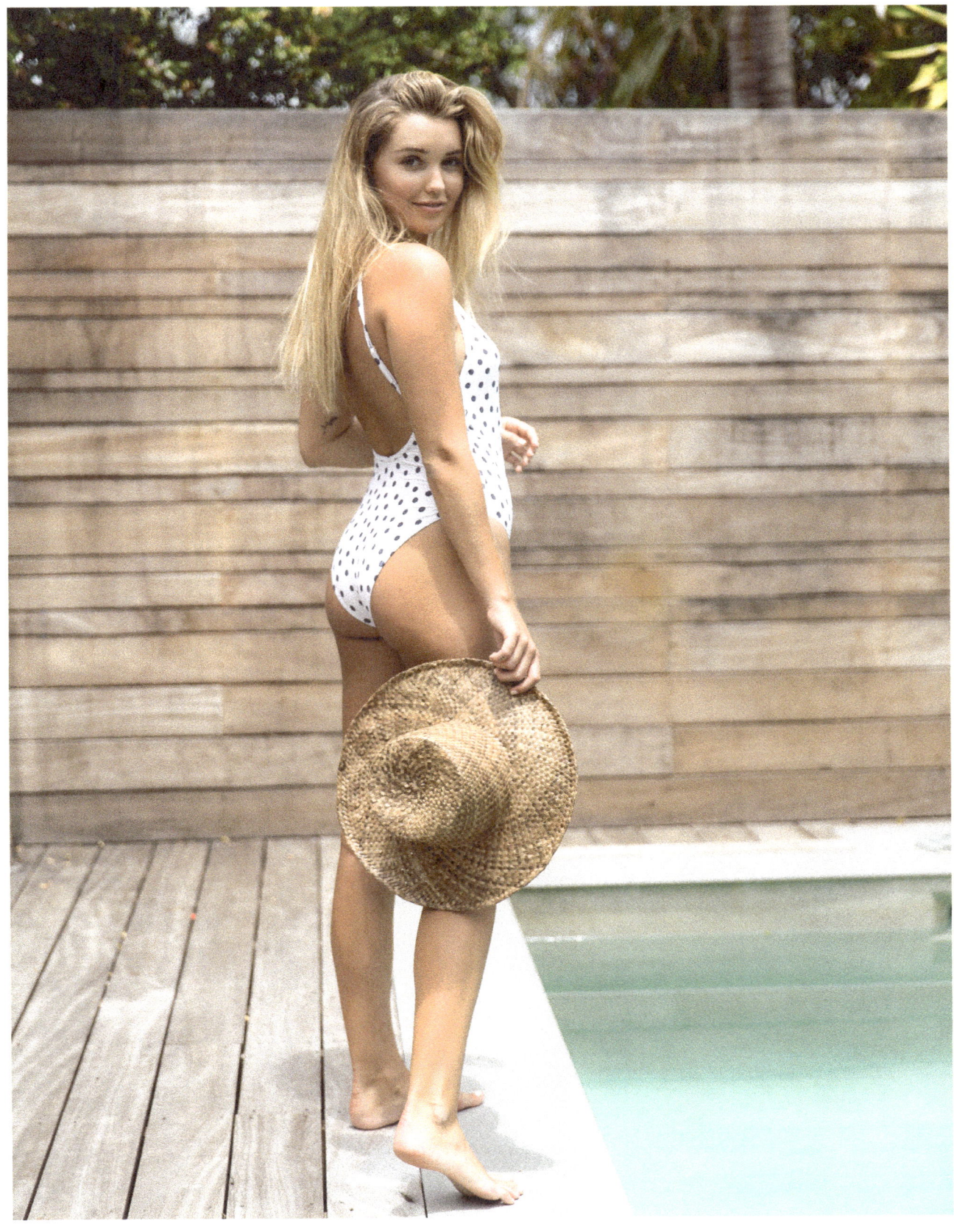

CHAPTER SIX

NATURE'S SECRETS
TO RADIANT BEAUTY

The Acid-Alkaline Balance

The ACID-ALKALINE BALANCE

I can still remember my first introduction to acid and alkaline substances at school. It happened in science class. As naive children we were tricked into tasting bitter acidic products like vinegar, and then alkaline substances like baking soda in water (ah! Delightful). I could see the teacher snickering as we grimaced in distaste. From this real life experiment we learnt about the pH scale, which is used to measure the acidity and alkalinity in a substance. pH stands for the parts or the concentration of hydrogen ions in a substance. The pH scale ranges from 0 (which is very acidic) to 7 (which is neutral) then to 14 (which is extremely alkaline). The higher the pH, the greater the hydrogen ions in a substance, and therefore the better it is able to alkalise your blood.

The idea of the pH balance is not a new concept. It has been well researched and put into practice since the late 1800s. In 1931, Otto Warburg won a Nobel Prize for his research into cancer. He showed that cancer cells thrived in an acidic, low oxygenated environment and that healthy cells flourished in an alkaline, oxygenated environment. Every naturopath, nutritionist and scientist knows how important it is to maintain a slightly alkaline blood pH (or extracellular fluids) in the human body in order to maintain ideal health. This harmonious acid-base balance sits between 7.35 and 7.45.

In order to keep this balance, the body uses three self-preservation tricks:

1. It increases breathing and excretes carbon dioxide (acid) out via the lungs

2. It increases urination and excretes acids out via the kidneys

3. It uses a buffering system. To do this it borrows alkaline minerals like calcium, magnesium, sodium and potassium from bones, organs and tissues to counteract an acidic pH (which is not an ideal situation).

ACIDITY is not a friend of natural beauty. It creates huge amounts of inflammation, breaking down collagen and elastin in the skin. It weakens bones, reducing their symmetry and form. Acidity deoxygenates the blood, causing dull, lifeless skin and hair. When the blood pH is acidic it creates a perfect breeding ground for parasites, bacteria and yeast. This allows the yeast to have a party in the blood, and in their excitement, they excrete poisonous mycotoxins. These nasty substances cause fatigue, brain fog, skin rashes, headaches, nausea, bloating, liver overload and a general feeling of being unwell.

The pH scale ranges from 0 (which is very acidic) to 7 (which is neutral) then to 14 (which is extremely alkaline). The higher the pH, the greater the hydrogen ions in a substance, and therefore the better it is able to alkalise your blood."

MY SECRET ALKALISING JUICE

2 celery sticks, with tops

3 kale leaves

A handful of alfalfa sprouts

A handful of spinach

1 lemon (use a little skin)

½ cucumber

1 tablespoon of chlorophyll liquid (to increase alkalinity)

1 tablespoon of an organic super greens (barley grass, wheatgrass, spirulina)

Place the vegetables through a cold pressed juicer. Mix chlorophyll and super greens in at the end.

Other signs to look out for include:

- Bumps on the tongue
- Burning on the tongue or in the mouth
- Chemical sensitivity
- Coated tongue
- Cold hands and feet
- Dry skin
- Dry stools
- Excess mucous
- Fatigue
- Fluid retention
- Fungal infections
- Frequent sighing
- Gout
- Headaches
- Heartburn
- Itchy skin
- Low libido
- Memory loss – cloudy thinking
- PMS
- Rashes
- Recessed eyes
- Rheumatic pains
- Sleeping problems
- Sore and aching joints
- Sore muscles
- Strong smelling urine

Health conditions linked to high acidity include acne, cardiovascular problems, osteoporosis, chronic candida, scleroderma, diabetes, kidney stones, gallstones, poor immunity, premature ageing, weak bones, bone spurs, back problems, low energy and parasite, yeast or virus overgrowth. As Otto Warburg pointed out, even conditions like cancer may thrive in an acidic environment.

ACIDITY OFFENDERS

Diet is one of the biggest factors driving beauty-robbing acidity in the body. A food's acid-alkaline balance is determined by the amount of alkaline or acidic minerals found within it. The best-known alkaline minerals are calcium, magnesium, sodium, potassium, manganese, copper and zinc. The acidic minerals are chlorine, iodine, silica, phosphorus and nitrogen. Some foods can seem acidic (like lemons and limes), but when they are broken down by the body, they create an alkaline ash, which makes them alkaline. The more foods we eat that are alkaline, the greater we contribute to creating a more alkaline and balanced blood pH. The other major driver of high acidity is STRESS. Overactive adrenal glands produce high cortisol and aldosterone. This creates a domino effect, causing the body to excrete magnesium and potassium, the two most important alkaline minerals.

Other causes include:

- Respiratory problems resulting in high carbon dioxide in the blood
- Diabetic ketoacidosis
- A high intake of drugs and substances like alcohol, aspirin, iron and others
- A loss of bicarbonates and other minerals through diarrhea
- Worry, resentment, anger and negative emotions

ACID and ALKALINE BEAUTY CHART

HEALTHY ALKALINE FOODS & SUBSTANCES		NEUTRAL OR MILDLY ACIDIC OR ALKALINE		VERY ACIDIC FOODS & SUBSTANCES	
CONSUME LOTS		**CONSUME MODERATELY**		**LIMIT INTAKE**	

VEGETABLES (Healthy Alkaline)

All sprouted beans and sprouts	Garlic
Alfalfa sprouts	Garlic
Artichokes	Kale
Asparagus	Kamut grass
Barley grass	Lettuce
Basil	Leeks
Beets	Onions – all
Broccoli	Parsley
Brussels sprouts	Peas
Cabbage	Radish
Capsicum	Red cabbage
Carrots	Rhubarb
Cauliflower	Rocket
Cayenne pepper	Spinach
Celery	Sea vegetables
Chives, collards	Seaweed
Comfrey	Spirulina
Cucumber	Taro
Dandelion greens	Turnips
Endive	Zucchini
Green beans	

DAIRY (Neutral)

Butter – unsalted – neutral	Cows milk raw – neutral
Oils and fats	
Most are neutral	

FRUITS – SLIGHTLY ALKALINE

Apples	Mango
Apricots	Orange
Banana	Peach
Blackcurrants	Pear
Blueberries – mild acid	Pineapple
Cantaloupe	Plums – mild acid
Cherries	Pomegranate
Coconut	Prunes – mild acid
Cranberries – mild acid	Raspberry
Currants	Red currant
Dates	Rosehips
Grapes	Strawberry
Mandarin	(not watermelon)
(not papaya)	

GRAINS (Neutral)

Wild rice – mild alkaline	Amaranth – mild alkaline
Quinoa – mild alkaline	

ANIMAL PRODUCTS (Very Acidic)

Beef	Ocean Fish
Chicken	Organ meats
Eggs	Oysters
Lamb	Pork and Bacon
Liver	Rabbit
Lobster	Veal
Mussels	

DAIRY (Very Acidic)

Buttermilk	Cream – raw is neutral
Goats cheese	Hard cheese
Ice-cream	Homogenised milk
Vegan cheese	

GRAINS (Very Acidic)

White processed foods	Biscuits
White bread	Rice, white, basmati
Wheat bread	Spelt – mild acidic
Rye bread	Cous cous – mild acidic

NUTS AND SEEDS (Very Acidic)

Peanuts

FRUITS

Avocado	Lime
Lemon	Nectarine
	(not tomato)

ORGANIC GRAINS AND LEGUMES

Buckwheat – sprouted	Soy beans
Lentils – sprouted	Spelt
Lima beans	Tofu
Navy beans	White beans
Soy lecithin	

NUTS AND SEEDS

Chestnuts	Sesame seeds
Flaxseeds	Brazil nuts
Almonds	

CONDIMENTS

Apple Cider Vinegar	Baking Soda

EMOTIONS

Happiness and joy	Deep breathing
Meditation	

DRINKS

Alkaline water – pH above 7.2	Cold pressed green juices
Coconut water	

NUTS

Hazelnuts
Macadamia
Walnuts

FISH

Freshwater fish

BEVERAGES

Coconut milk

OTHER

Sauerkraut

EMOTIONS

Anger	Resentment
Bitterness	Stress
Jealousy	Worry

SWEETENERS

Artificial sweeteners	Fructose
Barley malt syrup	Honey – processed
Beet sugar	Malt Sweetener
Brown rice syrup	Milk sugar
Chocolate	Molasses
Dried sugar cane juice	White sugar
Sugar	

CONDIMENTS

Ketchup or Tomato Sauce	Soy Sauce
Mayonnaise	Vinegar – processed
Mustard	Yeast

BEVERAGES

Beer	Alcohol
Coffee	Soft drinks, sports drinks
Fruit juice – packaged	Wine
Tea – black	

OTHER

Canned Foods	Monosodium Glutamate - MSG
Processed Foods	Hydrogenated fats/ trans fats
Dried Fruits	

- MOST ALKALINE FOODS EVER
- MOST ACIDIC FOODS EVER

ALKALINE BEAUTY TIPS

1 **LEMON and LIMES** are superb alkalising fruits that enhance hydration and kickstart a sluggish metabolism. Drink at least one glass of naturally alkaline or hydrogen-infused water on rising with ½ a freshly squeezed lemon or lime.

3 **A COLD PRESSED GREEN JUICE** is a great addition to an alkalising diet. My fav choices are kale, alfalfa sprouts, broccoli, asparagus, celery, mint and lettuce. Drink straight away to prevent oxidation. Try my secret alkalising juice.

5 **VITAJUWEL** crystal water bottles contain specific healing crystals sourced from all over the world. These crystals change the energy structure of the water increasing its hydration, healing and beauty properties. If you don't believe this, read the book *The Hidden Messages in Water* by Japanese researcher *Masaru Emoto* to understand the proven science behind the energy of these crystals.

7 **FERMENTED FOODS** are definitely vital to many people's digestive health and beauty. However, they are not alkaline, so if you are finding it difficult to alkalise simply moderate your intake of these.

2 **GREENS** are alkalising superstars – they contain abundant alkaline minerals to increase our health, energy and vitality. Why not try having a green salad with every meal OR a yummy alkalising green smoothie for breakfast? Include my top seven alkalising foods (see page 108)

4 **OMEGA 3** essential fatty acids can reduce inflammation, increase hydration and dramatically enhance skin, hair, nail and digestive health. If you include lots of oily fish, avocado, organic nuts and seeds and a good Omega oil like hemp, sacha inchi or Udo's oil you are sure to glow with vitality.

6 **ALKALINE, HYDROGEN**-infused water is the ideal water to drink for superb health. Alkaline water should contain a natural balance of alkaline minerals and a pH of around 8.5 to 9.5 with a negative ORP value to increase its antioxidant effects. I use a whole house filtration system and an UltraStream. I also often infuse water with hydrogen generator to make 'hydrogen beauty water'. For more information on these great products, check out my websites at www.wholistichouse.co or www.katrinaellis.com.au.

8 **SPROUTS** are incredibly alkalising – throw some yummy sprouts into your salads, juices or green smoothies to boost up your alkalinity.

9 AVOID the **EIGHT ACID NASTIES**: a HEAVY RED MEAT INTAKE, SUGAR, PROCESSED FOODS, FRIED FOODS, ARTIFICIAL COLOURINGS and PRESERVATIVES, SOFT DRINKS and STRESS.

10 **MEAT-FREE** days are easy to do and can definitely play a role in reducing high acidity.

11 **80% ALKALINE to 20% ACID** forming foods is the ideal balance for incredible health.

12 **SLEEP** is essential for healthy oxygenation and therefore maintaining a good pH balance. When you fall into deep sleep, the majority of healing occurs, including a shift in blood pH.

13 **ORGANIC SUPER GREEN**S like chlorella, wheatgrass, spirulina, barley grass or blue-green algae are the perfect addition to an alkaline diet. Be careful when buying these, as many companies buy fake organic certification from China, yet their products are not certified organic.

14 **BREATHE** deeply! Breathing is a superb way to release toxic carbon dioxide and inhale pure oxygen for increasing blood alkalinity. Learn great deep breathing techniques to bring more oxygen into your belly.

15 **NEGATIVE** emotions like worry, resentment, anger, bitterness, jealousy and stress can drive up acidity ten times more than any food. Find your happy space by practicing yoga, tai chi, meditation, exercise, deep breathing and other relaxation techniques.

16 **ABSORPTION is the FIRST STEP.** It is important to check for any signs of low stomach acidity (which most people have), and if so, to boost it. Low stomach acidity stops the body from absorbing alkaline minerals correctly. For tips to do this look in 'digestion - seeds of life force'. Be careful with taking bicarb of soda over a long term, as it can cause internal calcifications if you do not balance other alkaline minerals.

HYDROGEN – THE ULTIMATE BEAUTY WEAPON

The human body is around 70% water. If the water put into it is acidic – below 7.0 (tap water, reverse osmosis, most bottled waters etc.), the body will try to buffer this acidity by stealing alkaline minerals like calcium, magnesium and potassium from the tissues, bones and cells. This creates rapid ageing, collagen destruction, disease and illness. One way to combat this is by drinking water rich in alkaline minerals. Another clever way is by infusing hydrogen into your water through using a hydrogen water generator.

Hydrogen is the most abundant and smallest molecule on the earth, containing only one proton and one electron, so it has the ability to travel into any part of the body. Molecular hydrogen has strong antioxidant properties that help to stop cytotoxic oxygen radicals that cause premature ageing of the skin, as well as diseases. When you infuse hydrogen into water and remove the oxygen, you create pure healing water that can be drunk or used externally to create incredible skin hydration as well as reduce collagen breakdown.

HYDROGEN is the FUEL of LIFE. One cup of hydrogen water is equivalent to the antioxidant value of 76 carrots, 1000 apples and 1500 bananas. No wonder I love hydrogen so much!

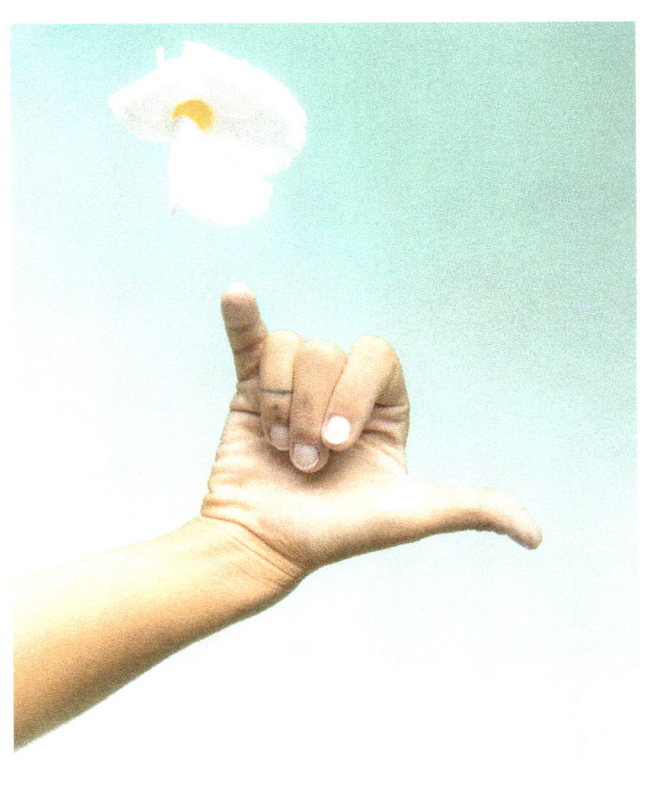

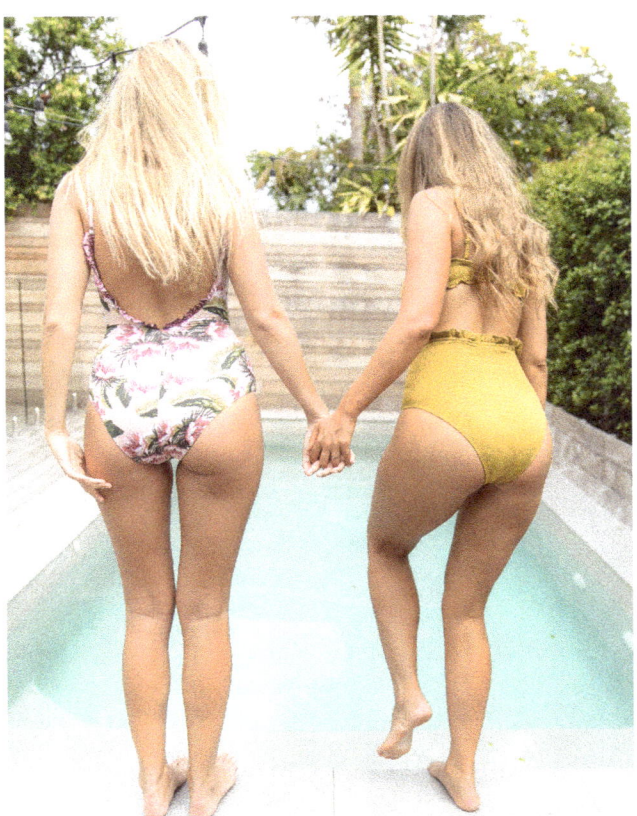

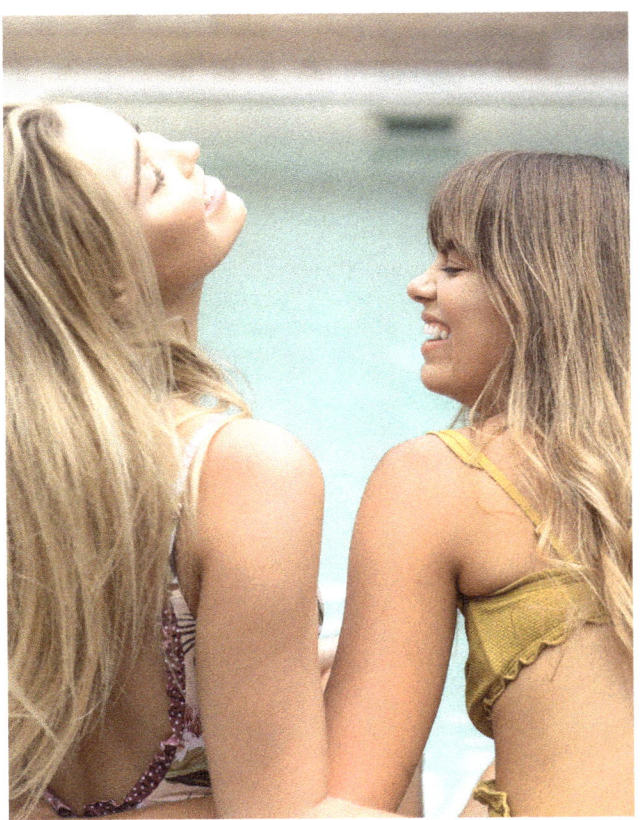

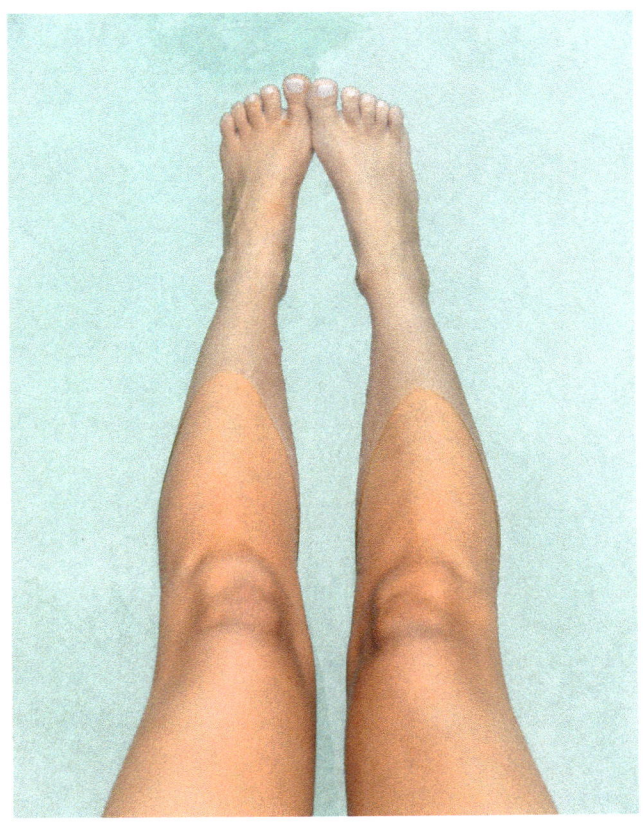

CHAPTER SEVEN

NATURE'S SECRETS
TO RADIANT BEAUTY

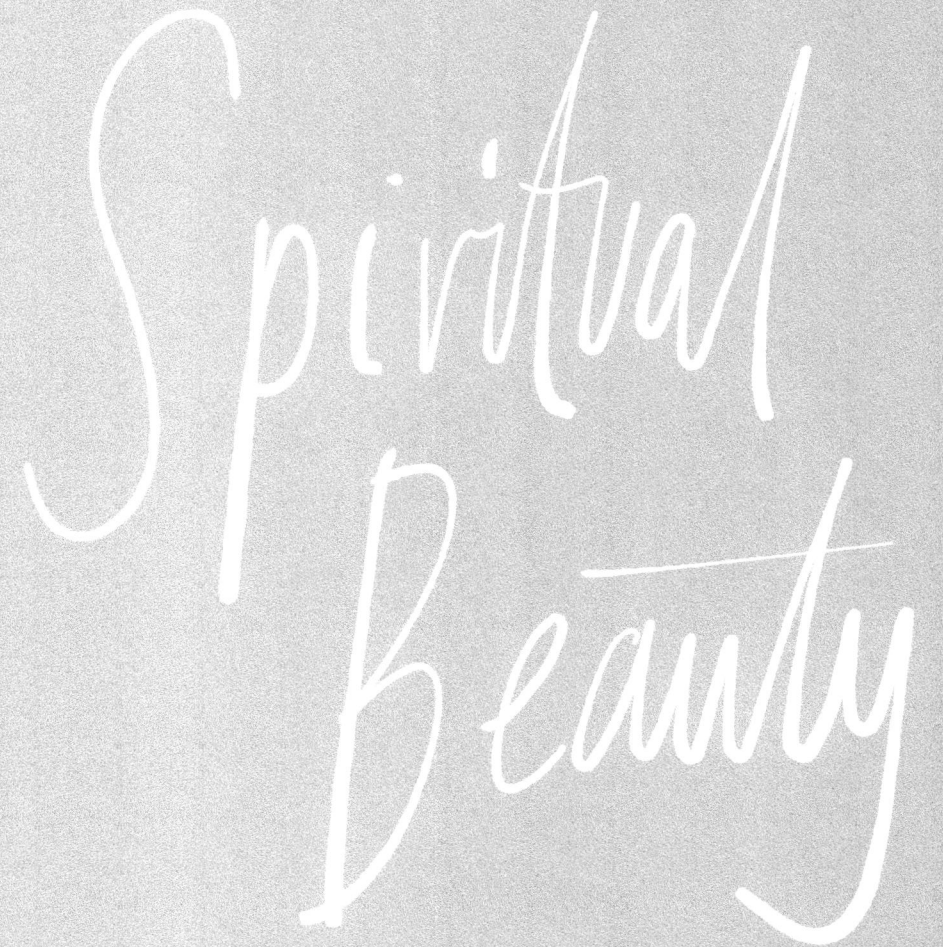

Spiritual Beauty

Happiness

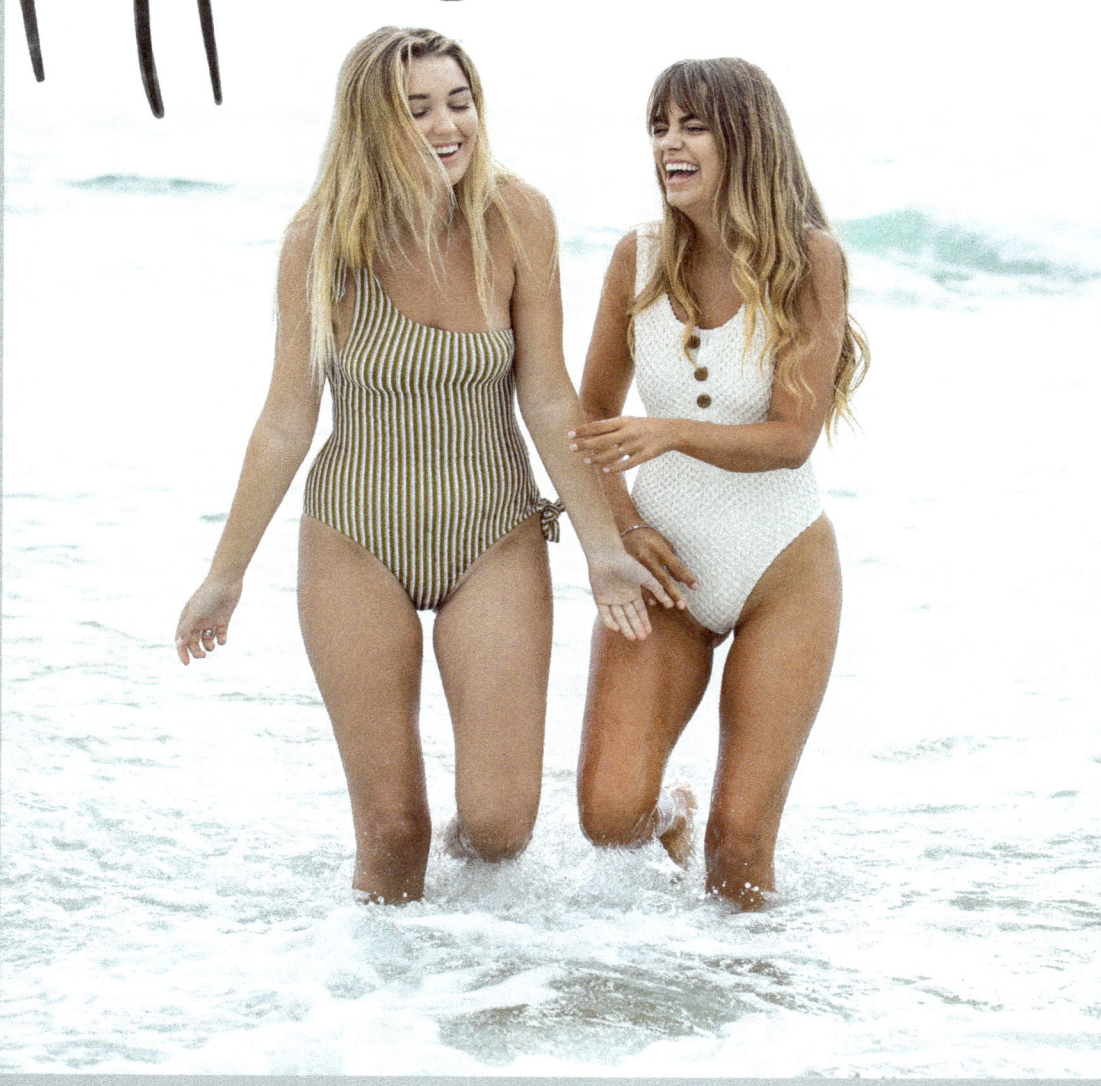

HAPPINESS IS THE SECRET TO ALL BEAUTY – AND THERE IS NO BEAUTY WITHOUT HAPPINESS.

Christian Dior

Christian Dior was onto something when he stated: 'Happiness is the secret to all beauty – and there is no beauty in this world without happiness'. Who would have thought that a fashion designer who lives in a materialistic world could have expressed such a poignant truth about the secret to natural beauty?

Since time began, scholars and mystics have been practicing and teaching the art of attaining happiness. Sadly, our quest to achieve this in today's world has become clouded. Overemphasis on the need for money, possessions and social status has made many believe that true happiness lies ONLY in attaining MATERIAL POSSESSIONS or SOCIAL STATUS in the form of an expensive car, a fairytale partner, a large bank account and more.

In the quest to attain these material possessions, we still seek the same end goal – that is, to be happy! Because, when we feel happy on the inside it is easy to reflect a radiant beauty on the outside. But happiness is so much more than a feeling. Countless studies have now proven that when people are truly happy they have lower stress hormones, better immunity and therefore a much better quality of life. If these scientific discoveries are true, then why are there still so many unfulfilled people in this world?

Is it because we still believe that inner happiness is only measured against what we have and our popularity in society? After all, this is what advertising is constantly selling us; images of beautiful, content people in perfect relationships. It's implied that this is all because of using an expensive skin cream to look younger or due to driving a luxury car that most of us can't afford. But at least, as the advertisement promises, this got them the life they had always desired.

So how is it possible to find inner happiness if we measure our happiness against what we don't have? These material possessions are wonderful to attain, yet they are nothing unless you are already content inside. Attaining happiness and therefore inner beauty is so simple and it is completely up to you. Below are some powerful, yet very straightforward happiness tips to help you find inner joy and in the process, radiant beauty.

7 SEVEN STEPS TO INNER HAPPINESS & RADIANT BEAUTY

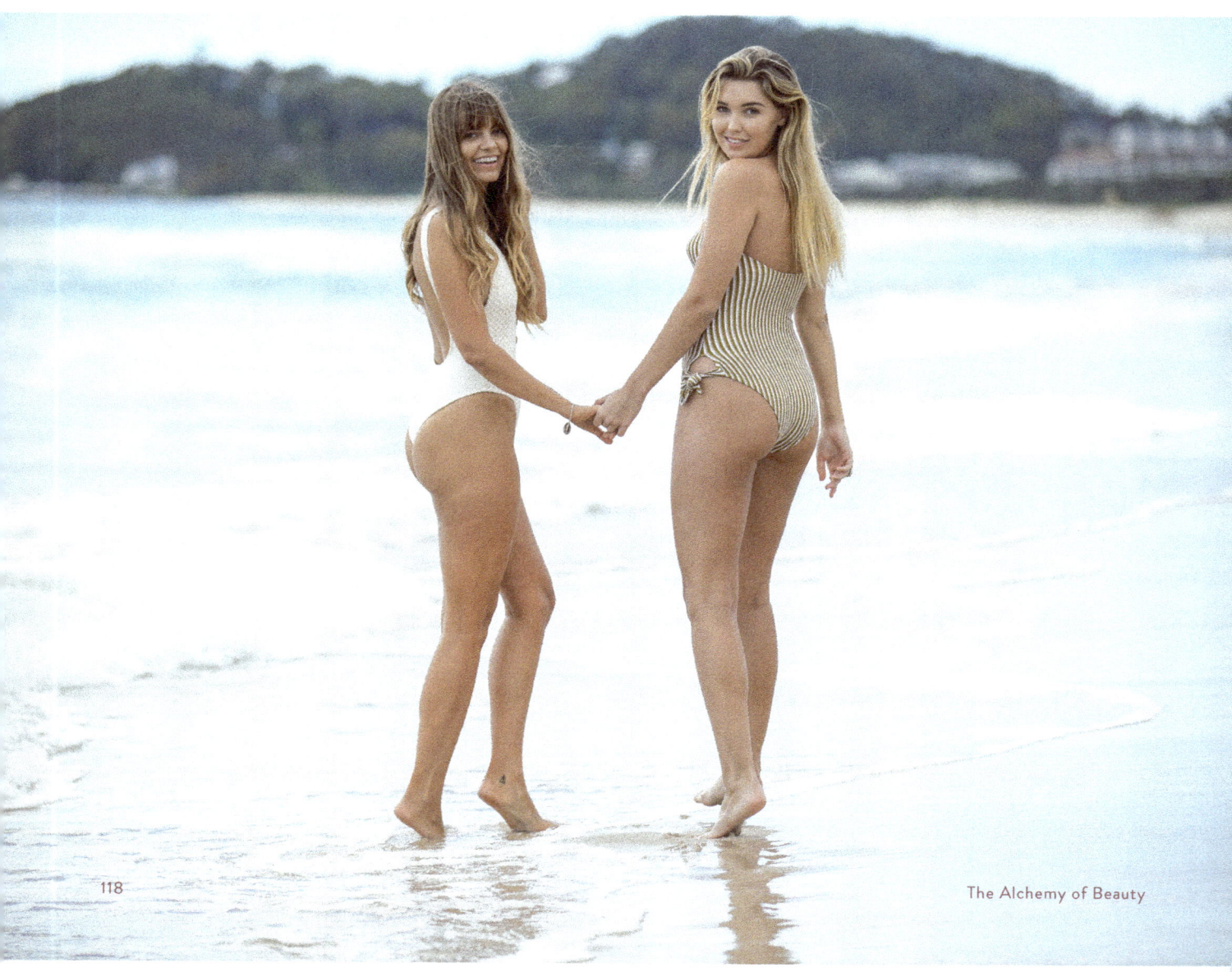

STAY PRESENT in the MOMENT

I know you have heard the saying 'LIVE in the NOW' over and over in hundreds of spiritual books, but, it is no wonder these teachers keep reinforcing this fact as it is perfectly valid in the quest for happiness. Unhappy people do not to live in the present. Their minds are always anticipating future events or reminiscing about past happenings, and this affects their ability to feel joy for what is already beautiful in their life right NOW! Have you ever found yourself racing through crazy thoughts in your mind, like 'I will be happy when I make more money, I will be happy when I meet the perfect man, I will be happy when I pay off my house,' and so on? Most of us have fallen into this pattern at some stage. The problem with this kind of negative thinking is that it takes us out of the now and focuses our dominant thoughts on what we don't have rather than gratitude for what we already have.

Buddhists have known this since time began. They call the practice of staying present in the now 'mindfulness'. Sadly, in today's society most of us are programmed to live life like a rat on a wheel – darting towards the search for more material possessions to hopefully fill the void of discontentment within our souls. Yet once we attain that particular object, our heart isn't quite as fulfilled as we thought and the search for more fulfillment begins again. This constant search for more money or material possessions is driven by the EGO and it can never create a true feeling of inner happiness. Inner happiness is already present within our lives. We just have to look around at our children, our family, our friends, nature and our own ability to give to feel this.

True beauty emanates from staying present in the moment and feeling gratitude for all that you have in your life right now. This inner feeling of gratitude creates a magical energy that reflects to the outside as authentic spiritual beauty.

Spiritual Beauty Trick 1: *One of the best ways to learn to stay present in the now is to practice 'mindfulness'. Mindfulness is when you concentrate on exactly what is happening in your life right now or exactly on what you are doing. For example, if I am sweeping the floor, I am 100% focused on the broom, the floor and the act of sweeping, rather than drifting into mindless thoughts of the past or present. You can use little reminders to help you stay present in the moment. For example, if you tie a red string around your wrist and every time you start to slip away from the present, the string will remind you to stay focused on the now.*

Another simple trick is to focus on your breath. As soon as your mind starts to wander into thoughts of the past or present, begin to concentrate on your breath. Breathe in and out deeply and start to count your breaths slowly. Only focus on your breath. I guarantee it will shift you back to the present moment.

If you find yourself still drifting into the past or present, say the following positive affirmation in your head or out loud 'I forgive the past, I release the future and I celebrate my life right now'.

2 YOUR MIND is your GREATEST BEAUTY TOOL

As humans we have close to 60,000 thoughts racing through our heads everyday and 80% of these are often negative. These thoughts are intensified by negative images in the media. If you watch the nightly news or read the newspapers countless stories of death, murder, bombings, extortion and betrayal are posted every day. Just imagine what that is adding to your 60,000 thoughts. On top of this, negative advertising attempts to convince us that we are not happy with our lives, or unworthy, by portraying images of 'perfect' people smiling, in the hope that we will spend our money on an expensive skin cream or cosmetic procedure to find the happiness we have been seeking. As a female in today's world, it is easy to be swayed by these picture-perfect images, but it is important to remember that most of them are false illusions that try to tell us that we are not pretty, slim or young enough, This does not mean they are true! Over 80% of imprinted thoughts are incorrect. I love this old Cherokee Indian legend about the battle going on inside of our minds.

An old Cherokee was teaching his grandson about life. "A fight is going on inside me," he said to the boy.

"It is a terrible fight and it is between two wolves. One is evil – he is anger, envy, sorrow, regret, greed, arrogance, self-pity, guilt, resentment, inferiority, lies, false pride, superiority, and ego." He continued, "The other is good – he is joy, peace, love, hope, serenity, humility, kindness, benevolence, empathy, generosity, truth, compassion, and faith. The same fight is going on inside you – and inside every other person, too."

The grandson thought about it for a minute and then asked his grandfather, "Which wolf will win?"

The old Cherokee simply replied, "The one you feed the most."

If we constantly feed the evil wolf negative thoughts, then this is reflected in the image we radiate to others and the manifestation of our lives. Yet if we feed the good wolf kind thoughts and acts of compassion and gratitude then we radiate an aura of love, beauty and happiness and ultimately live a beautiful life.

The American Indians knew what researchers in the field of neuroscience are only now just discovering. Whatever you focus your thoughts on shapes the road map in your brain to become your reality. If you constantly think negative thoughts that you are ugly, not perfect or overweight, then these neural pathways become stronger and those thoughts become habit forming. If you constantly focus on bills, you will attract more bills. If you focus on lack, you will attract more lack. The messages we put out and our emotional state linked to this is our point of attraction within life. Fear-focused thinking pulls us out of our alignment with positive energy disconnecting us from the universal source of attraction. Never focus on what you don't have – rather centre your attention on all of the beautiful things that you have in your life right now and you will attract more beauty and happiness into your life.

Spiritual Beauty Trick 2: Consciously notice your negative thoughts, by stepping back from yourself when this happens. These thoughts are out of alignment with your true happiness and joy. Ask yourself honestly 'how does this thought make me feel right now? If it makes you feel unhappy and uncomfortable then it is simply a lesson telling you what you don't want in your life. It is important to forgive this thought. Thank the thought for revealing this to you so you can consciously choose what you do want. What is the best thought attached to a beautiful feeling that you can think of right now. Ask the universe to take you towards this positive thought and feeling. It is important to thank the universe for guiding you towards the outcome of this positive thought and emotion. Remember, whatever you focus on becomes your reality, so if you have thoughts of fear, worry, lack or jealousy, forgive these thoughts and begin replacing with feelings and thoughts of hope, love, beauty and abundance and this will become your reality.

3 GRATITUDE is a MAGNET for MIRACLES

When my kids were little I would encourage them to play a gratitude game with me. I would ask them to say out loud, without thinking, three things they were grateful for in their lives. When we first started and they couldn't think of what to say, I would tell them 'maybe say that you are grateful that you were born with two legs to run' or 'that you are grateful that you have two parents who love you dearly'. When we first used to do this, they would always think of material things like getting a new bike or an ipad. Now my kids love this, because everything they have focused their gratitude on has manifested as the most beautiful gifts within their lives. It has taught them gratitude for the simple things they have and these simple things are so much bigger to them now.

The next time you look in the mirror, and you see lines or marks that you think are flaws, override this by thinking of the beautiful things about yourself. Think of the all of the kind things that you have done for someone, the smile you gave freely to a sad soul, the times you have touched someone's heart. See this AUTHENTIC KINDNESS as you look into your eyes. That way you will look past those beautiful so called 'flaws' and see nothing but compassion staring back at you. Practice gratitude daily and watch the magic unfold in your life. A grateful heart is a magnet for miracles.

Spiritual Beauty Trick 3: *Without thinking about it, in 60 seconds write down everything you are grateful for in your life right now. Practice this every morning when you wake up and in 28 days you will be surprised at how quickly your list grows and how much magic will enter your life!*

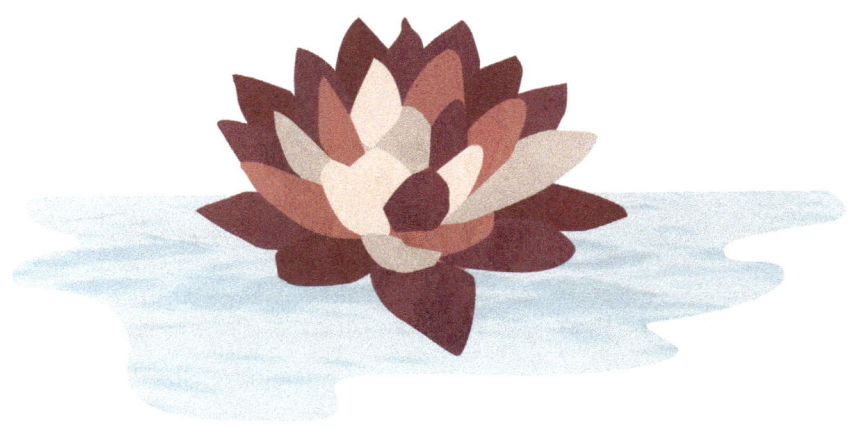

4 SELF-LOVE is your FRIEND

A very wise friend of mine always said to me 'never let a bad event or situation become your story'. What she was trying to teach me was 'no matter what perceived bad situations happen to us, we can either grow from them or fall victim to them and make them our story. If we make them our story, we will never blossom in life'. A victim believes the past and its events have a greater control over their life than the present. When you take on the victim role, you begin to blame others for your position in life. No one else is responsible for your happiness. Dwelling in drama will simply act as a chain that blocks you from experiencing true happiness in life. If you do not like something, change it and if you cannot change the situation, change your attitude towards the situation. We can choose to be a victim in the world we see or we can choose to perceive our difficult experiences as a catalyst for incredible change. Positive emotions can unlock the chains that have trapped us from experiencing alignment with the universal energy source. Make feeling great a priority in your life.

All of our attitudes and thoughts are displayed to the world in our facial expressions. We begin to look physically how we think and feel. If we think negative, stuck thoughts and see life as a struggle, this will show as etched lines of hardship on the face. If we practice smiling and laughing every day and realise that every lesson is an opportunity to grow, the lines that etch your face will be beautiful, happy lines of joy.

Spiritual Beauty Trick 4: Practice this powerful exercise to imprint a more beautiful self-image and to build your confidence. Stand in front of a mirror and look at yourself. Look deeply into your eyes and continue to stare into them. Now think of all of the beautiful things you have done for others in your life. Let go of any negativity or bad comments said to you that have affected your ability to love yourself. Now say the powerful words I AM and follow with something you love about yourself, like:

I am Smart.   I am Strong.

I am Caring.   I am Beautiful.

Continue saying this with passion and feeling. Focus your thoughts on beautiful images of yourself as you look in the mirror and continue to imprint these with positive emotions. Eventually this inner change will create radiant beauty on the outside. Smile often, laugh as much as you can and be happy. This is one of the secrets to becoming more beautiful in every way.

The Alchemy of Beauty

5 PRACTICE KINDNESS and COMPASSION

Being kind to ourselves and showing compassion for others will ignite positive change in our lives. It is easy to compliment someone, to smile at a sad soul or to help someone that is in need. Showing kindness without expecting anything in return is a perfect opportunity for spiritual growth. In today's society, it is not unusual to experience unkind judgments or to have someone gossip unfairly behind your back. As we know, GREAT MINDS discuss IDEAS, AVERAGE MINDS discuss EVENTS and SMALL MINDS discuss people.

When a person talks about another person in an unkind way it is simply showing to the world they are not content with their own lives. My beautiful, confident daughter experienced this kind of judgment at the age of nine. Many other children I know have gone through similar experiences. Often this doesn't originate from children, but rather from the role modelling of the parents. When my daughter was upset by the isolation and unfair words, I taught her to think kind thoughts about these people, as they are obviously discontent with their own lives. I also explained to her how important it is never to lower yourself to someone else's low vibration by retaliating in a similarly unkind manner. At night, we practiced gratitude techniques. Within six months she had a beautiful circle of the most kind-hearted and confident friends in her life, just like her. She did not make this her story. Together we made positive changes to alter her response to the situation to bring about happiness again. Practice kindness, even in the face of adversity, and beauty will always shine through.

Spiritual Beauty Trick 5: *If you want to raise your beauty vibration, think of someone that has harmed you or done you wrong. Now imagine, hugging that person and an aura of golden light surrounds you both as you smile. Forgiveness and practicing kindness towards our enemies is a powerful tool for spiritual growth.*

6 LIVE your TRUE LIFE PURPOSE

It is important to have the courage to follow your bliss by doing something that is meaningful in life. This will also give you the opportunity to increase your self worth. Finding and living your true purpose allows you to connect with the 'oneness of creation' that is completely separate from your ego. When you work in your purpose, you are serving humanity and this allows your spiritual beauty to shine from the inside. When you meet people who live and follow their life purposes, they radiate a special, magnetic energy that is impossible to replicate in any pill or potion. Life purposes can be completely different for everyone. Yours could be 'being a great mum' or 'saving animals' or becoming a healer, as long as what you choose to do fills your heart with happiness and joy then you have found your purpose.

Spiritual Beauty Trick 6: *This is a really old, but simple and effective technique for helping you get in touch with your true passion or purpose in life. Immerse yourself in a quiet space. Now grab a piece of paper and write at the top 'What is my life purpose?' 'What fills me with passion?'. Begin to jot down anything that comes to your head. It could be dancing, yoga, teaching, traveling, writing – anything. Eventually when you write something and think about it, that particular role will evoke an emotion in you creating a vibration or resonance in your heart. When you feel this special energy, it is your soul telling you, this is the right direction to take.*

7 Immerse yourself in NATURE

The more beauty you see within people and nature, the more beauty you can project into the world. Throughout life, we will always encounter 'visually beautiful people', but when you get to know their personalities and they speak unkind words about others, suddenly your original perception of their beauty is transformed into a vision of ugliness. Beauty is not all about physical symmetry and perfection as many people believe – it is much deeper than that. The more kindness, love and harmony that a being can resonate, the higher their beauty vibration will become. Our inner spirit and consciousness is the mirror by how we project radiant beauty to others. One of the easiest ways to get in touch with this is by immersing ourselves in the wonder of nature. It is important to take the time to feel beauty in everything – nature, sounds, colours and people. This appreciation will imbue you with a beautiful radiance.

Spiritual Beauty Trick 7: _Try immersing yourself in nature. You may want to visit a waterfall, climb to the top of a mountain, sit on the beach or even go for a surf. Soak up the beauty around you – look at the colours, listen to the sounds and take in the smells. Stay present in the moment and feel a deep love and appreciation in your heart for the beauty surrounding you. The more you do this, the happier you will feel and the quicker you will reflect beauty into your outside world._

An empathetic heart creates an energy that cannot be captured in a skin cream, pill or potion – it is a divine healing vibration that radiates pure beauty to the outside. If you take care of your spiritual beauty by practicing kind acts, smiling, laughing often, following your purpose, centering your mind, appreciating nature and eating spiritually healing foods – it will reflect in your expression and energy on the outside.

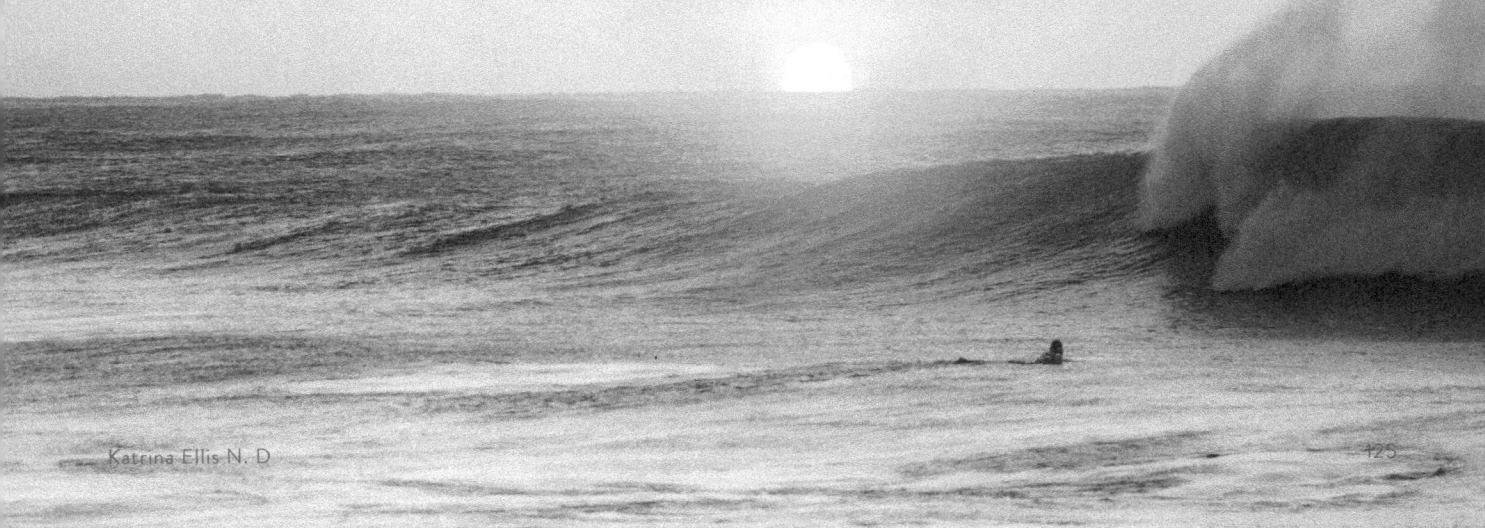

BEAUTY AFFIRMATIONS

Afirmations will make you feel beautiful, no matter how old you are. Real beauty emanates from the inside out, but unfortunately in some, it cannot shine because of a muddled cloud of the wrong thoughts, words, life experiences and social conditioning. If we cleanse our mind of negative thoughts our real inner beauty can shine through and reflect to the outside. Affirmations focused on inner beauty and happiness are a powerful tool to help with this.

When we hold onto bad thoughts of lack, anger, jealousy, sadness, and greed or wish bad things for others, it causes chemical changes in the body that not only drives disease, but also creates unattractive lines on the face. Likewise, if you think happy thoughts and wish for good things for others (even if they are not very nice people) then your facial lines will reflect this, radiating an attractive magnetic beauty.

Affirmations help purify and restructure the electrical potential of our brains. The word 'affirmation' comes from a Latin word that means to 'strengthen or steady'. Affirmations help to strengthen our ability to attain what we desire to manifest. They are a perfect way to rewire our brain towards a positive and desirable outcome.

It is important to believe in your affirmations and have no doubt of its outcome, otherwise the universe will not answer your prayers. Try to repeat the powerful affirmations below at least a few times daily. I love to do these in the morning when I am spiritually realigning and setting myself up for the day. I find a beautiful morning routine coupled with these affirmations is a powerful way to align yourself with positive change. As you say these out loud, feel the beautiful joyful emotion linked to attaining these dreams and these mantras will become your reality.

I radiate beauty from the inside out

I am a natural being of light and happiness
I start my day with positive thoughts and energy
I am proud of my beautiful body, mind and soul
I am healthy, glowing and vibrant
I am having fun today
I am kind, compassionate and beautiful in every way
Being beautiful is a breeze – I just think beautiful thoughts
and it shows on my face
Nothing holds me back
Every day my inner grace shines more beautiful than the day before

I seek beauty in ordinary things

My body is calm and my mind is clear

I am the architect of my own life so I choose to attract happiness every day
I am brimming with positive energy and overflowing with joy

I am a river of confidence
My thoughts are positive and my life is abundant
I am supported by the universe to manifest all of my dreams
Every day I radiate beauty, charm and grace
Happiness is my choice and today
I choose to be HAPPY
ALL IS WELL

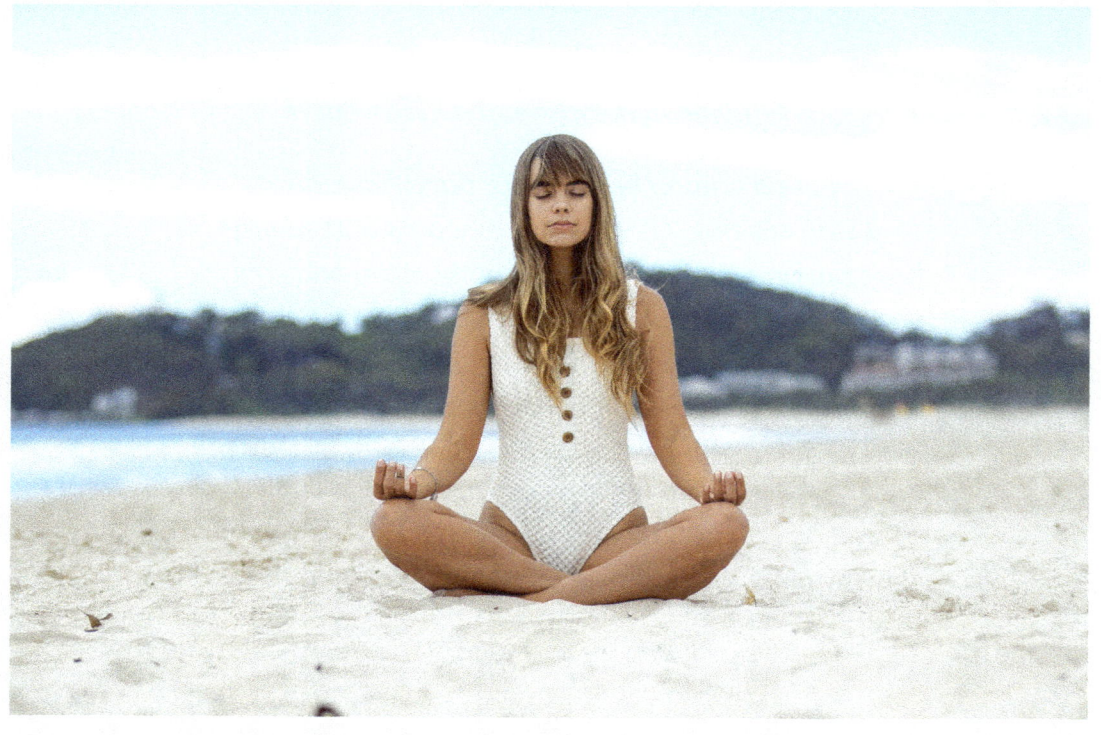

BREATHING EXERCISES FOR BEAUTY AND HAPPINESS

I have been practicing yoga for almost twenty-five years, with seven of these early years teaching in Thailand. Yoga is an ancient Indian practice that helps to improve and attain incredible health while also encouraging relaxation and strength within the mind. It is one of the ultimate keys to enhancing metabolism and encouraging weight loss. Since I first began, I have started most days with 'salute to the sun', which incorporates a number of powerful postures that can move stagnant blood oxygenating and rejuvenating cells, organs and tissues. I was planning to include my favourite yoga asanas for beauty within this book, but there are already thousands of wonderful books and yoga sites that show these in detail. So instead, I have included three of my favourite deep breathing exercises to enhance happiness, beauty and health on every level. Breathe and enjoy!

BHARAMARI
HUMMING BEE BREATH

Sit in a comfortable cross-legged position.

Inhale through both nostrils and then start breathing out through your lips making them vibrate (they should be loosely closed) – you will feel them tingle as you breathe out.

You should be making the sound of a buzzing bee as you breathe out.

Continue to do this improving your out breath each time.

Beauty Powers: I absolutely love the humming bee breath and I do this while walking on the beach. I feel all of the toxins eliminating as I do this, and it gives my face, cheeks and lips the best natural exercise to improve their structure and texture.

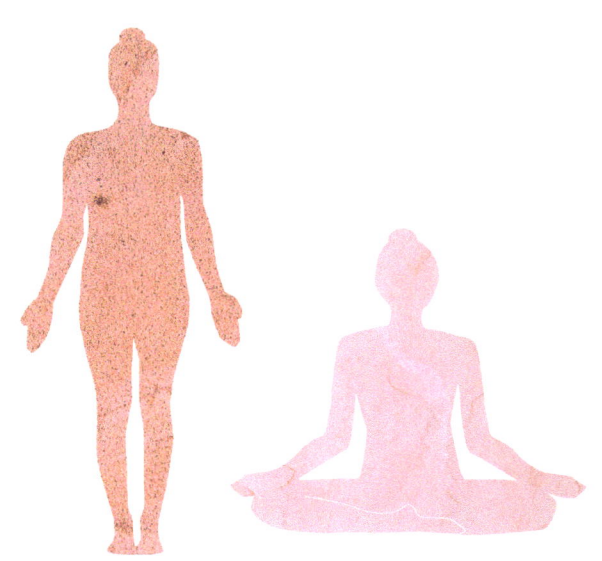

KAPALABHATI
CLEANSING BREATH

1.   Stand with your feet close together and your arms hanging by your sides.

2.   Take a deep breath, hold, then purse your lips as if you want to whistle.

3.   Now start exhaling forcefully, little by little.

4.   Do not blow the air out as if you are blowing out a candle and do not puff your cheeks. Keep the cheeks hollow.

5.   Rest, then repeat several times a day.

Beauty Powers: This is the perfect breathing exercise to strengthen the lungs and to remove acid wastes via the breath.

ANULOM VILOM
ALTERNATE NOSTRIL BREATHING

1.   Sit in a comfortable sitting position. Use your right thumb to close off the right nostril.

2.   Inhale slowly through the left nostril. Pause for a second, now close your left nostril with your ring finger and release your thumb off your right nostril.

3.   Exhale through your right nostril and then inhale through your right nostril. Pause.

4.   Use your thumb to close off your right nostril and breathe out through your left nostril. Do this a few times and increase the amount of repetitions as you learn to do this more and more.

Beauty Powers: This beautiful breathing technique restores balance in the brain, improves sleep, calms the nervous system and increases positivity and balances both sides of the brain and body. It is also the perfect way to cleanse the lungs and remove acid wastes.

Recipes

Alchemy of Beauty Recipes

152

202

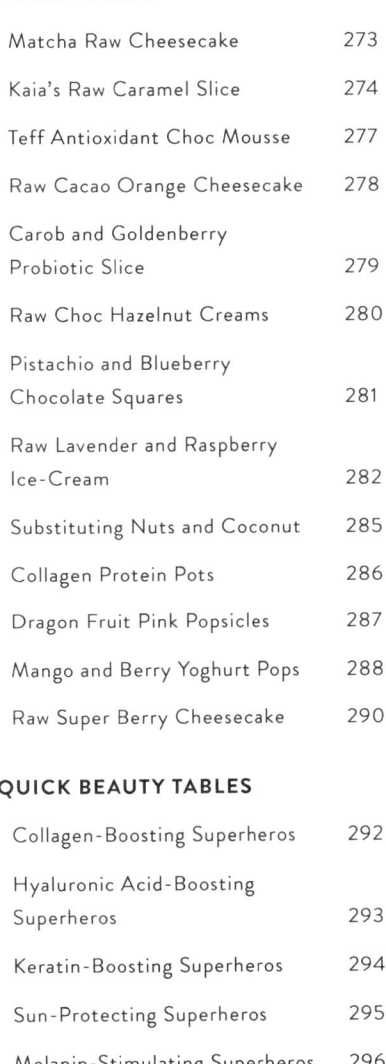

266

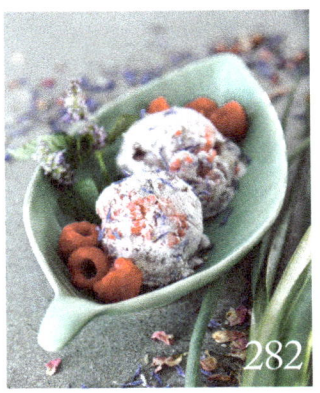

282

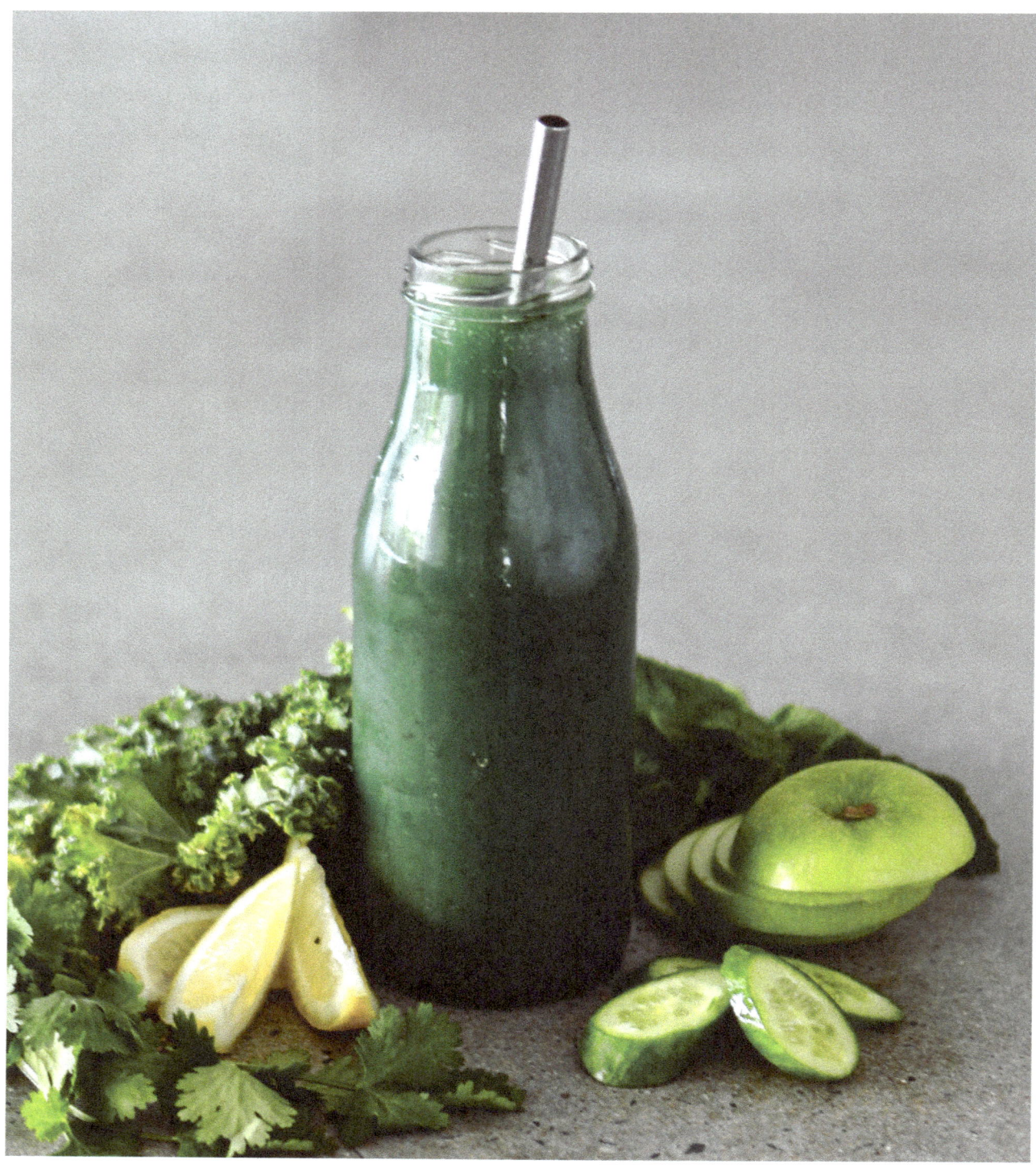

Raw BEAUTY JUICES

Garden Green Detox

MAKES 2 CUPS

INGREDIENTS

8 Romaine lettuce leaves (or mixed lettuce)

½ cup of baby spinach or English/Tuscan kale

A small handful of cilantro or coriander

2 celery stalks, with tops

2 green apples

¼ beetroot

1 lemon, use a little skin

2cm of fresh ginger

METHOD

1. Place spinach, lettuce and parsley in the cold pressed juicer followed by celery, apples, beetroot, ginger and lemon. Add a little alkaline water if needed.

Superfood Powers

Romaine lettuce, beetroot, parsley and spinach are rich sources of chlorophyll, silica, sulphur and B vitamins to purify the blood, lymphatics and kidneys. For extra cleansing add an organic green powder rich in barley grass, wheatgrass and spirulina.

Collagen Boost

MAKES 2 CUPS

INGREDIENTS

¼ green cabbage, sliced

2 kiwifruit, skinned

¼ whole pineapple, cut into pieces

1 red pepper

A handful of broccoli florets

¼ cup of raspberries

1 tablespoon of pure MSM or collagen powder

METHOD

1. Place all of the ingredients, except MSM and collagen, through a cold pressed juicer. After blending, add MSM or collagen powder and drink within twenty minutes.

Superfood Powers

Cucumber skin is full of silica, which stimulates collagen and hair growth. Kiwifruit, red pepper and pineapple are rich sources of Vitamin A and C to knit the skin's matrix while reversing sun-induced skin damage. To boost collagen even more, add some marine or vegan collagen powder, pure Icelandic silica liquid or MSM to this super juice.

Super Hydration

MAKES 2 CUPS

INGREDIENTS

1 to 2 cups of coconut water

3 oranges

¼ watermelon

2 stalks of celery

¼ cucumber, with a little skin

2 cups of baby spinach leaves

METHOD

1. Put all of the fruits and vegetables through a cold pressed juicer, mixing the coconut water in at the end.

Superfood Powers

If your skin is feeling dehydrated, this is the perfect juice to nourish parched pores.
All of the ingredients in 'Super Hydration' contain huge amounts of electrolytes and water to rehydrate the skin, hair and internal organs making you glow from the inside out.

Fast as Grass Hair Juice

MAKES 2 CUPS

INGREDIENTS

4 carrots

2 green apples, skin on

A handful of Romaine lettuce or mixed lettuce

¼ cucumber, skin on

½ lemon, use a little skin

2 cm of fresh ginger

A handful of parsley

A handful of alfalfa sprouts

METHOD

1. Place all of the ingredients through a cold pressed juicer, juicing sprouts before carrots and apples.

Superfood Powers

This juice will make your hair grow as fast as grass. It contains a cocktail of hair growth nutrients like zinc, silica, biotin, iron and carotenes. For some extra growth potential, throw in some organic alfalfa powder.

Burn it up Beauty

MAKES 2 CUPS

INGREDIENTS

1 red grapefruit, peeled

2 leaves of Tuscan or English kale

2 bulbs of fennel

¼ fresh pineapple, chopped

5 cm chunk of turmeric

3 cm chunk of ginger

A little alkaline or purified water

METHOD

1. Place spinach, lettuce and parsley in the cold pressed juicer followed by celery, apples, beetroot, ginger and lemon. Add a little alkaline water if needed.

Superfood Powers

Romaine lettuce, beetroot, parsley and spinach are rich sources of chlorophyll, silica, sulphur and B vitamins to purify the blood, lymphatics and kidneys. For extra thermogenic fat burning add some garcinia cambogia or matcha green tea powder.

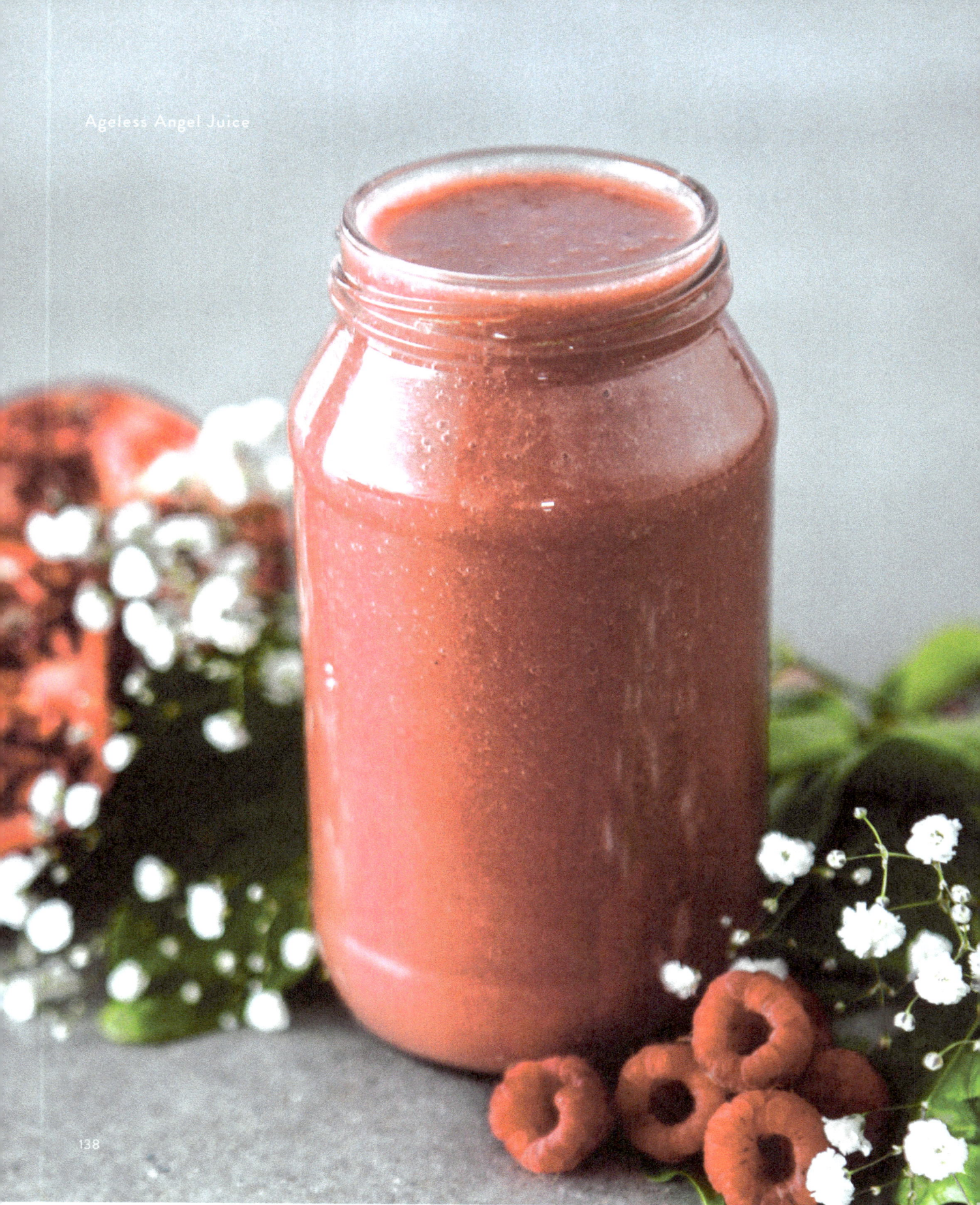

Ageless Angel Juice

Ageless
Angel Juice

MAKES 2 CUPS

INGREDIENTS

½ cup of strawberries

½ cup of blueberries

½ whole beetroot, diced

2 cm chunk of fresh turmeric (use ginger if you
do not have this)

2 green apples

½ lemon (use a little skin)

A small handful of mint

1 to 2 cups of alkaline water

METHOD

1. Put beetroot, apple, lemon, mint, turmeric and
    berries through a cold pressed juicer. Add alkaline
    water to dilute the juice.

Superfood Powers

These red and blue superfoods are packed full of Vitamin
A, C, folate, manganese and flavonoids to encourage the
removal of dead skin cells and the regeneration of new
ones. When you combine the healing properties of berries
and turmeric, you have a heaven-sent Angel Juice.

Flush
the Fluid

MAKES 2 CUPS

INGREDIENTS

2 cucumbers, with skin on

A handful of parsley

A handful of baby spinach

2 celery sticks, include some leaves

2 slices of watermelon

1 lemon

A handful of dandelion leaves
(if you can't find these, use parsley)

METHOD

1. Put all of the ingredients through a juicer,
    being sure to add some cucumber skin and
    celery tops for extra 'fluid flushing' potential.

Superfood Powers

All the ingredients in 'flush the fluid' are nature's best
natural diuretics. They contain all the perfect ingredients
to wash out trapped fluid, reducing cellulite and toxicity.

Beauty
in a Bottle

MAKES 2 CUPS

INGREDIENTS

¼ cup of blueberries

¼ cucumber with skin on

¼ purple cabbage, diced

3 to 4 carrots

A handful of spinach leaves

2 organic oranges, skinned

2 cm chunk of ginger

METHOD

1. Juice all of the fruits and vegetables together in a cold pressed juicer. Add a little alkaline water if you need to dilute this.

Superfood Powers

This juice is a liquid vitamin pill, as it contains every nutrient needed for optimal health. The berries are rich in Vitamin C and flavonoids, the pineapple is a powerful anti-inflammatory that reverses skin damage and cucumber and cabbage are packed full of Vitamin A, C, folate and B vitamins to regenerate dying skin cells. No wonder this juice is called 'Beauty in a Bottle'!

Tummy
Tonic

MAKES 2 CUPS

INGREDIENTS

1 pear

2 green apples

2 cm chunk of ginger

2 small fennel stalks

¼ fresh pineapple

A handful of mint

METHOD

1. Put pears, apples, fennel, pineapple, ginger and mint through a cold pressed juicer adding water to achieve the perfect consistency.

Superfood Powers

All of the ingredients in this tummy tonic are super high in natural electrolytes and prebiotics to aid constipation, bellyaches and bloating.

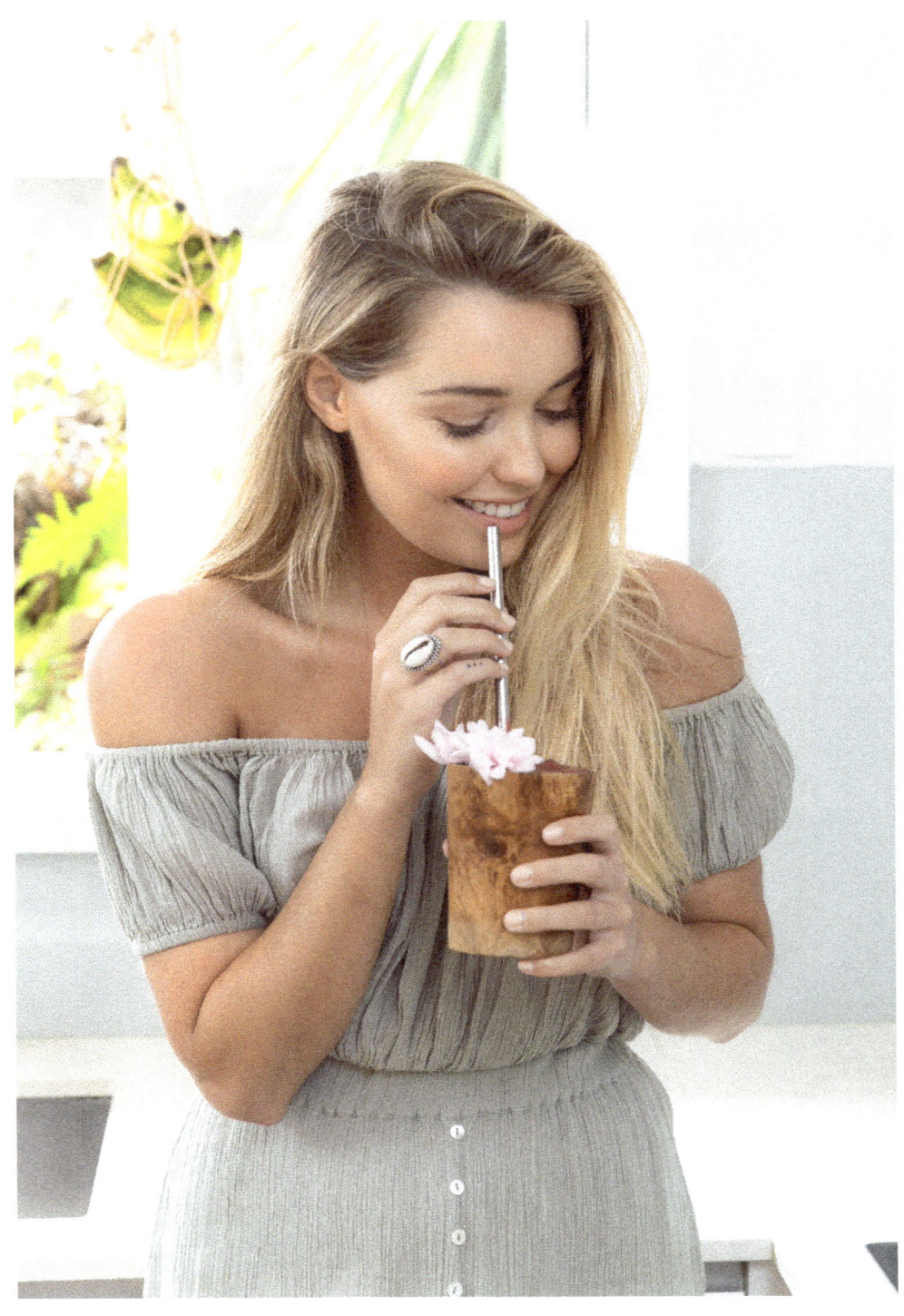

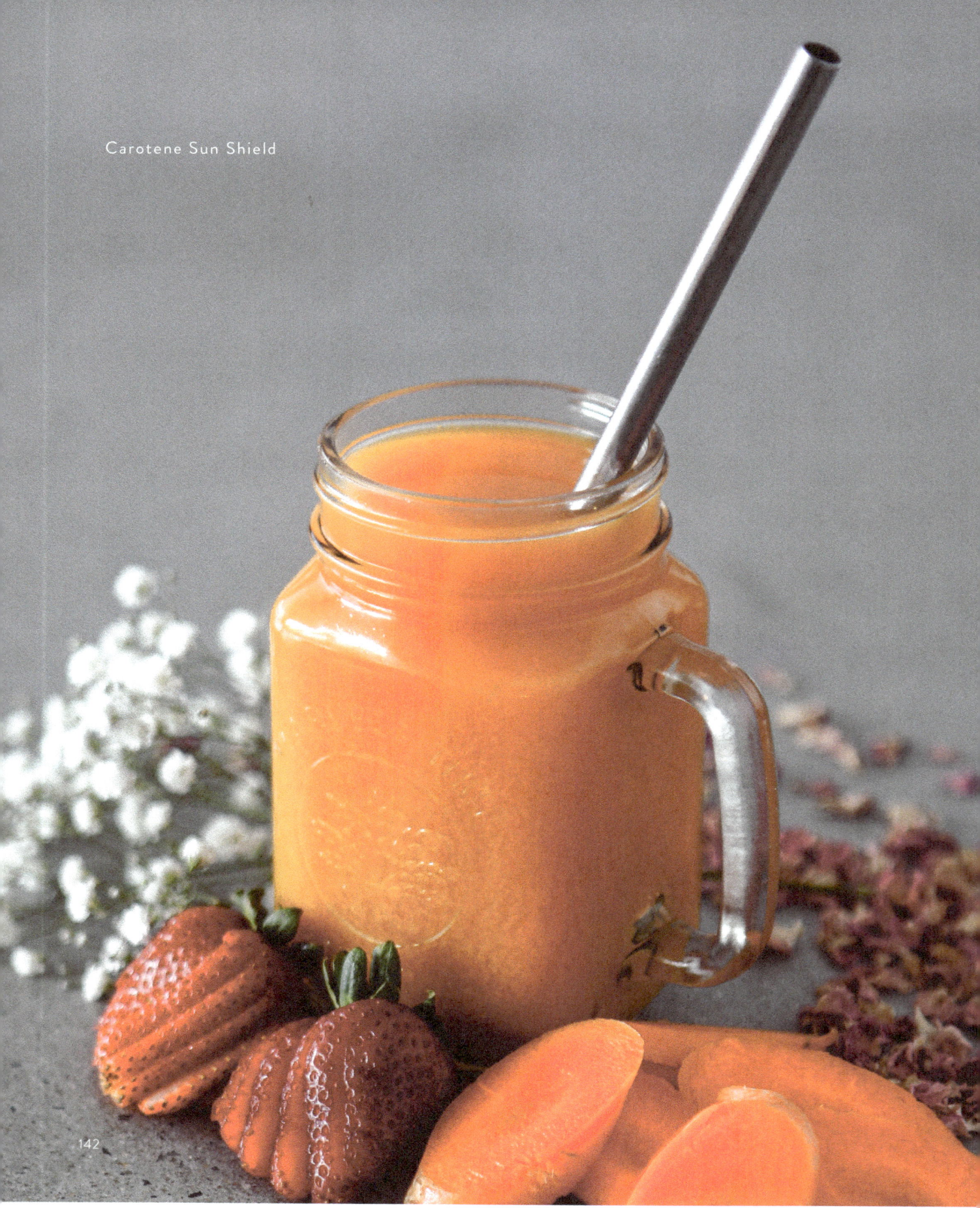

Carotene Sun Shield

Carotene Sun Shield

MAKES 2 CUPS

INGREDIENTS

4 to 6 carrots

2 mangoes, peeled

6 to 8 strawberries

½ red capsicum

3 leaves of Tuscan or English kale

Water

METHOD

1. Put carrots, mangoes, strawberries, capsicum and kale through a juicer, adding water to achieve the perfect texture.

Superfood Powers

This juice is incredibly rich in beta-carotene, zeaxanthin, alpha-carotene and lycopene. These super nutrients offer the skin protection against dangerous UV rays that can cause skin cancer and advanced ageing.

Happy Liver Flush

MAKES 1 TO 2 CUPS

INGREDIENTS

1 whole lemon or lime (keep a little skin)

2 stalks of lemongrass

¼ beetroot

6 small radish

2 fresh garlic cloves, minced or juiced

2 to 3 green apples

2 tablespoons of organic flaxseed oil (I love Stoney Creek or Melrose)

METHOD

1. Put all of the ingredients through a cold pressed juicer (except the flaxseed oil) and add a little lemon or lime skin for extra cleansing properties. Now stir in the oil.

Superfood Powers

This alkaline cleansing drink combats an acidic blood pH. The pectin and sulphur found in the lemon and apples removes heavy metals and toxins via the bowel and liver. Flaxseed oil improves gallbladder function and helps to dissolve nasty gallstones. This is a perfect bowel and liver cleansing juice that can be drunk daily.

SUPER BEAUTY SMOOTHIES & Drinks

Resveratrol Treat

MAKES 2 GLASSES

INGREDIENTS

¼ cup of blueberries

¼ cup of raspberries

¼ cup of strawberries

1 pomegranate, (cut in half, bang on the back with a knife to get seeds out)

1 cup of purple or red grapes

¼ purple cabbage

2 cups of purified water

1 tablespoon of Macqui berry powder (or an organic berry mix)

METHOD

1. Place all of the ingredients in a food processor or blender with a little ice. If grapes are out of season, leave them out.

Superfood Powers

This resveratrol-rich shake helps to stimulate cellular proteins in the skin (known as sirtuins) which promotes a longer cell life. It improves the health of the mitochondria, preserving energy while protecting against heart disease and cancer. To achieve extra beautifying qualities in this drink, add a high quality, organic berry mix.

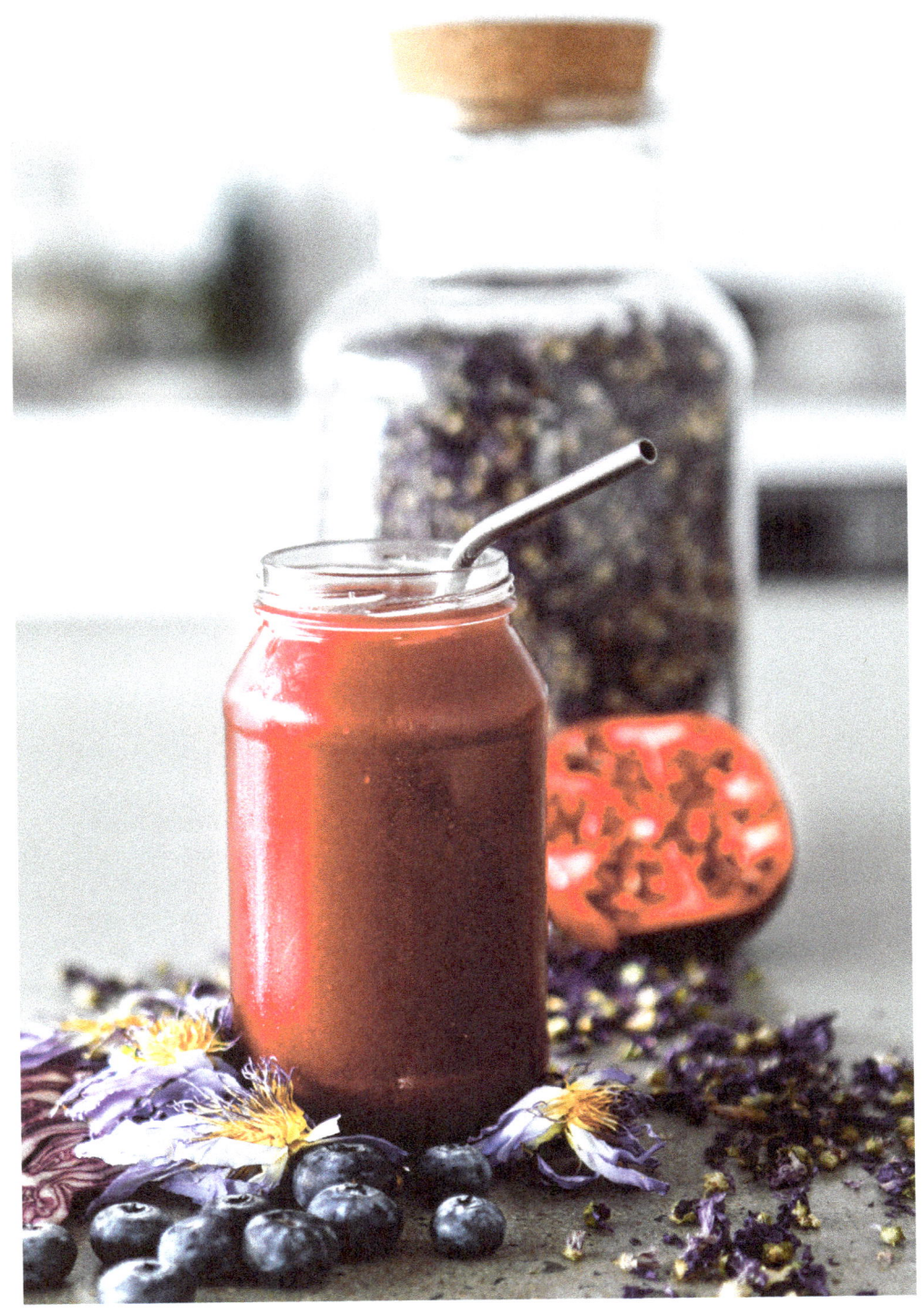

Avocado Beauty Express

MAKES 2 CUPS

INGREDIENTS

½ ripe avocado

2 cups of fresh pineapple

A handful of baby or English spinach

1 cup of watercress or kale

1 tablespoon of hemp seeds

2 tablespoons of an Omega oil (flaxseed, hemp, sacha inchi or avocado oil)

2 cups of alkaline water or 1 cup of coconut water

A handful of mint

METHOD

Blend the pineapple, greens and avocado, adding enough water to achieve the right consistency. Slowly add hemp seeds and Omega oils. Drink this beauty express within twenty minutes of making.

Superfood Powers

The rich monounsaturated oils found in the avocado and hemp seeds and the high amount of chlorophyll, Vitamin A and E found in the leafy greens are perfect for skin hydration and sun protection. Adding extra omega oils enhances this smoothie's skin hydrating properties.

Papaya Pigment Potion

MAKES 2 CUPS

INGREDIENTS

1 red or pink grapefruit

¼ red papaya

1 lime, use a little skin

2 oranges, use a little skin

2 small apricots (if in season)

1 to 2 cups of alkaline water

Ice

METHOD

If you want a more liquified smoothie, juice the grapefruit, orange, apricots and lime first. Then throw this mix into a blender with the paw paw and citrus skins or simply just blend all of the ingredients with water.

Superfood Powers

Grapefruit and papaya both contain Vitamin C, bromelain and alpha hydroxy acids to help reduce skin pigmentation. The citrus skin contains limonene to stop free radical damage and to smooth out a muddled complexion.

Skin Candy

MAKES 2 CUPS

INGREDIENTS

1 pomegranate (cut in half and hit on the back to get seeds out)

½ cup of raspberries

1 cup of spinach leaves

1 cup of Romaine or mixed lettuce

A handful of mint

1 frozen banana

2 cups of alkaline or purified water or 1 cup of coconut water

METHOD

Cut the pomegranates in half and bang them on the back with a large knife. All of the seeds will fall out. Place them in the blender along with the other ingredients and blend until smooth.

Superfood Powers

This smoothie is full of powerful antioxidants, polyphenols and minerals which will add a rosy glow to your cheeks. It contains Vitamin K, gingerols, silica and bromelain which help to strengthen the hair and nails too.

Glowing Green Smoothie

MAKES 2 CUPS

INGREDIENTS

6 to 7 leaves of Romaine lettuce (use mixed lettuce if you cannot find this)

1 cup of cabbage

A handful of broccoli florets

¼ fresh pineapple

½ lime (use a little skin)

3 cm chunk fresh ginger

2 glasses of purified or alkaline water

Ice

METHOD

Blend all of the ingredients together in a food processor, Vitamix or Thermomix with a little ice. If you want a thinner consistency, juice the pineapple and lime first and then blend with the rest of the ingredients.

Superfood Powers

This smoothie is packed full of chlorophyll, carotenes, Vitamin A and C and plenty of minerals to nourish dry skin, making you glow from the inside out. I often add a super green powder mix like Pure Synergy, Green nutritionals, Vitamineral Green or Green Vibrance.

Matcha Milkshake

MAKES 2 CUPS

INGREDIENTS

1 frozen banana

1 tablespoon of coconut flakes or meat

1 ½ cups of almond, hemp, coconut or hazelnut milk

2 teaspoons of organic Matcha powder
(depending on how strong you like it)

1 tablespoon of flaxseed meal

A handful of pumpkin seeds (preferably activated)

1 tablespoon of quinoa flakes (optional)

METHOD

Whizz the banana in the blender with coconut flakes, milk, Matcha, flaxseed and quinoa. If you want this sweeter, add a little monkfruit, maple syrup or Medjool dates. Pour into two glasses and sprinkle some fresh Matcha on top. To power this up with extra antioxidants, add fresh turmeric or raspberries.

Superfood Powers

If I'm feeling tired, I often whip up this Matcha shake to perk up my energy. Matcha Green tea is a cancer-fighting polyphenol rich superfood. It can increase telomere length, reverse skin damage and protect against skin cancer.

Electrolyte Elixir

MAKES 2 CUPS

INGREDIENTS

2 cups of coconut water

1 mango (if not in season, use frozen mango pieces)

¼ cucumber, with skin

1 cup of mint leaves

1 cup of baby spinach leaves

1 cup of kale

METHOD

Place all of the ingredients into a blender with a little ice and blend until smooth. If mango is not in season, replace with banana.

Superfood Powers

Magnesium, sodium, potassium and calcium are natural electrolytes that help to keep the body hydrated during summer months, or when you are ill. When the body is hydrated the skin takes on a luscious glow.

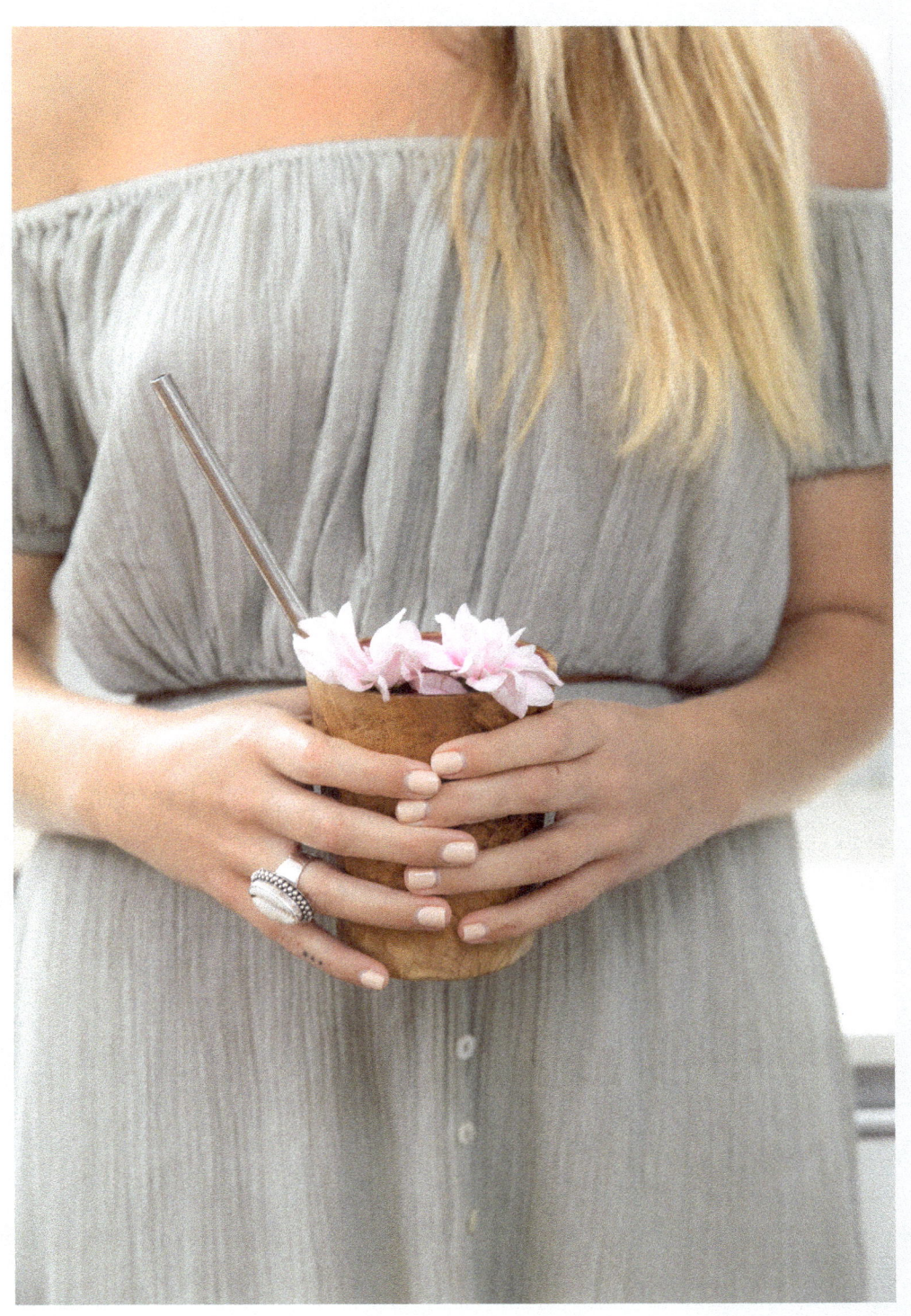

Maca Malt

MAKES 2 CUPS

INGREDIENTS

1 cup of hazelnut, almond or coconut milk

1 tablespoon of pure cacao or cacao nibs

2 tablespoons of organic, cold pressed coconut or hemp oil

1 tablespoon of organic, hulled hemp seeds

1 tablespoon of golden Maca powder

1 frozen banana

½ teaspoon of vanilla

METHOD

Place all of the ingredients into a blender with ice and extra water if needed. When you get a nice, smooth mix pour into two glasses and garnish with cacao. If the strawberries are not in season, use organic frozen berries instead.

Superfood Powers

Cacao and strawberries are super high sources of polyphenols which protect against harmful UV rays and encourage skin cell renewal. Maca balances the endocrine glands making it useful with hormone, energy and adrenal balance.

PUMP up your BEAUTY SMOOTHIE

By adding certain superfoods to your smoothies you can pump up their healing potential. Some of my fav all-time beauty boosters include:

MSM – MSM or methylsulfonylmethane, is an organic sulphur compound derived from the earth's rain cycle. It builds healthy keratin and collagen, which gives you strong hair, skin and nails. It also helps with joint flexibility detoxification, inflammation and digestion.

Organic Berry Mix with Açai, Macqui and other berries – All organic red, blue or purple berries are rich sources of polyphenols like lycopene and resveratrol. These powerful substances can protect against sunburn, skin damage, eye problems, and cancer and even improve the lusciousness of your hair.

Organic Supergreens – Wheatgrass, Barley Grass, Spirulina & others – organic greens increase the production of superoxide dismutase (SOD). SOD is a powerful antioxidant that protects a cell's mitochondria against free radical attack that can cause premature ageing, chronic fatigue, cancer and other diseases. These super greens are rich sources of chlorophyll which detoxifies heavy metals and provides oxygen to the colon for a happy gut.

Collagen – Collagen is naturally high in GAGS – anti-inflammatory substances that can fix leaky gut, improve bone, tooth and nail strength and help to build our own collagen, leading to beautiful skin.

Pearl Powder – This is made from crushed pearl shells. It helps to stimulate a powerful enzyme known as SOD which stops wrinkle formation, age spots and pigmentation. It is very good for reducing melanin production in the skin and reducing freckles and blemishes.

Schisandra – The beauty-enhancing qualities of schisandra have been revered for thousands of years in China. It can assist with stress, depression, virility and skin health. I often add 'BEAUTY BLEND' by Superfeast to my smoothies as it contains schisandra and pearl powder to make your skin glow with vibrance.

Blue-green algae from the Klamath Lake – one of the best natural protein sources in the world, contains over 40 minerals and plenty of chlorophyll which improves digestion, detoxification, energy and mental happiness. A perfect protein source for vegans.

When buying superfoods, it is important to make sure they are organic, ethically sourced, created without high heat and free from contaminants and heavy metals.

Supermodel Skin

MAKES 2 GLASSES

INGREDIENTS

3 cups of mixed lettuce

½ small tub of alfalfa sprouts

1 cup of baby spinach leaves

1 frozen banana

1 to 2 green apples (preferably juiced)

2 celery stalks

¼ cup of pumpkin seeds (activated are best)

½ lemon, with some rind

Superfood Powers

This supermodel smoothie contains lots of Vitamin A, C and E, manganese, folic acid and zinc, which boosts collagen, elastin and keratin production.

METHOD

Juice the apples and lemon and add to a blender with greens, pumpkin seeds, sprouts, banana and a little water to get the perfect texture. Pour into two glasses. If you do not have a juicer, simply blend all of the ingredients, adding more water to get the right texture.

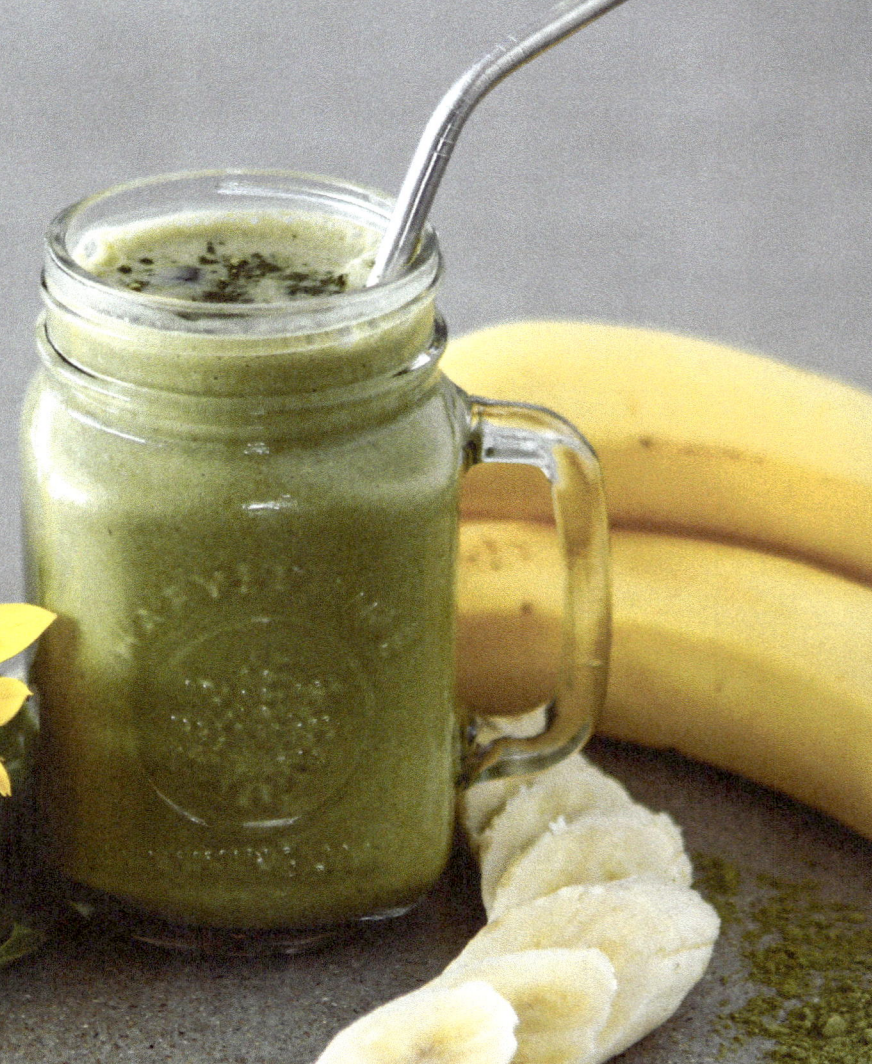

Fresh Complexion

MAKES 2 CUPS

INGREDIENTS

1 cup of coconut, almond or hemp milk
or coconut water

½ chopped mango, chilled

½ cup of raspberries

½ cup of organic Greek yoghurt (another option
is sheep or coconut)

1 tablespoon of organic wheat germ

1 tablespoon of flaxseed meal

1 cup of purified or alkaline water

METHOD

Blend all of the ingredients until smooth, adding
more water to get the perfect texture.

Superfood Powers

This smoothie is full of powerful antioxidants, polyphenols
and minerals which will add a rosy glow to your cheeks. It
contains Vitamin K, gingerols, silica and bromelain which
help to strengthen the hair and nails too.

Glowing Turmeric Milk

MAKES 1 CUP

INGREDIENTS

2 cups of coconut, almond, hemp or another milk

1 tablespoon of coconut, sacha inchi or hemp oil

1 tablespoon of turmeric paste/powder

¼ teaspoon of black pepper

A pinch or cinnamon powder (or cinnamon quills)

1 teaspoon of raw, activated honey, coconut nectar or monkfruit syrup

METHOD

1. Heat up your milk and slowly add the rest of the ingredients, besides the oil. Mix in the oil and natural sweetener when you have the perfect temperature.

Superfood Powers

The world is now aware of the superhuman healing powers of turmeric. Curcumin, found in turmeric, is a potent ant-inflammatory and anti-cancer agent that can reduce depression, boost immunity, detoxify the liver and stop melanin loss, therefore reducing skin pigmentation. By adding a little cayenne pepper to this milk you can also boost your metabolism and burn stubborn tummy fat.

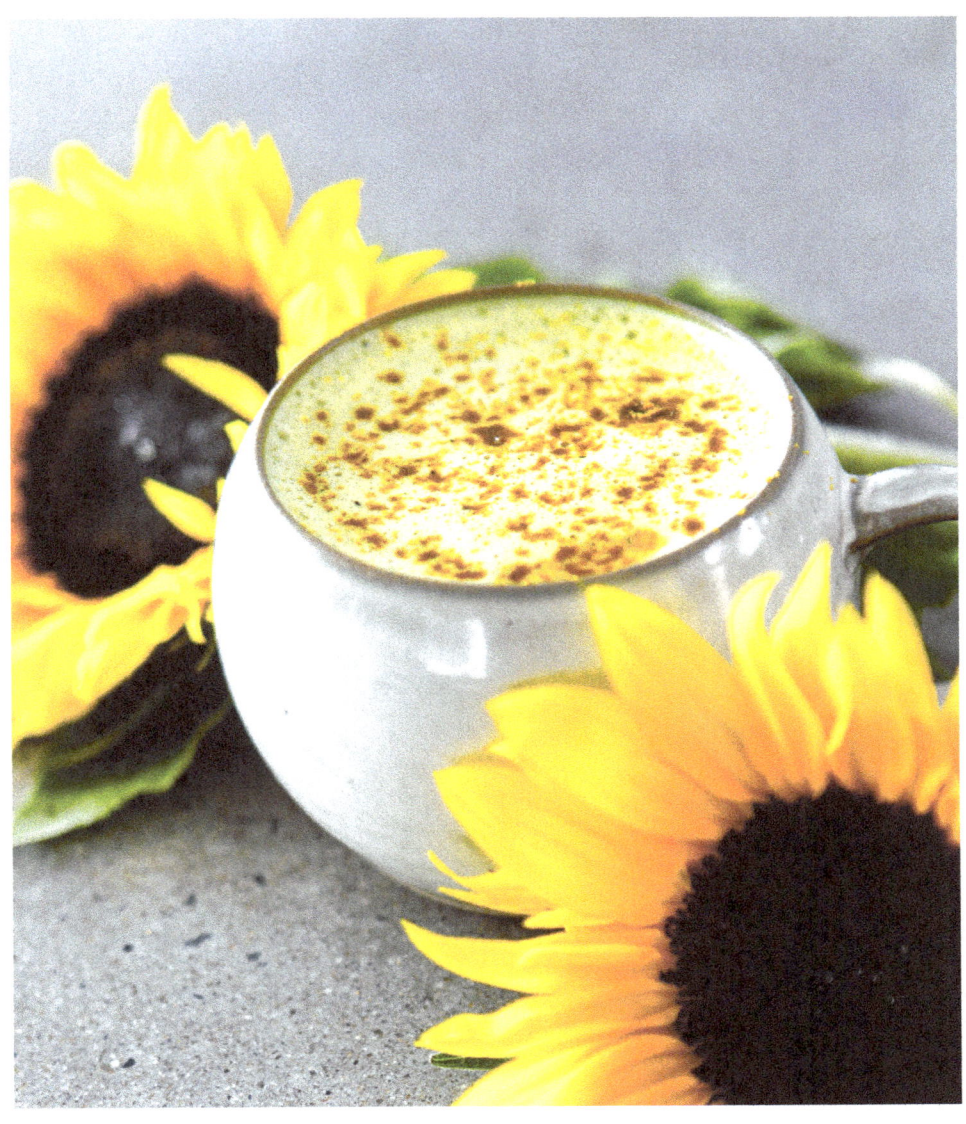

FERMENTED GOODIES, SAUCES BEAUTY & Dips

Coconut Kefir Super Drink

There are two types of kefir grains that you can use to make kefir drinks – milk-based kefir grains or water grains. I love to use the water grains to make my kefir. It makes a sweet, fizzy drink that children really love. It's very easy to change the flavour by adding different fruits or juices. The basic recipe is:

INGREDIENTS

¼ cup of dyhydrated water kefir grains (there are lots of different sources online)

¼ cup of natural sugar (the kefir eats this)

1 cup of coconut water or water

METHOD

1. Add the sugar to a jar or bottle and then add the coconut water. Stir well to dissolve the sugar.

2. Add the kefir grains and then cover with a lid or material cloth and let this sit in a dark, warm place for 24 to 48 hours.

3. After 48 hours it should start bubbling. Then drain the grains off and keep the kefir drink in the fridge.

4. To change its flavour and healing properties, you can add lemon, ginger, turmeric, galangal, hibiscus and other superfoods while fermenting.

Superfood Powers

Kefir is an ancient fermented drink that is an amazing natural prebiotic. It nourishes the gastrointestinal tract with healthy flora, which ensures great digestion and therefore beautiful skin, hair and nail health.

TIPS

The type of sugar you choose to ferment with the grains will change the taste and fizz of your kefir drinks. Rapadura sugar (sugar cane juice that is pressed) makes for a stronger flavour; refined white sugar makes a sweeter kefir; brown sugar (white sugar with molasses added) makes a stronger kefir; and raw sugar makes a less sweet water kefir.

Unfortunately, natural sugars like coconut palm sugar, maple syrup, honey, agave and others do not work with kefir grains well. Many people are concerned about making drinks containing sugar. However, don't be concerned as the sugar is eaten in the fermentation process anyway. Kefir drinks do contain small amounts of alcohol.

Glowing Skin Jam

INGREDIENTS

¼ cup of organic chia seeds

¼ cup of freshly squeezed lemon juice

1 to 2 cups of mixed berries (blueberries, strawberries etc.) – frozen are okay too

4 tablespoons of maple syrup or 1 teaspoon of monkfruit syrup (if you want it sweeter)

1 tablespoon of Açai powder or ½ packet of frozen Açai

2 tablespoons of Agar Agar (to thicken)

METHOD

1. Mix chia and lemon juice together and leave to soak for 2 hours. Blend the berries and natural sweetener.

2. Place this mix in a pan and cook for around 10 minutes on a low heat and then set aside to cool. In another pan, heat up 1 cup of water to 2 tablespoons of Agar or kuzu until it dissolves.

3. Stir this mix into the cooling fruit mixture until it thickens. This yummy jam will keep in the fridge for at least one week.

This jam tastes tastes great on toasted sourdough, buckwheat or teff pancakes or with nut yoghurt. If you are eating 100% raw, pre-soak chia seeds in water (let them swell) and then blend with the rest of the ingredients.

Superfood Powers

This jam is packed with protein, Omega oils, polyphenols and Vitamin C to nourish collagen, reverse pigmentation and protect against UV-related sun damage to the skin. Agar is a natural fibre derived from red algae. It has no calories, no sugars and no carbohydrates, making it perfect for weight loss diets.

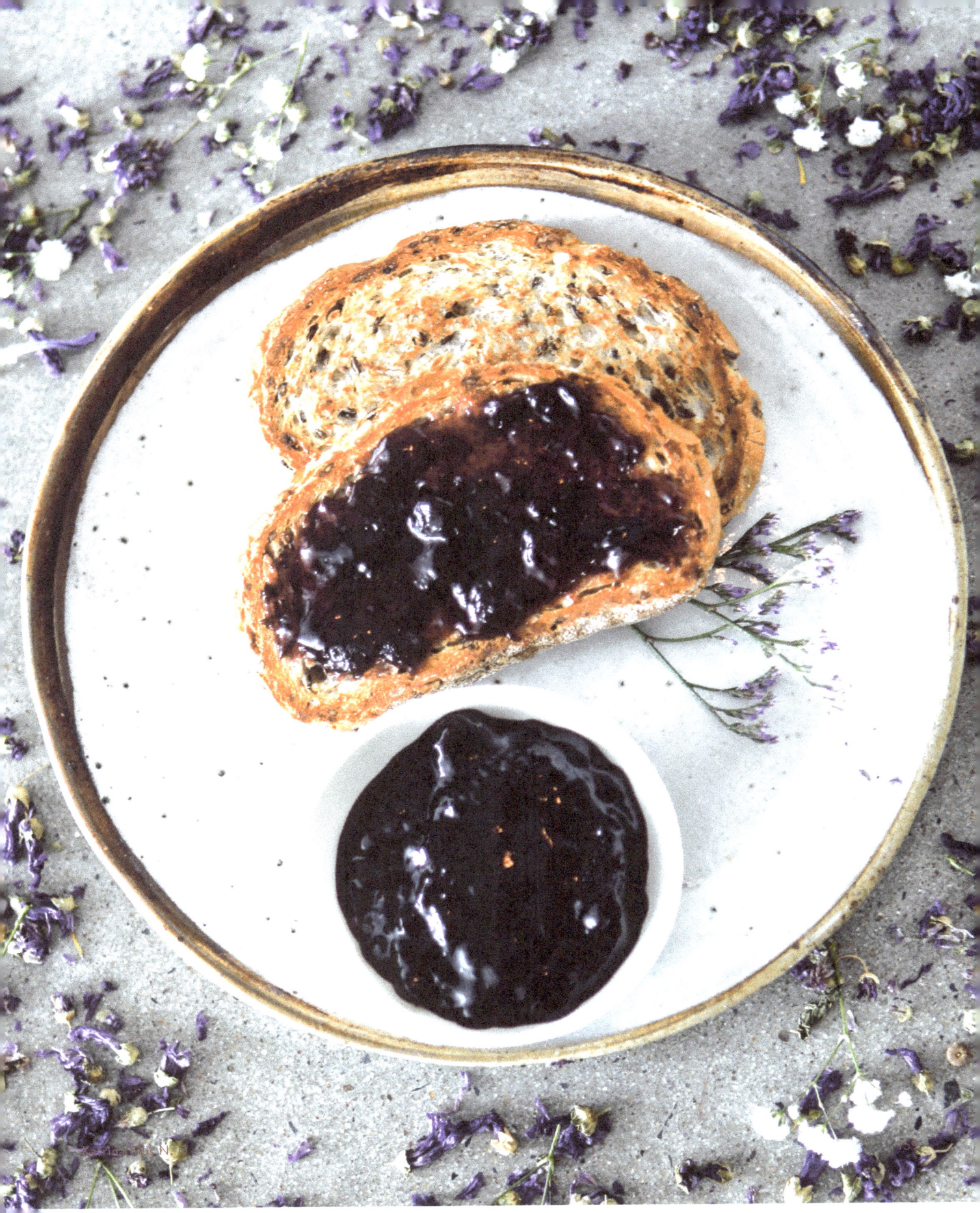

Sun Protection Salsa or Sauce

MAKES 1 BIG JAR

INGREDIENTS

3 to 5 truss or Roma tomatoes

1 pomegranate (cut in half and hit on the back
to get seeds out)

1 small purple onion (peeled and chopped)

4 to 6 garlic cloves, peeled

1 long red chilli pepper, diced

1 red capsicum, diced

½ cup of coriander or 1 tablespoon of coriander seeds

¼ cup of basil

2 limes, juiced

½ teaspoon of cumin

½ teaspoon of paprika

1 teaspoon of Himalayan salt

2 tablespoons of extra virgin olive oil

METHOD

1. Place tomatoes, pomegranate, garlic, onion, chilli, coriander, capsicum and basil in a food processor and pulse, keeping slightly chunky.

2. Transfer to another bowl and add lime juice, paprika, olive oil, cumin and salt.

3. If you want this to be a sun protection tomato sauce, blend all ingredients until smooth adding four tablespoons of Apple Cider Vinegar, four tablespoons of tomato paste and a little more olive oil.

Serve fresh with chopped vegetable sticks, home-made blue corn chips or dehydrated crackers.

Superfood Powers

Tomatoes and pomegranate are amazing sources of lycopene, a flavonoid that can give the skin up to 3 times more sun burn protection. When you add chilli peppers, red capsicum and olive oil you can get an added 20 per cent protection against the sun's harmful rays.

Oriental Anti-Ageing Pesto

MAKES 1 JAR

INGREDIENTS

A big handful of basil

A big handful of coriander

1 stalk of lemongrass

3 garlic cloves, peeled

2 tablespoons of brown rice vinegar,
coconut vinegar or mirin

4 limes, juiced

1 cup of pine nuts or hazelnuts (best when soaked
and dehydrated)

⅓ cup of hemp, olive, chia or macadamia oil

1 teaspoon of Celtic or Himalayan salt or
1 tablespoon of fish sauce

METHOD

1. Place all of the ingredients into a food processor and blend until nice and smooth.

2. If you want to pump this up with extra selenium, add a few brazil nuts.

3. If you want this pesto spicy, add 2 to 3 small red chillies.

Superfood Powers

This pesto is one of my favourite dips, as it has that beautiful Asian flavor with the added addition of lemongrass, lime and coriander.

Probiotic Rich Kimchee

MAKES 1 GLASS JAR

INGREDIENTS

2 heads of Chinese cabbage, finely shredded

6 radishes, peeled and sliced into thin matchsticks

5 carrots, peeled and sliced into matchsticks

4 cm chunk of ginger, peeled and minced

12 garlic cloves, chopped

¼ cup of fish sauce (or fermented bean sauce
if you are a vegetarian)

½ cup of chilli paste or 6 whole chillies diced

¼ cup of fine sea salt

Basic brine to make kimchi (6 tablespoons of fine
sea salt and 2 litres of water. Dissolve half the salt in
warm water and then add the rest to cold water).

METHOD

1. In a bowl, combine shredded cabbage with radish,
   carrots, ginger, garlic, sea salt, fish or vegan sauce
   and chilli paste.

2. Place this mix into a fermentation jar, pounding
   vigorously after adding each amount is added. Liquid
   will seep up from the vegetable mix to eventually cover
   the vegetables. The liquid always needs to be at least
   2 cm below the lid, as the cabbage mixture will expand
   when it ferments.

3. Cover the top to make sure the vegetables stay below
   the brine. Leave this in a warm, dark spot in the
   kitchen to ferment for 5 days or more. Keep checking
   to make sure the brine covers the mix. When you love
   the taste of your kimchee, transfer to the fridge.

Superfood Powers

I love using kimchee in my breakfast salads, in beauty bowls, on scrambled eggs or tofu. Just like sauerkraut, kimchee is
a superb probiotic tummy tonic. Cabbage, carrots and radish are three of the top 'beauty anti-ageing' foods, making this
fermented mix ideal for boosting the health of your skin, hair and nails.

Turmeric Longevity Dip

This dip can be made into a beautiful salad dressing if watered down. I love turmeric. In my book Raw Addiction I created a cancer-fighting turmeric and pistachio dip. This dip contains all the same healing properties, but is pumped up with even more disease-preventing and beauty benefits.

INGREDIENTS

1 big knob of fresh turmeric
or 2 teaspoons of turmeric powder/paste

⅓ cup of tahini or ½ cup of sesame seeds

⅓ cup of walnuts

2 garlic cloves or 1 teaspoon of garlic powder

2 limes, juiced

½ teaspoon of Celtic/Himalayan salt

4 tablespoons of coconut or rice vinegar

6 tablespoons of Apple Cider Vinegar (raw)

4 tablespoons of hemp, flax or pumpkin seed oil

METHOD

1. Soak nuts and seeds in water for two hours to soften and activate.

2. Place in a blender with turmeric, oils, tahini, lemon juice, garlic and vinegars. I always add a little extra vinegar and Celtic salt to season.

Enjoy with celery, bell pepper or carrot sticks.

Superfood Powers

Turmeric is a powerful anti-inflammatory food that can slow down skin ageing and cellular breakdown. Coupled with garlic and Vitamin E rich seeds and nuts, you have a perfect recipe for a youth-promoting super dip.

Rosemary Olive Tapenade

SERVES 2

INGREDIENTS

1 cup of black olives – pitted

½ Spanish onion, diced

2 to 3 garlic cloves, peeled

4 tablespoons of first cold pressed olive oil

1 fresh lemon, juiced

2 tablespoons of parsley

2 tablespoons of fresh or dried rosemary

Celtic salt and pepper for extra flavour

Method

1. I love my tapenades rustic, so if you are like me, simply pulse all of the ingredients quickly toget a rough texture.

This dip keeps for five days in the fridge and it goes beautifully with chopped vegetables, dehydrated crackers and many other foods.

Superfood Powers

Olives are true 'beauty superstars'. They contain nourishing Omega oils, Vitamin A, polyphenols, most B vitamins and other antioxidants which halt the free radical attack that causes skin ageing and disease. Rosemary is an anti-ageing herb that protects the brain against deterioration and memory loss. If you feel like a different taste, try swapping rosemary for basil or coriander.

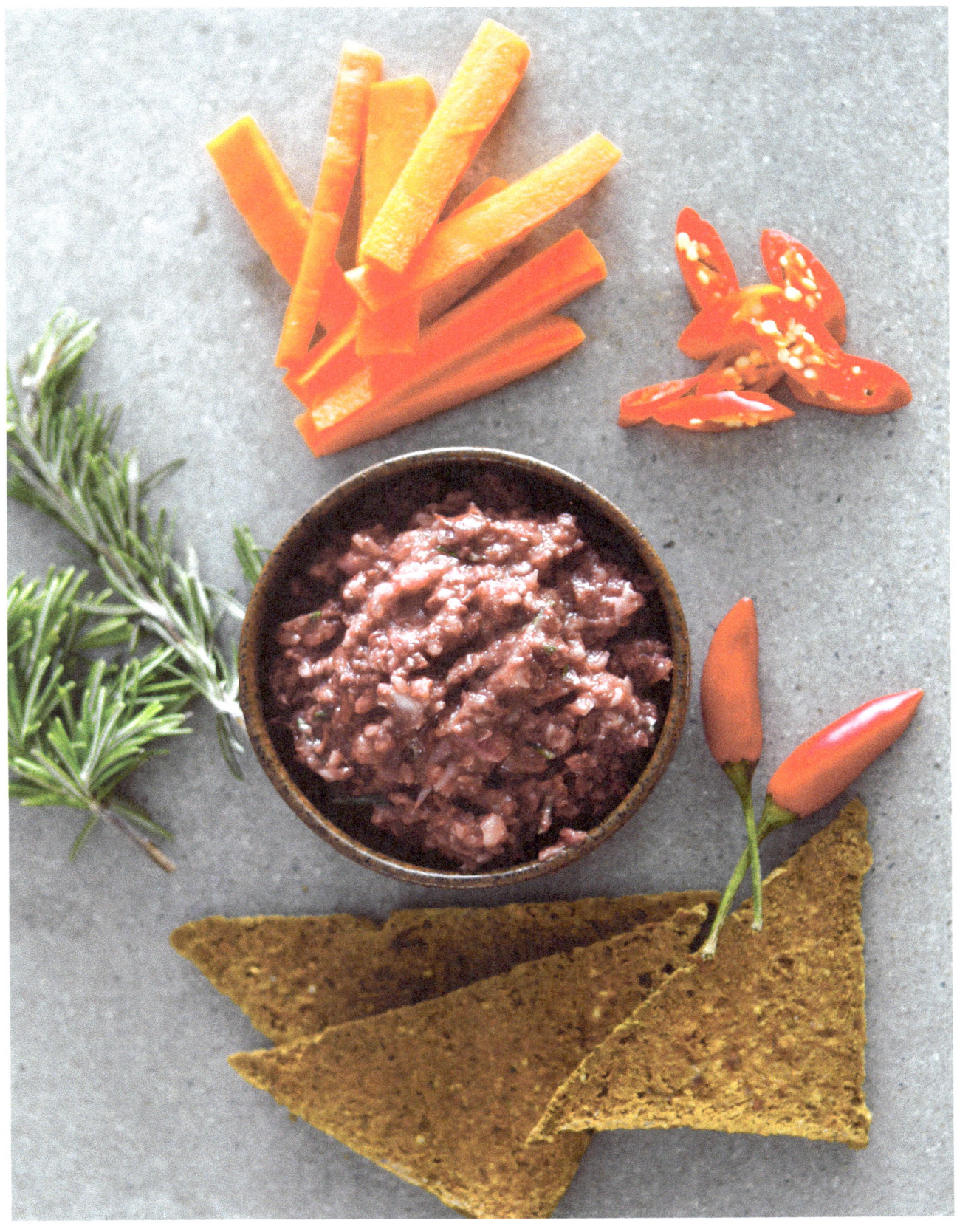

Fat Burning Jalapeño Sauerkraut

INGREDIENTS

4 heads of green cabbage
(you can use purple too)

½ cup of Himalayan or Celtic sea salt

Leave 6 of the large outer leaves of the cabbage aside

FERMENTING MIXTURE INGREDIENTS:

3 to 4 cups of purified water

2 big knobs of ginger, grated

½ cup of fine Himalayan salt

2 tablespoons of miso paste
(shiro or genmai)

4 jalapeño peppers, diced finely

METHOD

1. Shred your cabbage finely and place into a mixing bowl.

2. Then place all of the fermenting ingredients into a blender and mix until it is nice and creamy. Pour this over the cabbage mix. Now place the cabbage mix into jars and push down tightly, leaving a little space at the top. Make sure the liquid covers the cabbage.

3. Pack the cabbage leaves you put aside on the top of this and then cover. Leave this in the cupboard for 5 to 10 days.

4. Remove the top cabbage leaves and throw into the bin. Put the jars in the fridge. When the mixture bubbles this means all of the healthy probiotics are fermenting and you now have a super-healthy raw ginger, jalapeño sauerkraut.

Superfood Powers

Jalapeño peppers contain lots of capsaicin which help to speed up the metabolism and to burn stubborn fat. Ginger is an incredible circulatory stimulant that also has fat burning qualities. This beautiful, spicy sauerkraut is not only great for digestion, but perfect to add to salads every day.

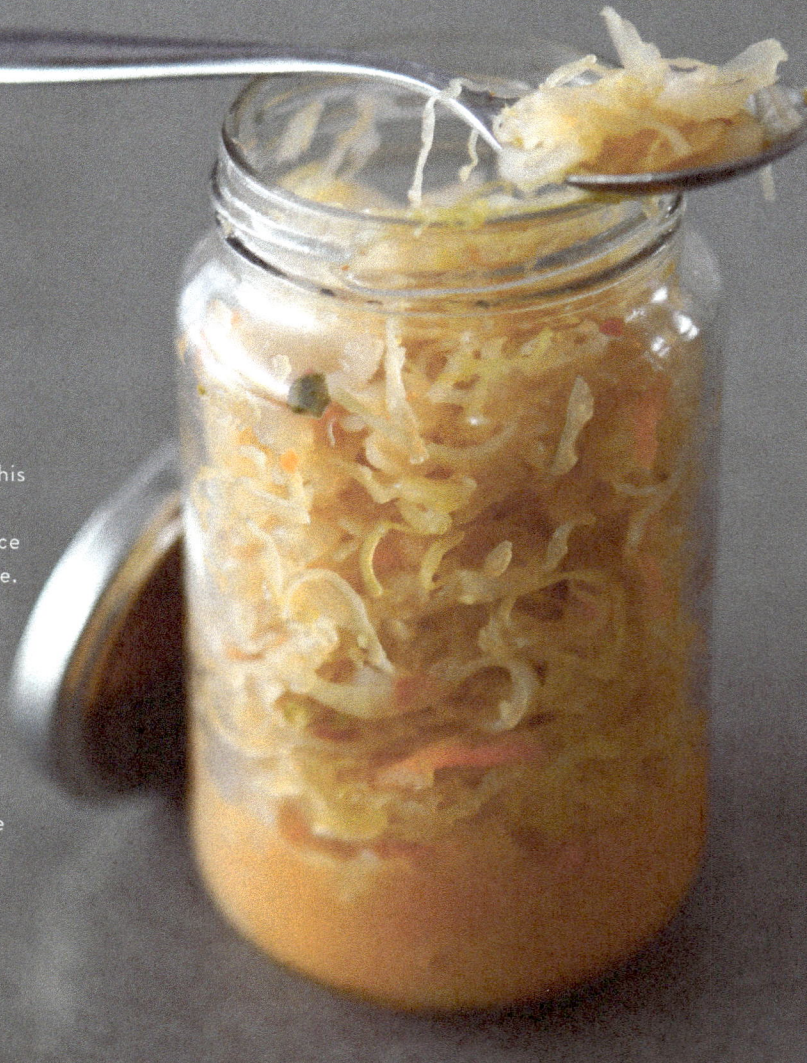

Eggplant, Miso and Wasabi Dip

SERVES 2

INGREDIENTS

3 small eggplants

3 tablespoons of shiro or white miso

¼ cup of tahini

1 whole lemon, juiced

4 tablespoons of organic, first cold pressed olive or hemp oil

¼ cup of pine nuts

2 garlic cloves peeled

1 teaspoon of horseradish paste or wasabi

METHOD

1. Prick your eggplants. Place them in the oven and roast at 180°C for 45 minutes to 1 hour. If you are following a raw diet, dehydrate these for 8 hours at less than 46°C or 115F.

2. When they are soft, scoop out the insides and place in a food processor with garlic, miso, wasabi or horseradish paste, lemon juice, oil, pine nuts and tahini.

Superfood Powers

Eggplant is a true beauty food as it contains an abundant amount of Vitamin C, anthocyanins and antioxidants to guard against skin damage, advanced ageing and even cancer formation. They are 97% water, which makes them perfect for keeping the body and skin hydrated. Pine nuts contain a chemical that suppresses the appetite, and tahini is a superb source of natural minerals, particularly calcium.

Beauty Sambal Sauce No#1

MAKES 1 SMALL JAR

INGREDIENTS

2 long, green chillies, halved, seeded and chopped

1 bunch of coriander

3 limes, juiced

3 Roma tomatoes

2 tablespoons of low-sodium fish sauce or Bragg's amino acid seasoning

2 spring onions or shallots diced

METHOD

1. Place all of the ingredients together in a blender and pulse until you get a slightly smooth consistency. This beautiful tasting sambal will keep in the fridge for one week. I really love this with eggs and salad in the morning for breakfast.

Superfood Powers

Sambal is used in most dishes in Indonesia and Sri Lanka. If made with the right ingredients, it is a pure 'skin treat' as it contains lots of Vitamin C, essential oils, minerals and vitamins which kill the bad bacteria, fungus and viruses that can cause poor digestion.

Beauty Sambal Mint Sauce No#2

MAKES ½ SMALL JAR

INGREDIENTS

A big bunch of mint leaves, chopped

½ red onion, finely chopped

1 big knob of ginger

2 long green chillies, halved, seeded and chopped

2 garlic cloves

1 teaspoon of paprika

1 fresh coconut scraped or 100 grams of coconut flakes

1 to 2 limes, juiced

Water, as needed

METHOD

1. Place all of the ingredients into a mortar and pestle and grind until smooth or alternatively pulse all of the ingredients in a blender. This sambal will keep for around 3 to 5 days in the fridge.

Superfood Powers

This delicious sambal is rich in anti-inflammatory compounds and anti-bacterial substances which helps to fight harmful parasites, fungi and bacteria. Mint helps to improve digestion, purple onion is rich in copper to promote skin elasticity and paprika helps to speed up the metabolism.

Turmeric Anti-Ageing Laksa Paste

MAKES 1 JAR

INGREDIENTS

1 long red chilli

8 cm of fresh turmeric or 2 teaspoons
of organic turmeric powder

4 cm chunk of ginger or 1 tablespoon of ginger powder

⅓ cup of almonds (preferably activated)

1 tablespoon of tamari

½ cup of coconut cream

3 spring onions

2 stalks of lemongrass

1 tablespoon of tamarind paste

1 tablespoon of lecithin granules

METHOD

1. Place all of the ingredients into a food processor and puree into a creamy paste. If you add lemon juice it will keep for at least one week in the fridge.

Superfood Powers

This delicious paste can be used with stir fries, curries, salads, as a dip or even in the breakfast salads. It is a powerful anti-ageing paste that reduces inflammation and stimulates the building of natural collagen. Turmeric is superb for nail, hair and skin health and ginger speeds up circulation helping to remove cellulite.

Red Chilli and Garlic Sauce

MAKES 1/4 JAR

INGREDIENTS

12 small red chillies, deseeded & diced

4 garlic cloves

6 tablespoons of rice or Apple Cider Vinegar

1 to 2 tablespoons of raw honey, monkfruit or maple syrup

1 teaspoon of Himalayan salt

Water to get the right texture

METHOD

1. You can either use a mortar and pestle and grind herbs adding liquids or place all of the ingredients in a Thermomix or food processor and blend until you get the perfect texture. I absolutely love this garlic chilli sauce. I add this to everything.

Superfood Powers

Chillies are super rich in Vitamin C and antioxidants to boost immunity, metabolism and energy. They are incredible little anti-inflammatory foods. When combined with Apple Cider Vinegar, you have the perfect weight-loss sauce.

Vegan Teriyaki Sauce

MAKES ¼ JAR

INGREDIENTS

4 tablespoons of shoyu, tamari or dark soy sauce

1 lemon or lime, juiced

4 tablespoons of rice or coconut vinegar or balsamic

1 teaspoon of ginger powder
or 1 tablespoon of grated ginger

1 teaspoon of garlic powder or 4 garlic cloves, minced

3 star anise

4 tablespoons of toasted sesame oil

1 tablespoon of maple or monkfruit syrup or raw honey

Water

METHOD

1. Place all of the ingredients in a pan, except for kuzu. Simmer for ten minutes to draw the flavor of the anise into the liquid. Stir kuzu into a glass of water and add to the teriyaki mix to thicken.

2. When it is nice and thick, pour into a large glass jar and store in the fridge.

Superfood Powers

I love teriyaki sauce, but unfortunately most brands are packed with colourings, high fructose corn syrup, caramel flavour and other nasties. This teriyaki sauce is super healthy and contains lots of beautifying ingredients. It goes perfectly with any salad, cauliflower rice, zucchini noodles, stir fried vegetables, beauty and poke bowls.

Raw BEAUTY BREAKFAST TREATS

Although these recipes are in a separate 'breakfast section' any of the other 'beauty creations' like the Super Smoothies or the Beauty Bowls can be used for breakfast. Starting the day with lots of green beauty foods, a good source of protein like quinoa, teff, organic eggs, salmon or tempeh and healthy Omega oils is a perfect way to get a steady stream of energy during the day without any blood sugar drops. If you are doing intermittent fasting, simply use these as a healthy lunch or dinner option.

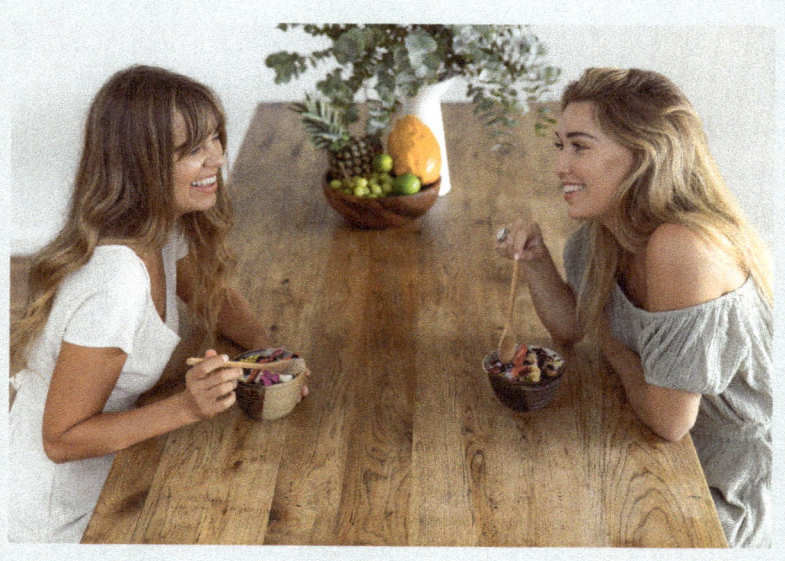

Probiotic Nut Yoghurt

MAKES 1 GLASS JAR

INGREDIENTS

2 cups of cashews (or any other nut or seed)

½ cup of purified water

½ cup of nut or coconut milk

1 teaspoon of cinnamon powder

½ cup of pitted dates

1 whole lemon, grated

2 teaspoons of multi-strain probiotic powder
(look for one with billions of bacteria)

METHOD

1. Soak nuts for 5 hours.

2. Dry and put into a food processor with water and milk, cinnamon, dates and lemon. Blend until creamy, then mix in a probiotic powder.

3. Place in a glass jar with a cheesecloth on top for 24 hours.

4. If yoghurt isn't firming up, dehydrate at 42°C for 7 hours until it thickens.

5. Alternatively, after blending you can heat in a pan with Agar Agar to thicken.

Superfood Powers

I like to add lots of multi-strain probiotic powders when I make yoghurts to get a higher, more broad spectrum 'friendly bacteria' count. This yoghurt is great for gut immunity, digestive and skin health.

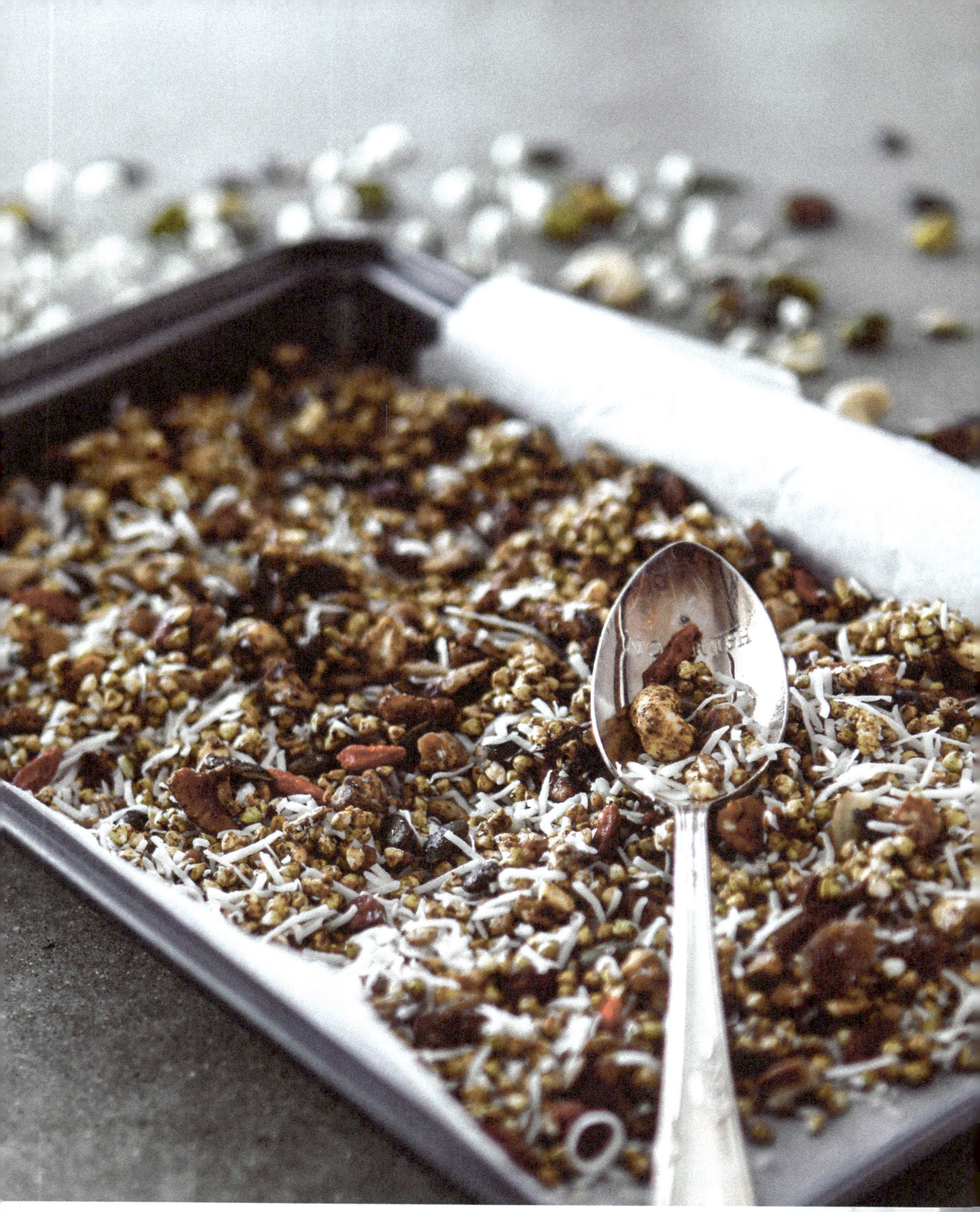

Energy
Flax Muesli

MAKES AROUND 2 TO 3 BOWLS

INGREDIENTS

½ cup of dried goji or goldenberries

4 to 6 organic dried figs, diced

½ cup of pumpkin seeds, finely diced

½ cup of sunflower seeds, finely diced

½ cup of macadamia nuts, finely diced

¼ cup of organic flaxseed meal or activated flaxseeds

½ cup of organic coconut flakes

½ teaspoon of organic vanilla powder

½ teaspoon of organic cinnamon powder

¼ cup of organic coconut oil

3 to 5 tablespoons of coconut nectar or maple syrup

METHOD

1. Put the finely diced nuts and seeds into a bowl and mix with a wooden spoon.

2. Now mix in diced figs, coconut flakes and berries.

3. In a separate bowl, mix the spices, coconut oil and natural sweetener.

4. Spread the nut, seed and berry mix onto a baking tray and then pour liquid mix over the top.

5. Place in the oven and cook on a low heat until golden or alternatively dehydrate at 45°C for a few hours or until cooked.

6. Remove from oven and break granola into pieces.

7. Store in a glass jar in the fridge. When you are ready to eat, serve in a bowl with a plant based milk, fresh fruit and a dash of coconut yoghurt.

Superfood Powers

This museli is an amazing natural bowel broom that can sweep impurities, bad hormones and heavy metals out of the colon. Flaxseeds are a phytoestrogen (a plant based estrogen) that guards against menopausal symptoms, hormone imbalance and breast cancer. The berries and figs in this grain-free granola contain lots of Vitamin C and antioxidants to promote energy, beautiful skin and optimal health.

Creamy Coconut Yoghurt

MAKES 1 JAR

INGREDIENTS

½ cup of coconut milk or cream

2 to 3 young coconuts

1 vanilla pod or 1 teaspoon of vanilla extract

1 whole lemon, juiced

½ cup of pitted dates

3 teaspoons of multi-strain probiotic powder

METHOD

1. Open the coconuts and pour out the coconut water. Take all the meat out of the coconuts.

2. Put coconut meat into a processor with dates, lemon, coconut cream or milk, vanilla bean and lemon juice.

3. Eat straight away or ferment into a yoghurt by adding probiotic powders.

4. Place in a jar, cover with a cheesecloth and put in a dark place for 24 hours. Wait for this to ferment and then place in the fridge. If it isn't thickening up fast enough, place in a dehydrator on 42°C for 7 hours.

Superfood Powers

Coconut yoghurt is a dairy free option that ensures you are getting lots of friendly probiotics for superb gut health. When your gut is healthy, so is your skin.

Kaia's Beauty Bowl

MAKES 2 BOWLS

INGREDIENTS

¼ cup of blueberries

¼ cup of raspberries

½ green apple, diced

2 cinnamon quills

2 star anise

1 tablespoon of pumpkin seeds

1 tablespoon of sunflower seeds

2 tablespoons of chia seeds

2 tablespoons of flaxseeds or flaxseed meal
(buy fresh or grind yourself)

METHOD

1. Place chopped apple in a pan and simmer on a low heat with some water, cinnamon quills and star anise. Let this poach for around ten minutes.

2. In a separate bowl, mix flaxseeds, chia and a little nut, seed or coconut milk. When apple is poached remove from heat, take out quills and anise and mix in chia and flax mix.

3. Place in two bowls and dress with coconut flakes, berries, pumpkin and sunflower seeds. If you want this sweeter, mix in a little maple, monkfruit syrup or erythritol.

Superfood Powers

This beauty bowl is packed with youth promoting polyphenols and flavonoids to help improve the beauty, hydration and elasticity of your skin. The rich omega oils found in the flax and chia seeds can reduce inflammation and nourish dry hair and nails.

Glowing Açai Bowl

It is now super easy to make Açai bowls at home simply by buying organic freeze dried Açai powder or by using frozen Açai and mixing this with other nutritious ingredients. Traditional Açai bowls are extremely high in sugar, so try making this low sugar version at home.

INGREDIENTS

2 frozen bananas

½ packet of frozen Açai or 2 tablespoons of Açai powder

¼ cup of almond, hemp or coconut milk

2 tablespoons of chia seeds (better if pre-soaked)

2 tablespoons of activated sunflower or pumpkin seeds

Extra berries (for added beauty qualities)

METHOD

1. Blend all of the ingredients (except for seeds) in a blender until creamy. Serve in a bowl or cup with fresh berries, seeds and cacao nibs.

Superfood Powers

Everyone knows of the healing properties of Açai. Açai is super rich in antioxidants like polyphenols. These flavonoids stop free radical attack to the skin, resulting in a more beautiful, glowing skin.

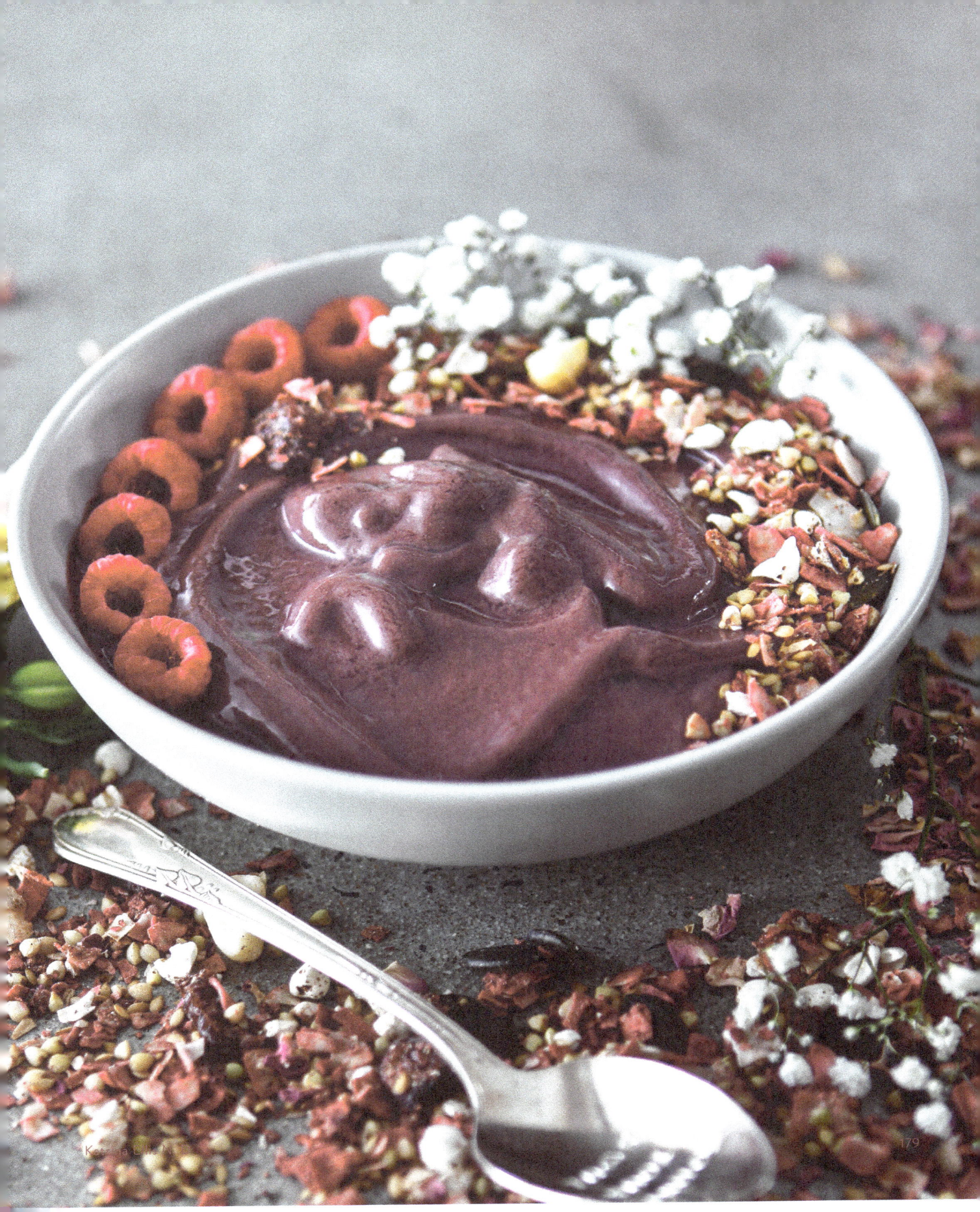

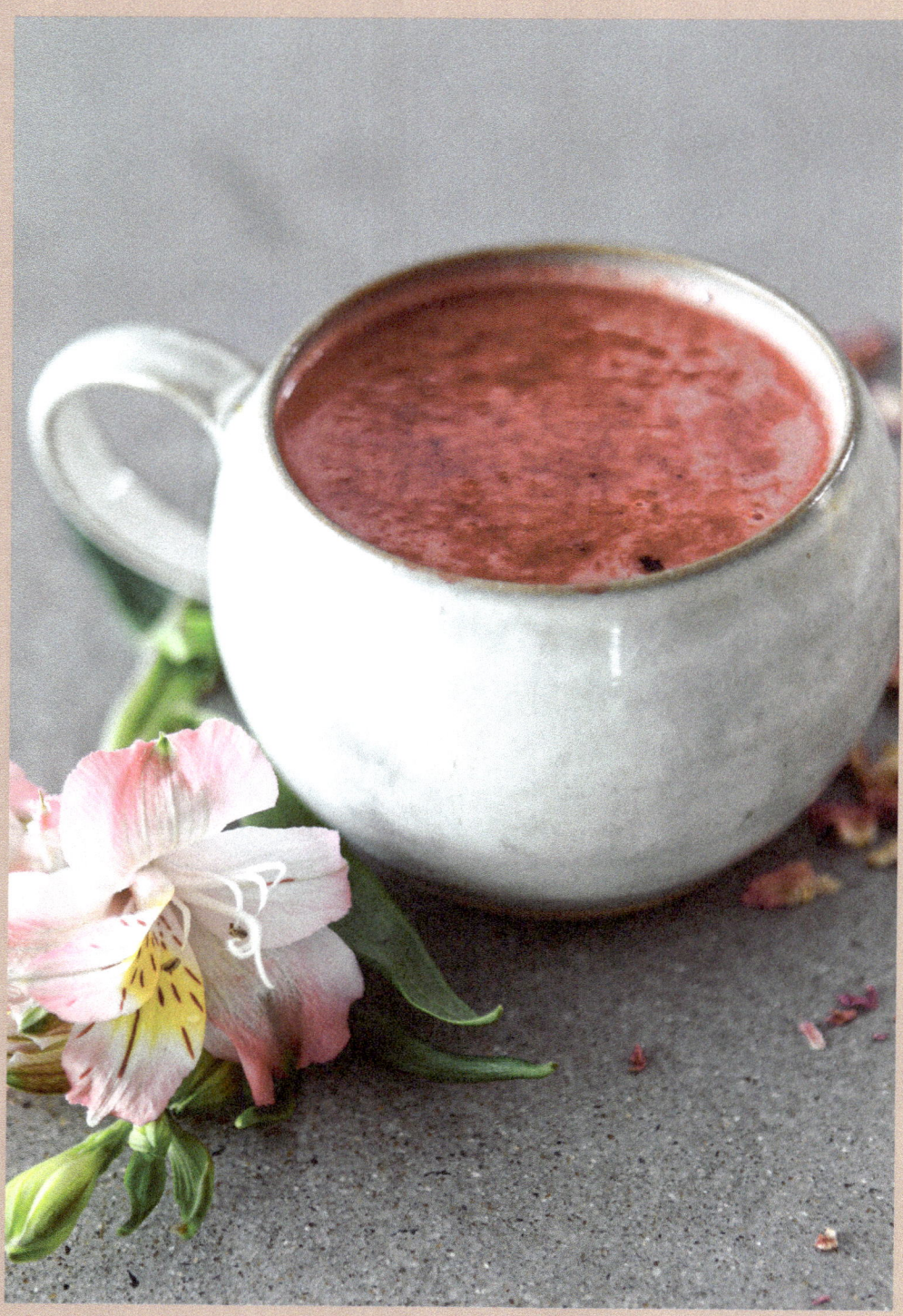

Chia Collagen Pots

SERVES 2

INGREDIENTS

1 cup of hazelnut milk (or macadamia,
hemp or coconut milk)

4 to 6 tablespoons of chia seeds

1 mango or ½ cup of berries

2 tablespoons of shredded coconut

2 scoops of collagen powder (there are some
great vegan options available)

METHOD

1. Mix together milk and 2 tablespoons of chia seeds.

2. Add in the collagen mix, stir and set aside
   until it thickens.

3. Peel the mango, chop up and whizz the chopped
   mango or berries, 2 tablespoons of chia seeds and
   2 tablespoons of water in a blender.

4. Divide the chia mix between 2 to 3 small pots and
   then pour the mango or berry puree over the top.
   Let this set in the fridge for 1 hour.

Garnish with shredded coconut and chopped hazelnuts.

Superfood Powers

Chia and hazelnuts are rich sources of protein, Omega oils, zinc, magnesium, B vitamins, folate, Vitamin C and E. These
nutrients provide great protection against age-promoting free radicals while helping to boost collagen stores.

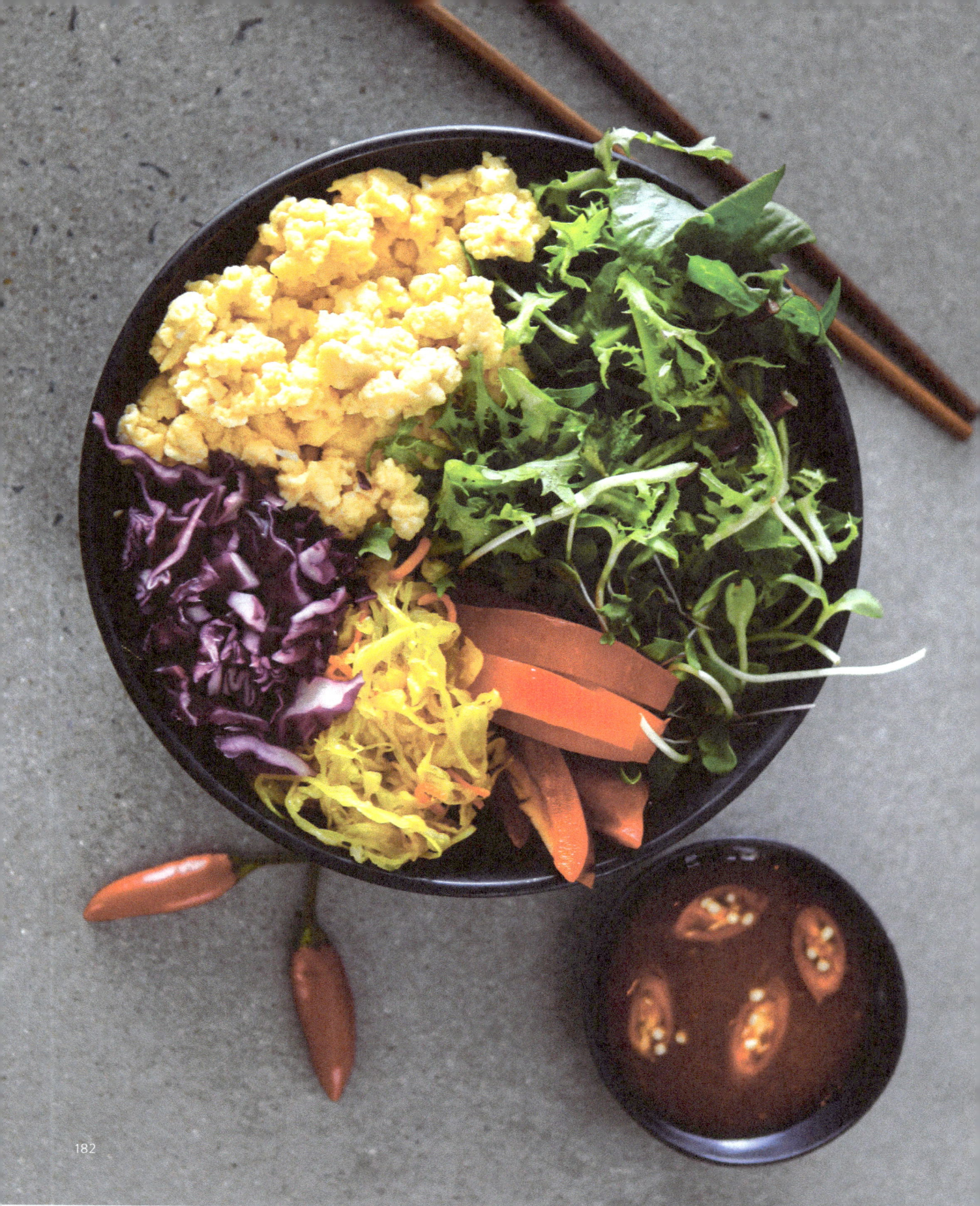

Raw Beauty Brekky Bowl No#1

SERVES 2

INGREDIENTS

SCRAMBLED EGGS

3 eggs

½ cup of nut milk

BOWL

A handful of parsley, diced

1 red capsicum, diced

2 tablespoons of kimchee

¼ purple or green cabbage, diced

3 cups of lettuce mix or Romaine lettuce

A handful of sprouts

2 limes, juiced

4 tablespoons of sesame seeds

A dash of rice or Apple Cider Vinegar

GARLIC CHILLI SAUCE

¼ cup of bird chilli (chopped and deseeded)

1 tablespoon of coconut nectar
or 1 tsp of monkfruit syrup

3 tablespoons of rice vinegar

a dash of Celtic salt

1 garlic clove diced

8 cherry tomatoes

METHOD

Place all the ingredients into a pan and heat, stirring until everything mixes well. If eating raw, simply pulse all of the ingredients until you get the perfect sauce.

METHOD

1. To make the chilli eggs: whisk eggs with chopped parsley, garlic chilli sauce and nut milk. Quickly cook in a pan with a little coconut oil or ghee and scramble as you cook. If you want it spicier, add more chilli sauce after eggs are scrambled.

2. To make the beauty mix, chop the lettuce and place in a bowl with sprouts, red capsicum and cabbage and sprinkle with sesame seeds. Cut an avocado in half and place any leftover chilli sauce inside the avocado and sprinkle vinegar over the top.

3. Add kimchee to each bowl and finish with the scrambled chilli egg mix.

Absolutely delicious!

Superfood Powers

This is a totally delicious and nutritious breakfast bowl. It contains around 20 grams of protein, lots of indoles to detoxify harmful chemicals, fermented foods to improve digestion and plenty of Vitamin A, C and E, to guard against dangerous age-promoting free radicals. What a yummy way to eat yourself towards more beauty and health!

Buckwheat Bircher

MAKES 2 BOWLS

INGREDIENTS

2 cups of activated buckwheat

A handful of coconut chips or flakes

½ cup of activated sunflower seeds, diced

½ cup of activated pumpkin seeds, diced

½ cup of activated walnuts, diced

½ cup of activated pecans, cashews or macadamia, diced

¼ cup of activated chia seeds

½ cup of dried blueberries, either puncture or put in hot water to break skins

¼ cup of dried pomegranate (cut in half, bang on the back and the seeds will fall out)

METHOD

1. If you are planning to dehydrate your own buckwheat, simply cover with water, celtic salt and a little apple cider vinegar and leave for 8 hours or overnight.

2. Rinse and spread on a tray and dehydrate on a low heat until dry.

3. To activate the nuts and seeds, do the same thing by soaking for 4 to 8 hours with apple cider vinegar and celtic salt, rinse and spread on a dehydrator tray and as a general rule heat at 105 to 150°F for 8 to 12 hours.

4. With berries and pomegranate, simply rinse, spread on a tray and dehydrate for a longer period. When ready, mix all of the ingredients together and keep in a glass jar in the fridge.

5. Serve with coconut, hemp or nut milk and more fresh berries.

Superfood Powers

Buckwheat is power packed with zinc, magnesium, Vitamin A and C, flavonoids and B vitamins to boost hair growth and to protect against skin ageing and wrinkles. When you add the antioxidant rich berries you have a true beauty bowl. If you are in a hurry, you can buy all of the ingredients already activated. Simply mix together and enjoy all of this bowl's youth promoting qualities.

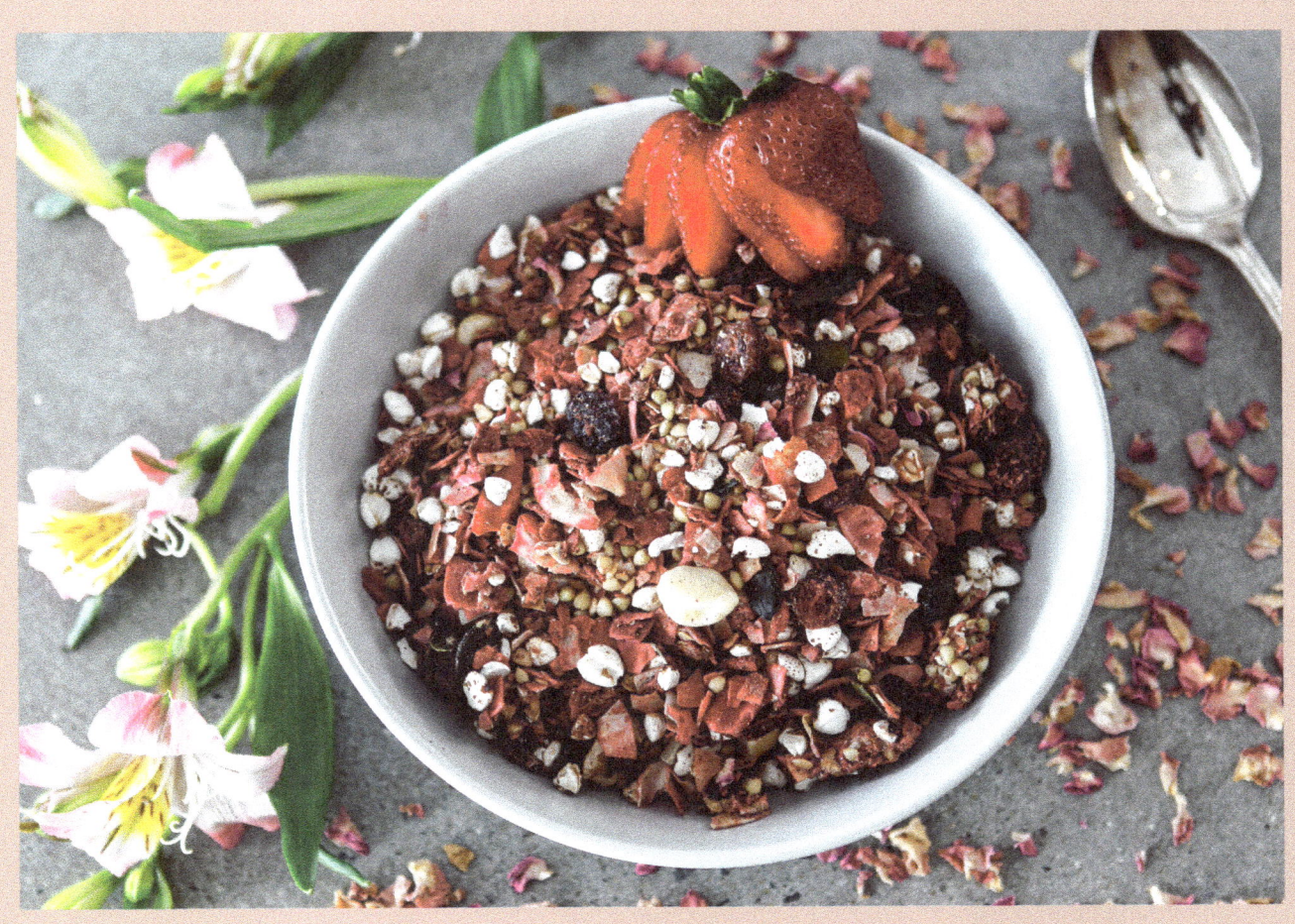

Green Quinoa Salad with Sambal Eggs

INGREDIENTS

½ cup of white or red quinoa, rinsed

1 cup of vegetable stock or broth (recipe in the soup section or make your own)

4 organic eggs

2 to 3 cups of kale

2 to 3 cups of silver beet or baby spinach leaves

¼ Lebanese cucumber, diced

8 Cherry tomatoes

2 tablespoons of Pumpkin seeds

DRESSING

4 tablespoons of toasted black sesame oil

2 garlic cloves, minced or diced

2 tablespoons of tamari or Bragg's amino acid seasoning

1 lemon, juiced

2 tablespoons of sambal paste (recipe in the condiments section)

METHOD

1. Put quinoa and stock into a saucepan, bring to the boil and then reduce heat to a simmer for around 15 minutes. Most of the liquid should be absorbed, set aside for 10 minutes.

2. If you are using eggs, boil or poach in another saucepan for a few minutes. Cool under running water and peel.

3. This breakfast salad can be served hot or cold. If you wish to eat this hot, heat the kale and spinach until slightly wilted in a pan with sesame oil, tamari, lemon juice and garlic and roll in the quinoa.

4. Alternatively, prepare salad mix fresh in bowls adding the cherry tomatoes, quinoa and diced cucumber.

5. In a bowl, mix sesame seeds, sambal paste, sesame oil and Celtic salt. Roll halved peeled eggs through this mix and place on salad mix. Serve with extra sauerkraut, lemon juice and sambal sauce.

Superfood Powers

I absolutely love this dish for breakfast. The sambal sauce contains lots of thermogenic ingredients to speed up the metabolism; the sesame oil protects the teeth against bacteria and improves liver health; and the pumpkin seeds are super rich in zinc which boosts immunity, energy and happiness levels.

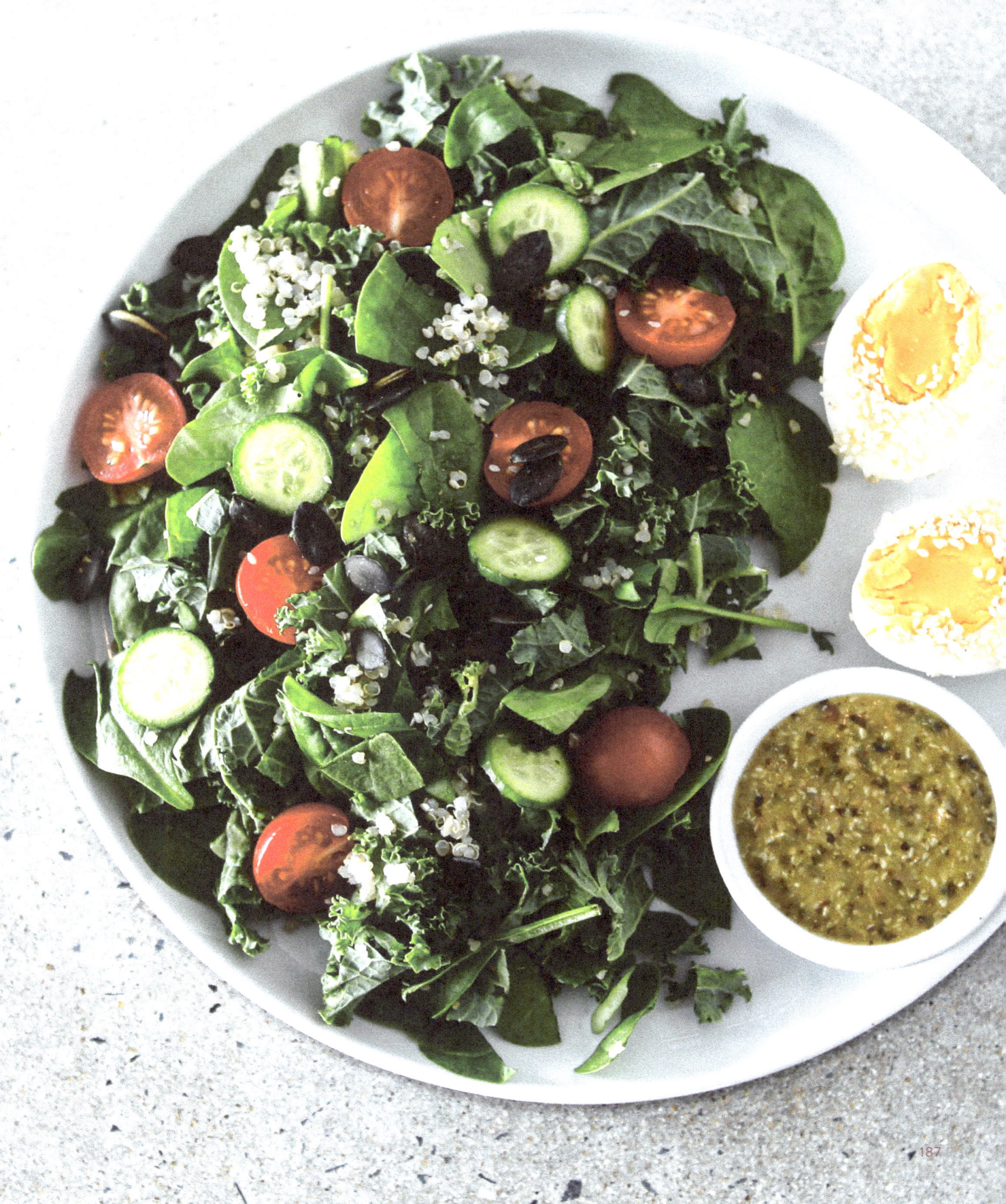

Gingered Kale Salad with Scrambled Tofu

SERVES 2

INGREDIENTS

SCRAMBLED TOFU

250 grams of organic tofu, crumbled (or tempeh)

½ brown onion, diced

2 garlic cloves, diced

Spice mix – 1 tsp of turmeric, 1 tsp of cumin, ½ tsp of cayenne or paprika

2 tablespoons of olive oil

A dash of tamari or Bragg's amino acids

SALAD

½ tub of mixed greens or rocket

A handful of kale or spinach, chopped

¼ purple cabbage, diced

½ avocado, cubed

2 tablespoons of pumpkin seeds (preferably activated)

2 tablespoons of sauerkraut

GINGER DRESSING

4 tablespoons of sesame oil, 1 knob of grated ginger or 1 teaspoon of ginger powder, 1 lemon juiced, 2 tablespoons of coconut or Apple Cider Vinegar

METHOD

1. To make the scrambled tofu, pulse or simply break up in your fingers and place in a bowl with oil and spices. Let this marinate.

2. When the tofu has soaked up these delicious flavours, quickly sauté or fry in a pan with onion and garlic for a few minutes or dehydrate if eating raw.

3. In a separate bowl or plate, place chopped greens, purple cabbage, avocado, sauerkraut and pumpkin seeds. When tofu is scrambled, either mix through salad mix or place on top and drizzle with the ginger dressing.

Superfood Powers

Organic tofu contains powerful isoflavones like genistein and daidzein which help to protect against many types of cancer and menopausal symptoms. Kale and cabbage contain indoles, Vitamin C and Vitamin K to remove toxins and harmful hormones while boosting collagen and elastin production.

Buckwheat and Enoki Breakfast Salad

MAKES 2 PLATES

INGREDIENTS

½ to 1 cup of Buckwheat (soak for a few hours)

A handful of enoki mushrooms (if you cannot find, use shiitake, black jelly or oyster)

3 cups of mixed greens

½ red capsicum, diced

½ packet of snow pea sprouts

1 small avocado, diced

A handful of coriander, chopped finely

Poached eggs (optional)

METHOD

1. Place 1 cup of buckwheat in a pan with 1½ cups of water and a little Celtic salt.

2. Turn to high to boil, then simmer for around 15 minutes or until all of the water is absorbed.

3. When your buckwheat is nice and fluffy remove from the heat. I also love dehydrating or toasting my buckwheat too for a different texture.

4. In a bowl, add chopped greens, avocado and sprouts. Sauté mushrooms in a frying pan with a little water and tamari and place on top of the greens and mix the buckwheat through.

5. If you need extra protein, add poached, organic eggs. Squeeze fresh lemon juice on the breakfast salad and add cracked pepper and shredded coriander. Yum!

Superfood Powers

Buckwheat is a great source of magnesium, manganese, quercetin, iron, zinc and copper – all amazing nutrients for improving the quality and texture of the skin. It is also a great source of the flavonoid rutin. Rutin helps to protect against capillary damage and improves blood flow to the skin and heart.

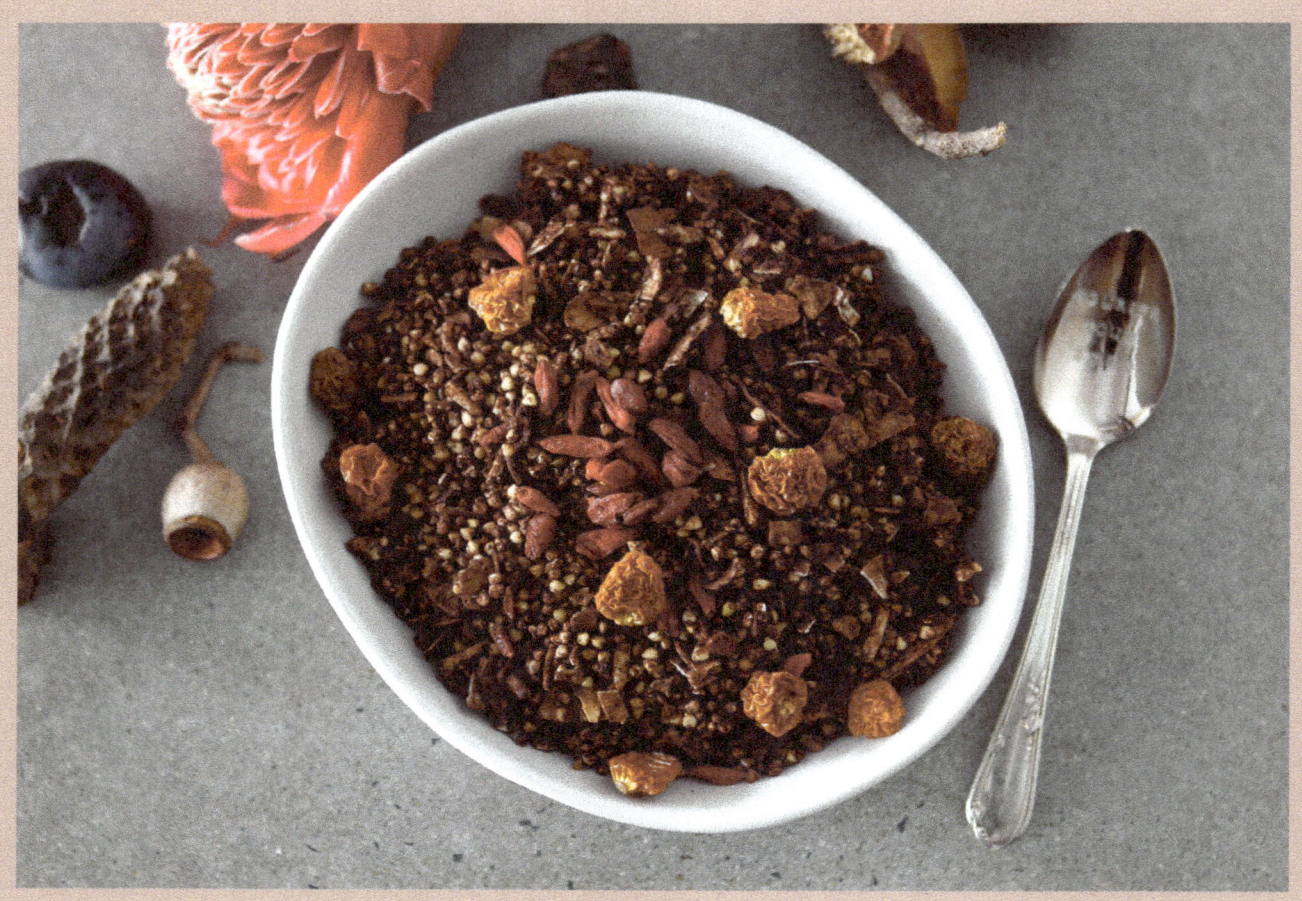

Keto Cacao Crunch

MAKES 1 JAR

INGREDIENTS

1 cup of shredded coconut

½ cup of flaxseeds

½ cup of almonds, chopped up

½ cup of pumpkin seeds

⅓ cup of chia seeds

⅓ cup of walnuts, cut into small pieces

¼ cup of pure monkfruit syrup (if following keto),
if not use maple syrup or coconut nectar

¼ cup of coconut oil, melted

1 to 2 tablespoons of cacao powder

1 teaspoon of vanilla

2 teaspoons of cinnamon

METHOD

1. Preheat oven to 180°C or use a dehydrator
   if eating raw.

2. In one bowl combine all nuts and seeds and coconut.
   In another bowl, combine monkfruit syrup, melted
   coconut oil, cacao, cinnamon and vanilla.

3. Line a tray with baking paper. Spread the nut and seed
   mix over the tray, then pour the cacao mix over this.

4. Bake for 45 minutes or until golden brown or
   dehydrate for 6 to 8 hours on a low heat if eating raw.

Superfood Powers

This is a super powerful ketogenic breakfast cereal. It is
low in carbohydrates, rich in protein and omega oils and
antioxidants which improves weight loss, raises energy
and strengthens the skin, hair and nails.

SENSATIONAL *Soups*

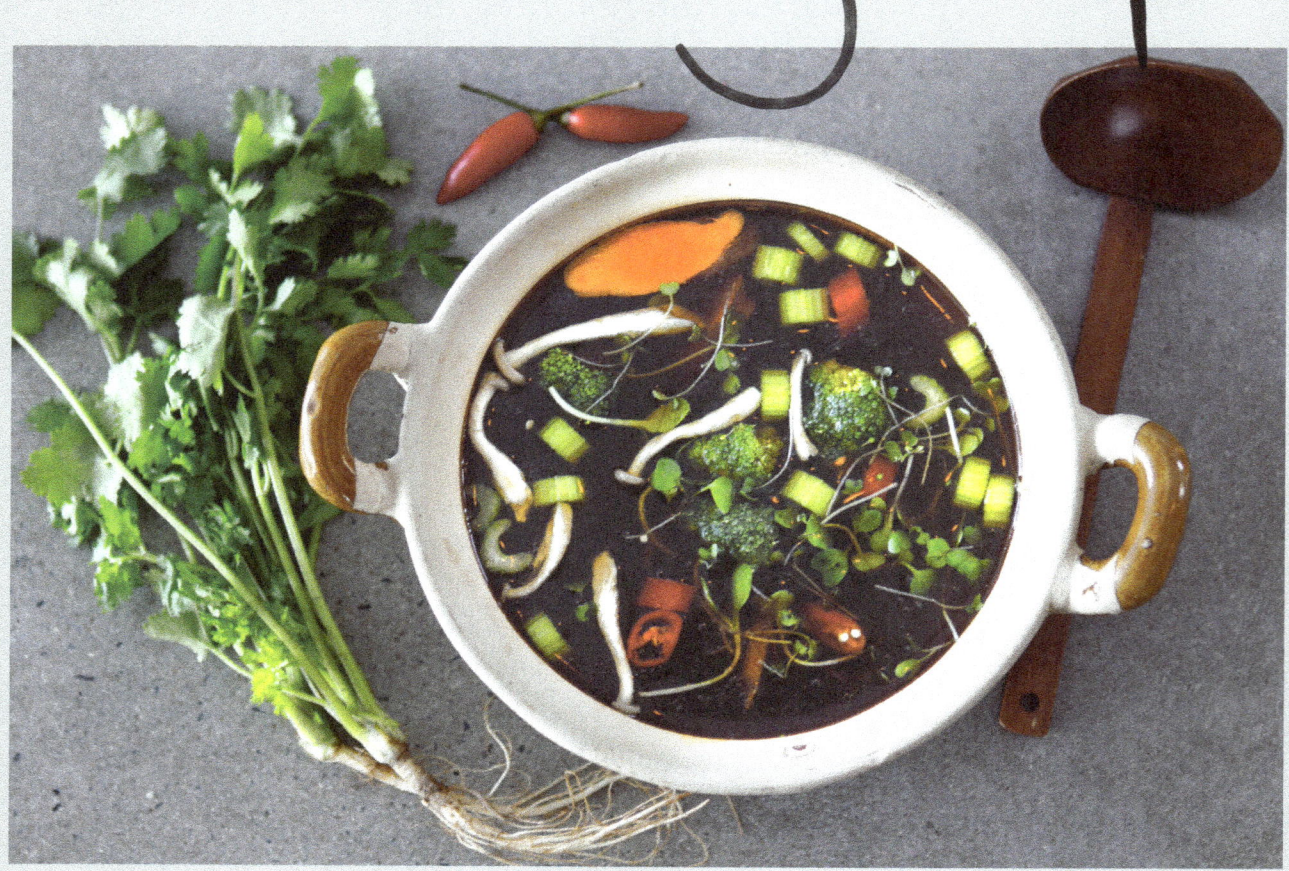

Rich Chicken Collagen Broth

INGREDIENTS

2 to 3 organic chicken carcasses
or 12 chicken and wing bones

2 leeks, trimmed and chopped

3 spring onions or scallions, chopped

4 garlic cloves, diced

1 celery stick, chopped

1 carrot, chopped

4 cm piece of ginger, peeled and grated

4 cm piece of turmeric, peeled and grated

1 teaspoon of black peppercorns

1 teaspoon of coriander seeds

1 teaspoon of fennel seeds

2 bay leaves

A small bunch of parsley

4 to 6 litres of water

METHOD

1. If using wing or thigh bones, preheat the oven to 180°C. Spread the bones on a large baking tray and cook for 30 minutes until crispy, then place the bones into a pot with the rest of the ingredients.

2. If using whole carcasses, get a knife and cut the skin off the chicken as much as possible. Then place the chickens in a large pot or slow cooker and add the rest of the ingredients.

3. Bring to the boil. Cover and reduce the temperature to a simmer and leave to cook for around 4 to 6 hours.

4. Skim the surface of the liquid to remove any fatty chunks and set the broth aside to cool.

5. Strain the broth through a colander and discard the vegetables.

6. Place in the fridge for at least 2 hours so it sets like a jelly.

7. This will keep in the fridge for around 5 days and in the freezer for 3 months.

8. Every time you want to make a soup simply heat broth and add vegetables or alternatively add to any dish to increase its healing properties.

Superfood Powers

This chicken bone broth is full of alkaline minerals like calcium, phosphorous, potassium and magnesium, which reduces acidity, strengthens the bones and improves gut health. It also contains lots of GAGS (glycosaminoglycans) – a natural anti-inflammatory that beautifies the skin and heals a damaged intestinal lining. Broths are also great sources of the amino acids glycine and proline to help knit connective tissues together.

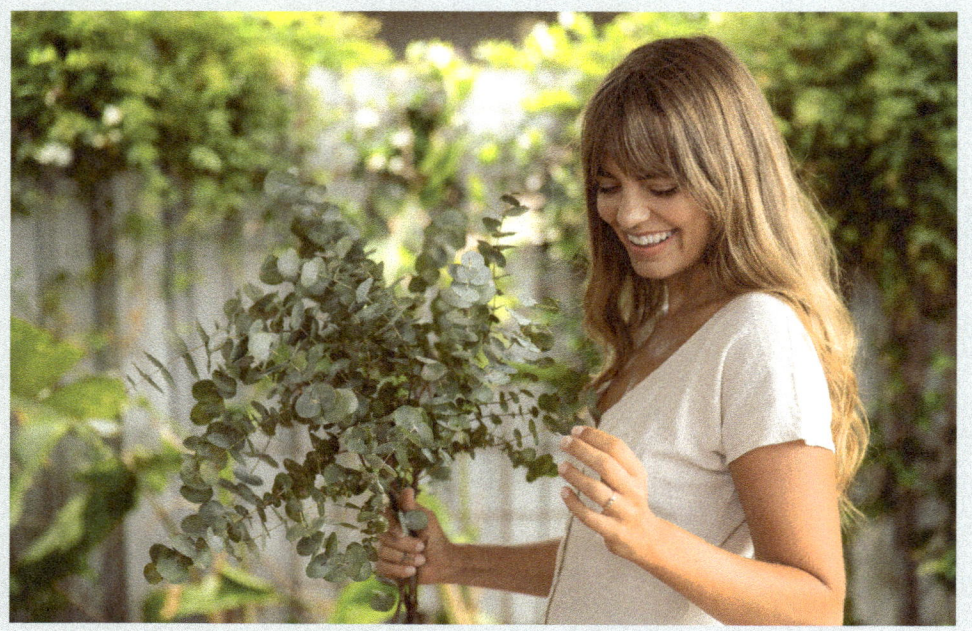

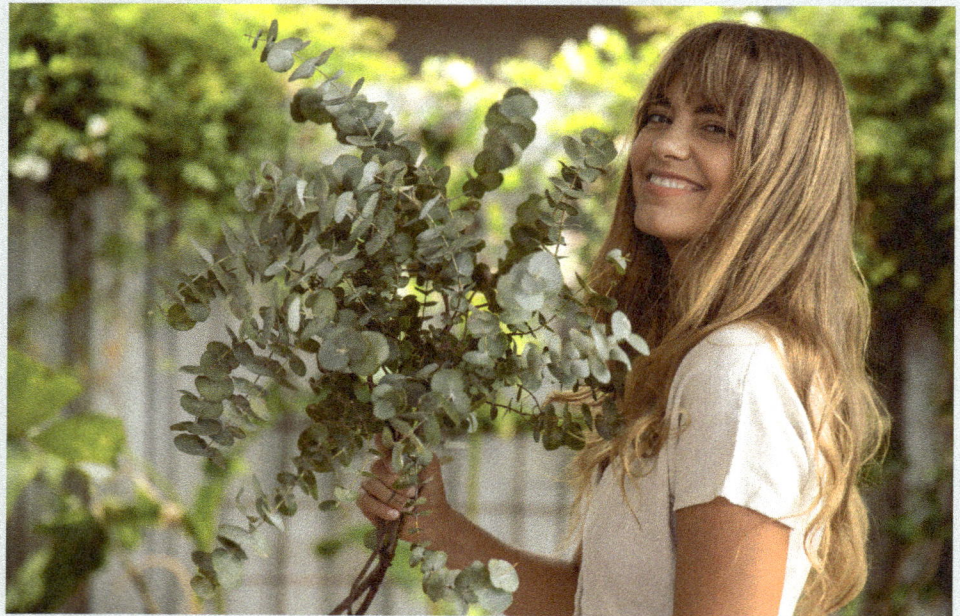

Super Collagen Marrow Broth

INGREDIENTS

2 kg of organic grass fed beef marrow bones or 2 chicken carcasses or fish bones

1 kg of meaty bones like ribs (optional)

½ cup of Apple Cider Vinegar (raw)

4 to 5 litres of filtered water

1 onion, chopped

3 celery stalks, diced

3 carrots, diced

3 to 6 garlic cloves, diced

6 cm chunk of turmeric

A handful of parsley

Celtic salt

METHOD

1. Place the bones on a tray and roast in the oven at 180°C for 30 minutes to bring out their flavor.

2. Then transfer into a large cooking pot and add the Apple Cider Vinegar and cold water. Let this sit for a while so the vinegar can draw the minerals from the bones.

3. Add enough water to cover the bones.

4. Add the chopped vegetables, bring to the boil and then for the next 2 hours, skim any scum that rises to the top. You will see less scum when using high quality, organic grass fed bones.

5. Reduce to a simmer, cover and cook for 24 hours for chicken bones, 48 hours for beef and 8 to 12 hours for fish bones.

6. In the last ten minutes, throw in some fresh parsley for extra minerals.

7. Let this cool and strain to make sure the marrow and gelatin is drawn from the bones to the broth.

8. Add Himalayan salt and Bragg's amino acid seasoning at the end.

9. Strain and store in glass jars in the fridge. A good marrow broth should turn to jelly and will store for around 5 days in the fridge or 3 weeks frozen.

Superfood Powers

This marrow broth is packed full of alkaline minerals, amino acids, anti-inflammatory substances like GAGS and other healing nutrients. It helps to seal up 'leaky gut', improves bone and tooth health, alkalises the bloodstream and builds a strong immunity. The GAGS are incredibly nourishing to the skin and provide the framework to rebuild the body's collagen matrix.

Lymphatic Detox Consommé

MAKES 1 BIG POT

INGREDIENTS

1 carrot, unpeeled

2 sticks of celery, with tops

2 beets with tops

1 medium potato, brushed

1 brown or white onion, chopped

A hand full of parsley, chopped

2 parsnips, chopped

A handful of spinach, chopped

1 medium sized zucchini, skin on, chopped

3 litres of purified water

A pinch of Celtic Salt

2 tablespoons of tamari

2 tablespoons of Bragg's amino acid seasoning

Seaweed like wakame (added at the end)

METHOD

1. Place all ingredients into a saucepan, bring to the boil and simmer on a low heat until the vegetables are cooked. This may take around 2 to 4 hours. Strain the vegetables out to get a beautiful clear liquid.

2. Store in a glass jar in the fridge and use as the perfect detoxification consommé.

Superfood Powers

This is an ancient detoxification recipe that was traditionally used as a healing tonic by all health practitioners and it is still used by naturopaths today. It is super rich in potassium and other minerals to purify the lymphatic system ensuring a beautiful, glowing skin and metabolism.

Carotene Antioxidant Soup

SERVES 3 BOWLS

INGREDIENTS

2 to 3 large sweet potatoes

3 garlic cloves, peeled and diced

1 small onion, diced

2 teaspoons of curry powder or curry leaves

1 teaspoon of turmeric powder

½ teaspoon of paprika

1 tablespoon of grated ginger or ginger powder

1 cup of chopped shallots or spring onions

1 teaspoon of Himalayan salt

3 cups of chicken/beef or vegan broth or water

METHOD

1. Chop up sweet potato and steam in a steamer to soften. In a pan saute' onions, ginger, garlic and shallots with a little avocado or olive oil or use your Thermomix if you have one.

2. Add the steamed sweet potato to the food processor with the onion mix and blend.

3. Slowly add bone or vegan broth or water, spices and Himalayan salt to get the perfect taste and texture.

4. Warm up in a pan. Serve in 3 to 4 bowls, with extra turmeric, black pepper and a little torn coriander.

Superfood Powers

This soup is absolutely delicious and packed full of carotene which adds a sparkle to the eyes, a glow to the skin and offers protection against harmful UV rays. Sweet potatoes help to make hyaluronic acid to plump up the skin and give it back its natural elasticity and softness. If you are following a ketogenic diet, replace sweet potato with carrot or pumpkin and if eating completely raw simply blend all of the ingredients and warm up in winter.

Vietnamese Broth with Kelp Noodles

SERVES 3

INGREDIENTS

2 to 4 cups of bone or vegan broth or water

3 star anise

2 cinnamon quills

4 cm of ginger, peeled and chopped into matchsticks

1 whole lime, juiced

2 teaspoons of fish sauce (if vegan – use tamari or Bragg's amino acid seasoning)

A small bunch of pak choi, chopped

1 tablespoon of mint leaves

1 tablespoon of coriander leaves

2 long red chillies, thinly sliced

A few drops of stevia or monkfruit syrup

1 packet of kelp, konjac or vegetable noodles

METHOD

1. Combine the broth or stock, ginger, star anise, cinnamon and chilli in a saucepan, bring to the boil. Reduce the heat and simmer for 10 minutes.

2. Add lime juice, fish sauce or tamari, natural sweetener and diced protein source (prawns, fish, grass fed beef, Shiitake or tofu) and return to the boil.

3. Now add pak choi or bok choy, cook for another few minutes and then remove from heat. If using kelp or shirataki noodles, place in another bowl with hot water to soften, then drain.

4. Put the noodles in the bowls, pour the soup over the top and garnish with torn mint, coriander and chilli.

Superfood Powers

I love Vietnamese food as it is totally delicious and very nutritious – after all look at the beautiful skin on Vietnamese women. These herbs contain powerful antioxidants which protect against UV-related sun damage, as well as anti-bacterial, anti-fungal and anti-parasitical qualities.

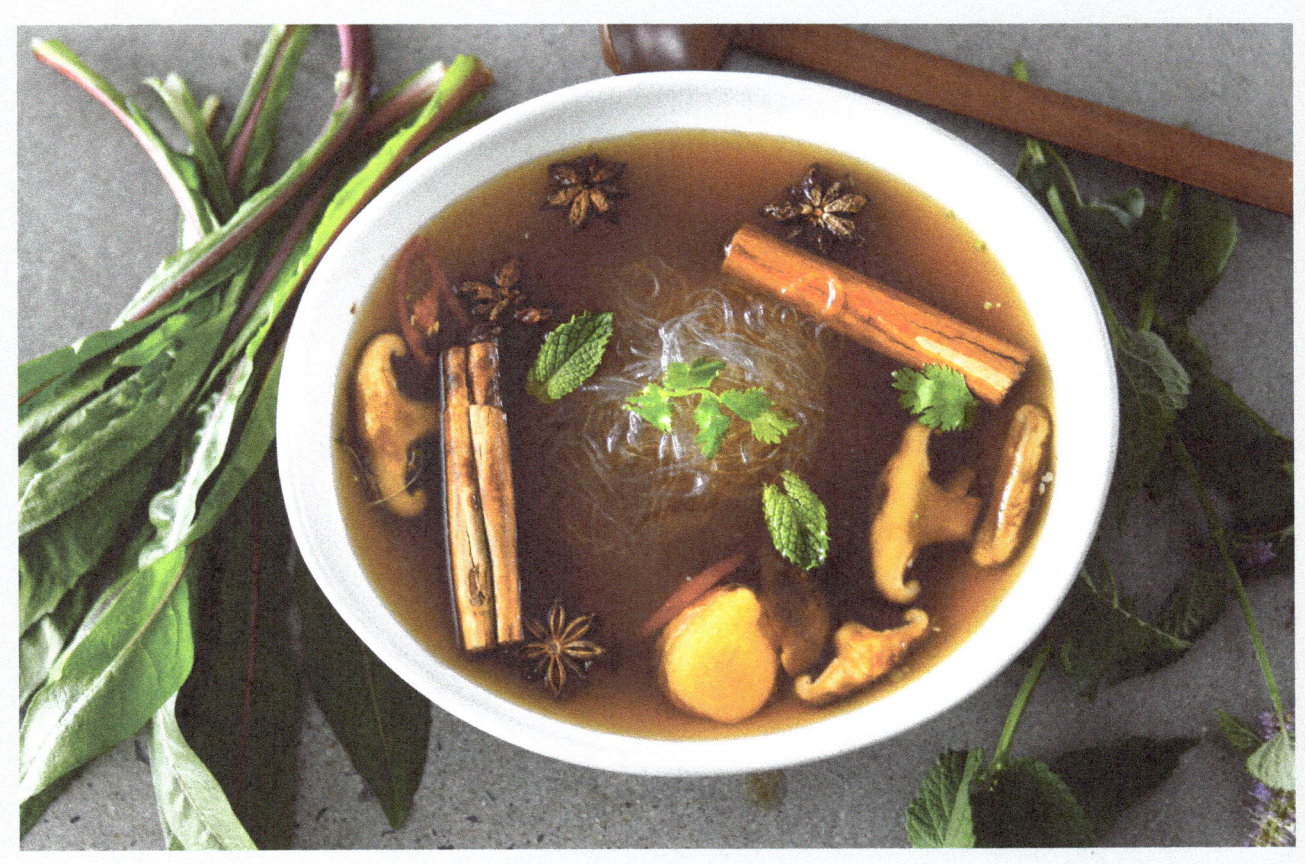

Beauty Beet Soup

SERVES 2 TO 3

INGREDIENTS

6 whole beetroots, peeled and diced

2 small sweet potato or carrots, peeled and diced

1 onion, diced

4 garlic cloves, diced

1 red chilli or 1 teaspoon of chilli flakes

2 tablespoons of tamari or shoyu

1 teaspoon of cumin

1 teaspoon of coriander seeds

½ teaspoon of celtic salt

4 tablespoons of Apple Cider Vinegar or coconut vinegar

1 litre of chicken or vegetable stock/broth or water

METHOD

1. Peel the beetroot and sweet potato or carrots, slice thinly and place in a pan with onion, garlic and olive oil.

2. Sweat the beet and sweet potato or carrots for a few minutes, then add broth or stock.

3. Continue to simmer with spices and add tamari, herbs, salt and vinegar.

4. Simmer for 15 minutes and then puree this mix in a food processor or Thermomix to make smooth and creamy.

5. If too thick, add some extra vegetable or chicken broth to dilute. I really love adding Bragg's amino acid seasoning to bring out the flavor in this soup.

Superfood Powers

Beetroot is one of the richest sources of polyphenols and Vitamin C to help reduce skin pigmentation. If you are low in iron, this is the perfect soup to boost your haemoglobin levels. Beetroot is also a fantastic lymphatic and liver cleanser that can really help stimulate hair growth.

Spicy Carrot and Parsnip Soup

SERVES 2 TO 3

INGREDIENTS

1 onion, diced

2 garlic cloves, diced

1 red chilli, diced

A handful of coriander, chopped

1 litre of vegetable or chicken broth/stock

4 parsnips, peeled and diced

2 to 3 carrots, peeled and diced

1 teaspoon of turmeric powder

1 teaspoon of cayenne or paprika

1 teaspoon of cumin

2 tablespoons of macadamia oil

Himalayan salt and pepper to taste

METHOD

1. Place a small amount of macadamia oil or ghee in a pan, quickly sauté onion, garlic and chilli.

2. When onions are soft, add parsnip and carrots.

3. Cook for a little longer, then add spices and stock or broth. If you want this soup creamier, feel free to add coconut cream or nut milk.

4. Simmer for thirty minutes or until vegetables are soft. Let cool for a few minutes, then place in a food processor and puree.

5. Serve in bowls with chill flakes, torn coriander and lime juice.

Superfood Powers

Parsnips are rich in Vitamin C, B1, B5, B6, K, E and the minerals calcium, copper, iron, manganese, phosphorous and potassium. They are also power packed with antioxidants that can guard against cancer, fungus, bacteria and inflammation. Parsnips help with the production of hyaluronic acid, a substance which helps to make skin youthful, plump and taut.

Turmeric, Pumpkin and Lentil Soup

SERVES 3 TO 4

INGREDIENTS

1 brown onion, diced

3 garlic cloves, finely chopped

2 stalks of celery, diced

1 kg of pumpkin, skinned and chopped

2 teaspoons of cumin

2 teaspoons of coriander seeds

1 tablespoon of turmeric powder or paste

1 teaspoon of Celtic or Himalayan salt

2 tablespoons of tamari or shoyu

1 cup of red or orange lentils

1 litre of vegetable stock or broth or water

½ cup of coconut cream (optional – but yummy)

METHOD

1. Pre-soak lentils overnight to break down its anti-nutrients. After soaked, place in a colander and wash several times.

2. In a separate pan, sauté onion, celery and garlic with a little water or stock and when soft add cumin, coriander seeds, turmeric, tamari and chopped pumpkin.

3. Add the lentils, water or vegetable/chicken stock, bring to the boil and then simmer for twenty minutes or until cooked. Add a little black pepper and more Celtic salt to season.

4. Divide the soup into bowls and serve with mint leaves and turmeric.

Superfood Powers

Pumpkin is super rich in skin beautifying vitamins & minerals like Vitamin A, C, E, magnesium, iron and zinc. Lentils contain important nutrients that can strengthen collagen, protect against dangerous free radicals and hydrate the skin, hair and nails.

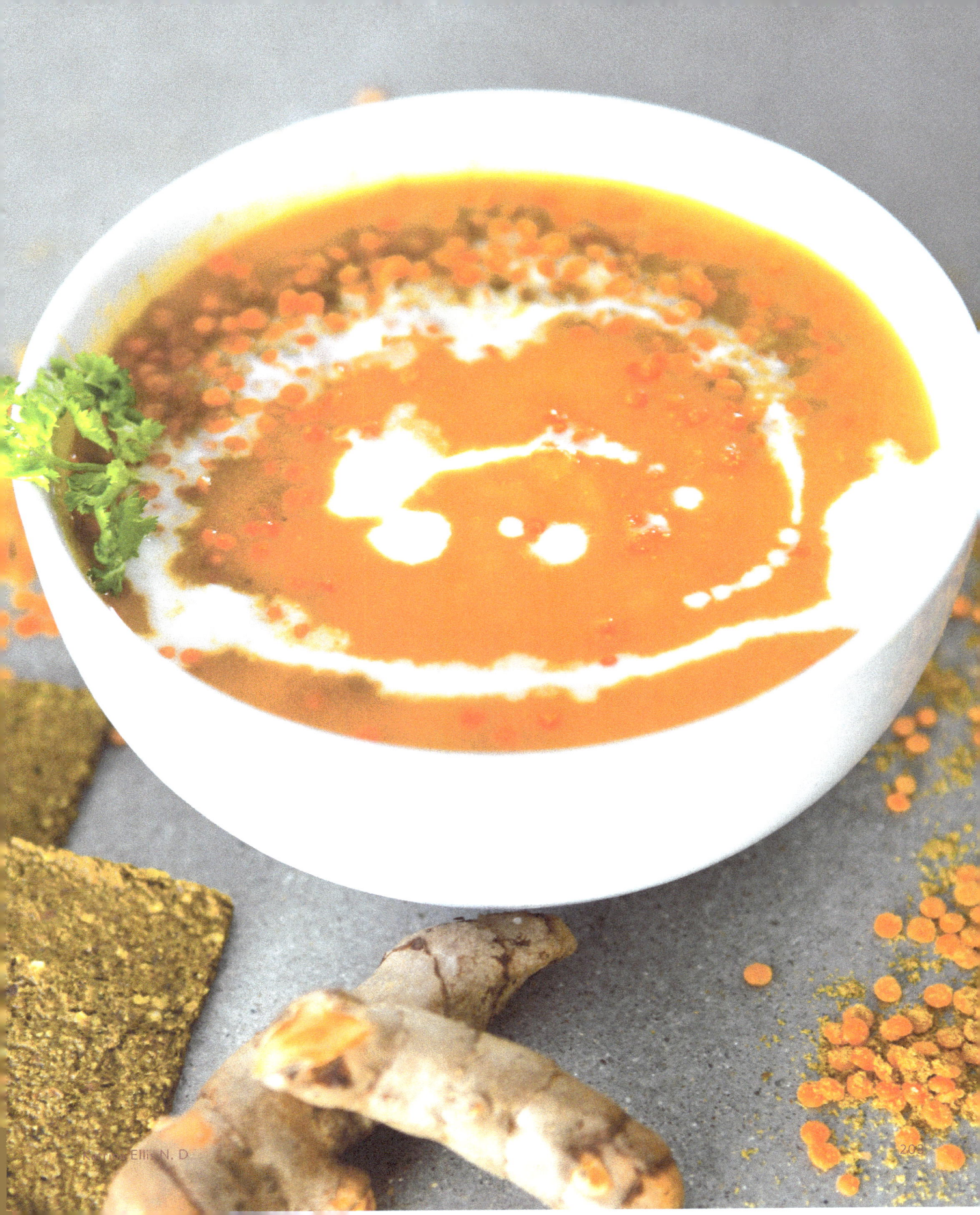

Thai Laksa with Konjac Noodles

SERVES 3

INGREDIENTS

A small packet of konjac noodles (or zucchini noodles if eating raw)

LAKSA PASTE

4 garlic cloves, peeled

1 small knob of ginger, diced

6 small red chillies, chopped finely

½ teaspoon of turmeric powder or fresh turmeric

1 small knob of galangal

1 tablespoon of cumin seeds or 1 teaspoon of cumin powder

2 sticks of lemongrass, sliced thinly

5 kaffir lime leaves, shredded

1 lime, juiced

1 tablespoon of shrimp paste (if vegetarian, use yellow bean or other fermented paste)

LAKSA

½ Chinese cabbage or pak choy, shredded finely

300 grams of firm organic tofu, cut into small cubes or 500 grams of uncooked King Prawns

1 cup of bean sprouts

½ bunch of Thai basil

1 can of coconut milk or cream

Purified water

METHOD

1. Process garlic, ginger, chilli, galangal, turmeric, coriander and cumin seeds, lemongrass, lime leaves and a little peanut oil until it forms a paste.

2. In a separate pan, bring coconut milk to the boil. When it starts to boil, stir in the laksa paste and a little maple or monkfruit syrup. Add the wombok or pak choy, tofu or prawns or any other vegetable.

3. Cook for a few minutes, adding water if needed and when ready remove from the heat. Pour into 2 to 3 bowls, and dress with sprouts and shredded coriander.

Superfood Powers

Laksa, when made with healthy ingredients, is one of the most nutritious pastes on the planet. When you combine galangal, ginger, turmeric, lemongrass and other Asian spices you have a pure skin-healing and regenerative paste. Its rich herbs and spices provide anti-inflammatory and anti-parasitical qualities as well as the ability to stimulate blood circulation, toxin removal and cancer protection.

Green Garlic Broccoli Soup

SERVES 3 PEOPLE

INGREDIENTS

6 cups of water or vegetable or chicken broth

2 large heads of broccoli, chopped

6 garlic cloves, diced (or fermented black garlic)

1 onion, diced

3 scallions or spring onions, diced

2 stalks of celery, chopped

A handful of parsley, diced

A handful of coriander or basil, diced

3 tablespoons of tamari

1 tablespoon of toasted sesame oil

1 tablespoon of rice vinegar

½ lemon, juiced

Celtic or Himalayan salt to flavour

Coconut cream (optional)

METHOD

1. In a pan, add a little oil and soften garlic, onion, spring onions and celery. As they begin to soften, add broccoli, stock, tamari, rice vinegar, lemon juice and spices.

2. Simmer for around 10 to 15 minutes or until broccoli still retains a beautiful green colour.

3. Now place all of the ingredients into a food processor or Thermomix and blend until you get the perfect consistency, adding more stock if you need. If you prefer a creamier soup, simply add less stock and more coconut cream.

Superfood Powers

Broccoli is a true superfood as it contains plenty of Vitamin A, C, E, B2, B3, B5, zinc, magnesium and other minerals to help boost hair strength, texture and resilience. An oil found in broccoli, known as erucic acid, can give hair a lustrous sheen. This soup is a pure cancer-protective, skin-reviving and hair nourishing beauty soup.

Collagen Vegan Broth

If you are a vegetarian, the thought of making a bone broth is horrific. But there are other ways. Seaweeds are amazing sources of natural minerals, vitamins and antioxidants which help to promote digestive health and collagen formation. Add in collagen promoting vegetables and miso for its prebiotic qualities and you have a healing, bone free collagen broth.

MAKES 1 BIG POT

INGREDIENTS

4 tablespoons of organic olive oil

2 brown onions, diced

4 shitake or enoki mushrooms, diced

2 cups of celery, finely diced

2 cups of carrots, diced

4 English spinach leaves, diced (or dandelion leaves if you can find)

1 beetroot (diced)

2 handfuls of Wakame, arame or hijike

¼ cup of Shiro miso paste

¼ cup of parsley, diced

¼ cup of coriander, diced

4 cm of ginger, diced

2 garlic cloves, diced

2 tablespoons of tamari or shoyu

12 cups of purified water

METHOD

1. Sauté mushrooms, garlic, onions and olive oil in a fry pan until soft. Put aside.

2. In a pot combine carrots, beets, celery, ginger and water, bring to the boil and then reduce to simmer.

3. Soak dried seaweed in hot water for a few minutes separately.

4. Once it expands, add to the carrot mix. Slowly add the mushroom mix, plus spinach, lemon juice, parsley and coriander.

5. Simmer for around 1 to 2 hours.

6. Stir in the miso paste at the end to ensure you do not kill the miso's live bacteria.

7. Add tamari or shoyu for extra flavour.

8. Drain off vegetables and store this liquid in the fridge for around 1 week.

Superfood Powers

I love making these algae broths. They are really pretty and absolutely delicious. I often add Apple Cider Vinegar towards the end with some Brewer's Yeast to pump up the B vitamins. Just like bone broths, this soup is high in collagen-type substances derived from the miso and seaweed which helps boost collagen, strengthen bones and improves digestive health.

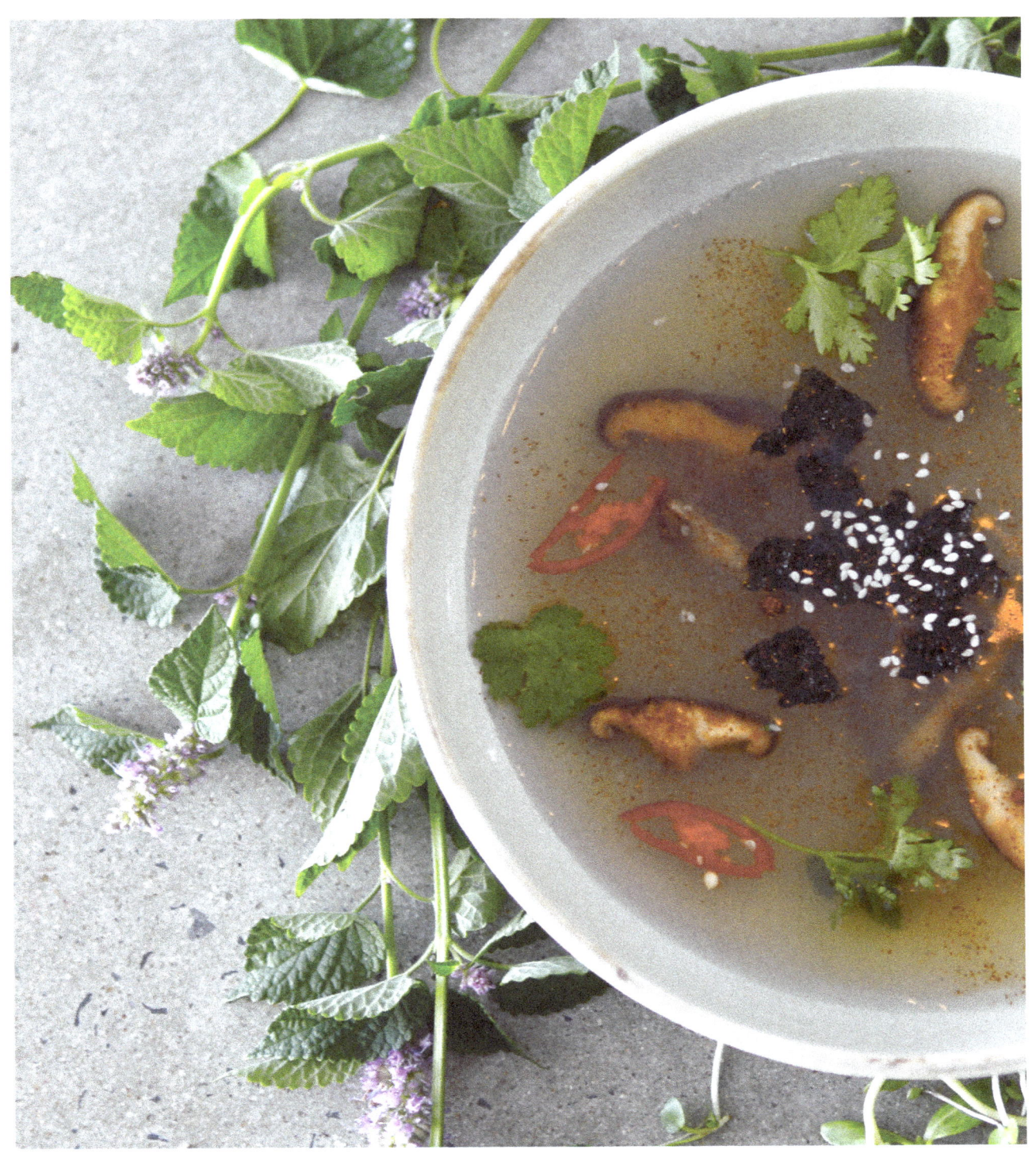

BEAUTY BOWLS & POKE PLATES

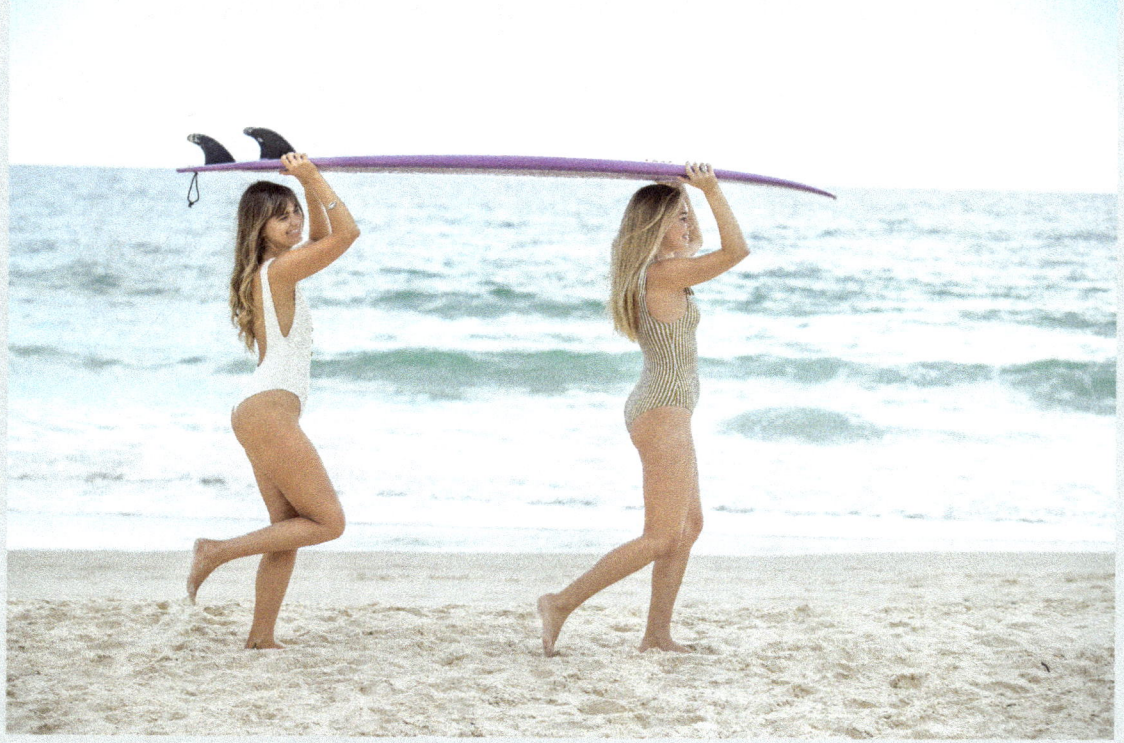

These beauty bowls are traditionally also called 'Buddha' or 'nourish' bowls. They are bowls of pure goodness and nutrition. They contain the perfect amounts of protein, fibre, antioxidants, minerals and vitamins to increase your vitality, enhance your wellness and improve the beauty and quality of your hair, skin, nails and mind.

Ahi poke plates or bowls are traditional Hawaiian dishes served with their local fish – Ahi tuna – which is why these are often called Ahi bowls too. However, you can make these with any local fish. They are often served with salad, brown rice and wakame. These bowls are super delicious and packed full of pure nutrition and youth-promoting nutrients.

Fermented Korean Poke

SERVES 2

INGREDIENTS

POKE MIX

2 slices of yellowfin tuna, cut into 2 cm squares

1 red onion

2 scallions or spring onions, diced

½ carrot, cut into matchsticks

A handful of coriander

¼ cup of pine nuts

2 tablespoons of kimchee

A handful of sesame seeds

MARINADE

2 tablespoons of Tamari

1 lemon or lime, juiced

4 tablespoons of toasted sesame oil

4 tablespoons of rice vinegar

2 garlic cloves, crushed

1 tablespoon of Gochujang (fermented chilli paste)

METHOD

1. Blend all of marinade ingredients together and pour over the tuna squares. Let this sit in the fridge for around 2 hours to cook.

2. When ready, mix with chopped salad greens, purple cabbage, thinly slice carrots and red onions and add pine nuts, sesame seeds and coriander.

3. Place kimchee in each bowl.

Superfood Powers

Tuna is super rich in anti-inflammatory omega 3 oils, vitamin B3, B6 and B12 and selenium. These nutrients are great for the heart, eyes, immune system, metabolism, bones and skin. Gochujang sauce is a fermented Korean chilli sauce made from soybeans, green chilli, rice powder and honey or sugar that is fermented over many years. This fermented paste is a superb gut healing tonic.

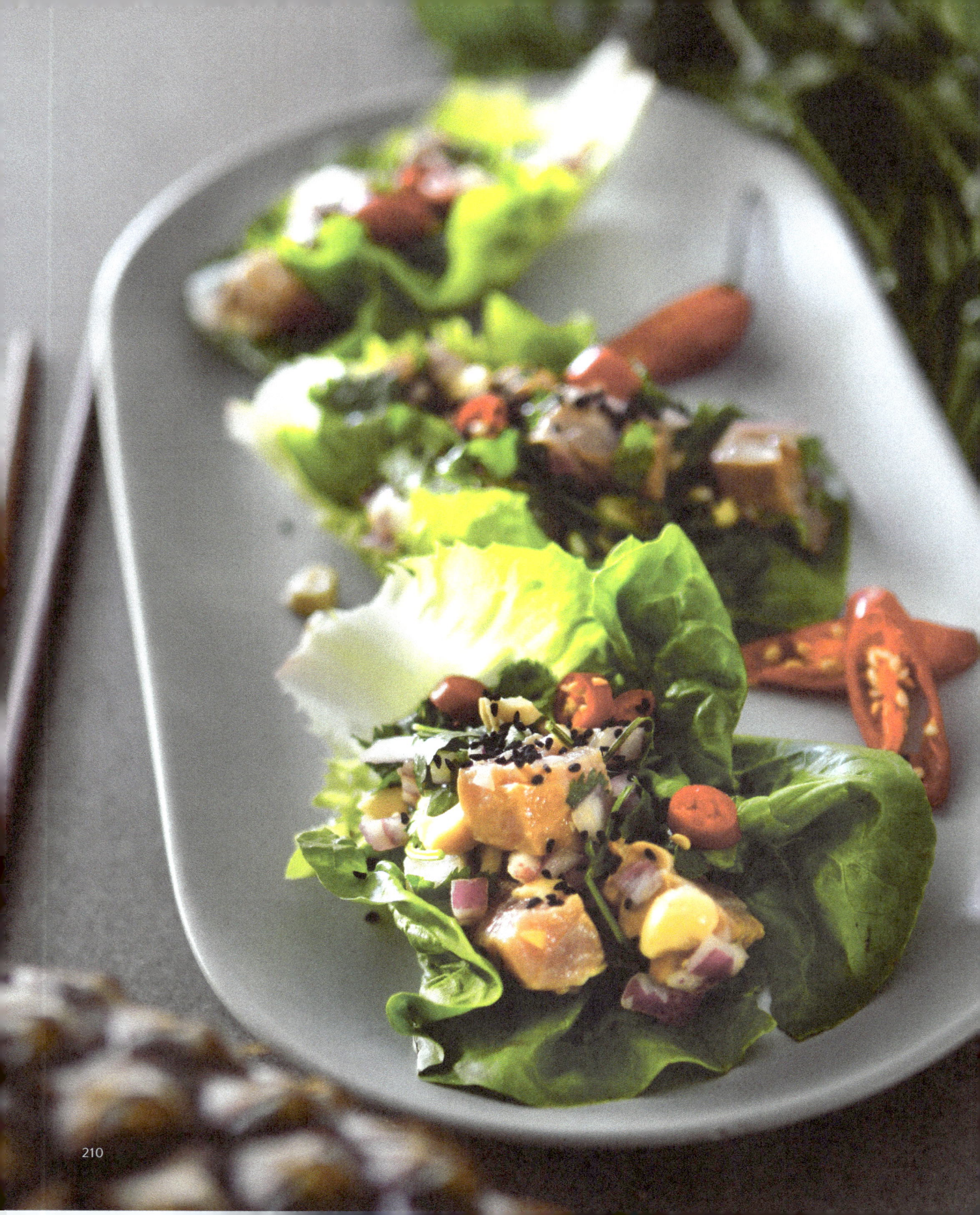

Hawaiian Ahi Poke Plate

SERVES 2

INGREDIENTS

POKE MIX

2 slices of A-grade yellowfin tuna, kingfish or another fish

A handful of coriander

¼ cup of macadamia nuts, diced

1 red onion, diced

Toasted nori or seaweed flakes

MARINADE

2 tablespoons of tamari

4 tablespoons of sesame oil

1 tablespoon of miso (I love shiro)

2 tablespoons of rice vinegar

1 fresh lime, juiced

1 garlic clove, finely diced

METHOD

1. Cut the fish into small 2 inch slices. Blend the marinade ingredients together in a blender and pour over the fish mix. Keep this in the fridge for 1 to 2 hours, covered.

2. When ready, place in lettuce cups with chopped coriander, red onion and macadamia nuts and sprinkle nori or toasted seaweed on top.

Superfood Powers

A nutritious Omega 3 and mineral rich beauty bowl that is particularly high in protein and iodine to enhance metabolism, encourage weight loss and to make hair and nails grow as fast as grass

Omega 3 Quinoa and Harissa Bowl

SERVES 2

INGREDIENTS

½ cup of quinoa to 2 cups of water

HARISSA DRESSING

2 teaspoons of harissa paste

1 lime, juiced

2 tablespoons of Apple Cider Vinegar (raw)

4 tablespoons of chia, pumpkin seed or hemp oil

A small amount of water

1 teaspoon of Celtic sea salt

¼ cup of tahini

SALAD INGREDIENTS

1 cup of kale

¼ purple cabbage, diced

¼ head of broccoli, steamed or raw

1 cup of lettuce mix, diced

½ avocado, diced

A handful of alfalfa or sunflower sprouts

A handful of walnuts

A handful of hemp or activated chia seeds

METHOD

1. Cold rinse quinoa to wash. Then place in a saucepan with plenty of cold water, bring to the boil and simmer for around 15 minutes or until fluffy.

2. To make the dressing, blend tahini, lime juice, harissa, salt, Apple Cider Vinegar, oil and a little water. Set aside.

3. In bowls, add chopped kale, lettuce mix, spinach leaves, purple cabbage, steamed or raw broccoli, quinoa, avocado and sprouts. Sprinkle with walnuts and hemp seeds and dress with lime and harissa dressing. Absolutely divine.

Superfood Powers

All of the vegetables, seeds and oils in this dish are very high sources of Omega 3 fatty acids. These oils reduce inflammation, hydrate the skin, prevent hair breakage and add a beautiful sparkle to the eyes. Quinoa is a brilliant source of protein, Vitamin A, zinc, magnesium, calcium and iron which boosts energy and weight loss and improves your skin tone.

The Alchemy of Beauty

Zucchini Noodle Beauty Bowl

MAKES 2 BOWLS

INGREDIENTS

2 tablespoons of pickled ginger

2 to 4 zucchini

6 small radishes, diced or shredded

8 to 10 green beans, chopped

A handful of broccoli sprouts

3 cups of rocket

½ cucumber, diced

½ cup of shiitake or other mushroom, sautéed quickly with tamari and lime juice

4 tablespoons of black sesame seeds

Wakame or seaweed flakes

WASABI DRESSING:

4 tablespoons of mirin or rice vinegar, 1 inch chunk of wasabi rhizome grated or 1 teaspoon of real wasabi paste, 6 tablespoons of toasted sesame oil and 1 lime juiced – mix well.

METHOD

1. Place zucchini, carrot, sweet potato, kohlrabi or any other vegetable into a spiraliser to make beautiful vegetable noodles.

2. Place the noodles into half of the wasabi dressing to marinate.

3. In 2 bowls, add rocket, diced radish, cucumber, green beans, capsicum and broccoli or snow pea sprouts.

4. Quickly sauté mushrooms and place in the bowls with noodles. Put pickled ginger on top with seaweed flakes, black sesame seeds and the rest of the wasabi dressing.

Superfood Powers

This is a pure vegan beauty treat super rich in Vitamin A and B complex, minerals, protein and oils to encourage healthy hair growth. The flavonoids found in this dish guards against sun-induced free radical damage that speeds up skin ageing and wrinkle formation.

Japanese Poke

MAKES 2 BOWLS

INGREDIENTS

POKE BOWL

2 large pieces of Ahi or mahi mahi or salmon, chopped into 2 cm squares

POKE MARINADE

2 to 4 tablespoons of toasted black sesame oil

2 tablespoons of brown rice vinegar or mirin

1 teaspoon of wasabi paste

1 teaspoon of grated ginger or ginger powder

3 limes, juiced

SALAD

1 bunch of watercress

½ cup of brown or organic Jasmine rice

6 small radish, shredded or diced

2 small carrots, shredded or made into matchsticks

250 grams of edamame, steamed and opened

1 tablespoon of organic, pickled ginger

Seaweed flakes

2 tablespoons of white or black sesame seeds

METHOD

1. Chop the fish into 2 cm squares and place in a bowl. Combine all of the marinade ingredients and pour over the fish mix.

2. Place in the fridge for around 2 hours to cook. In 2 to 3 bowls, place cooked rice, watercress, radish, carrot, edamame and ginger.

3. When the fish is ready, spread evenly into each bowl and mix with the salad ingredients. Dress each bowl with pickled ginger, sesame seeds and nori flakes.

Superfood Powers

Like all poke bowls, this dish is super high in Omega 3 oils. It contains fermented foods to enhance digestive health and watercress to remove bad hormones protecting against cancer. Organic edamame beans are one the most powerful beautifying foods in the world.

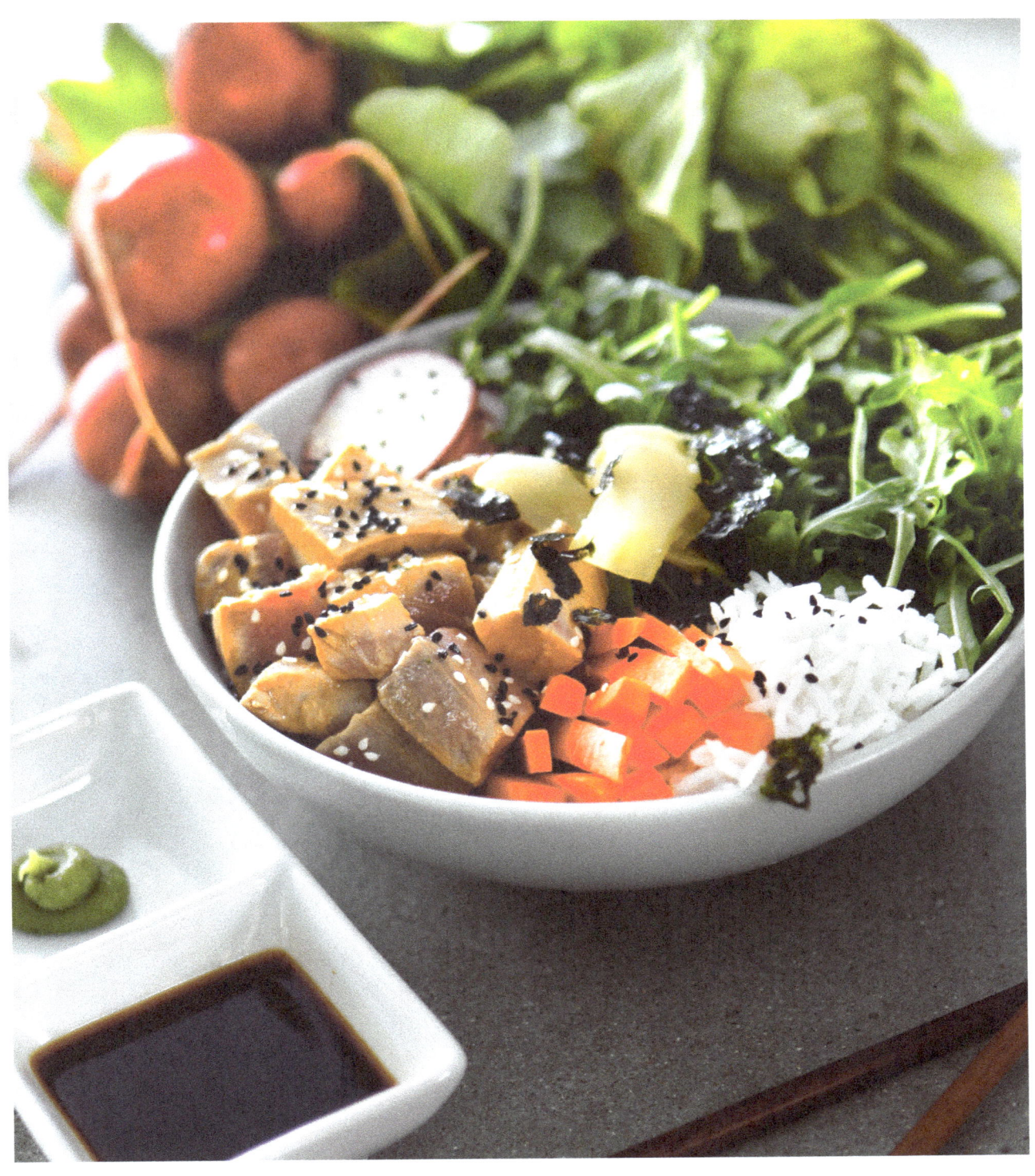

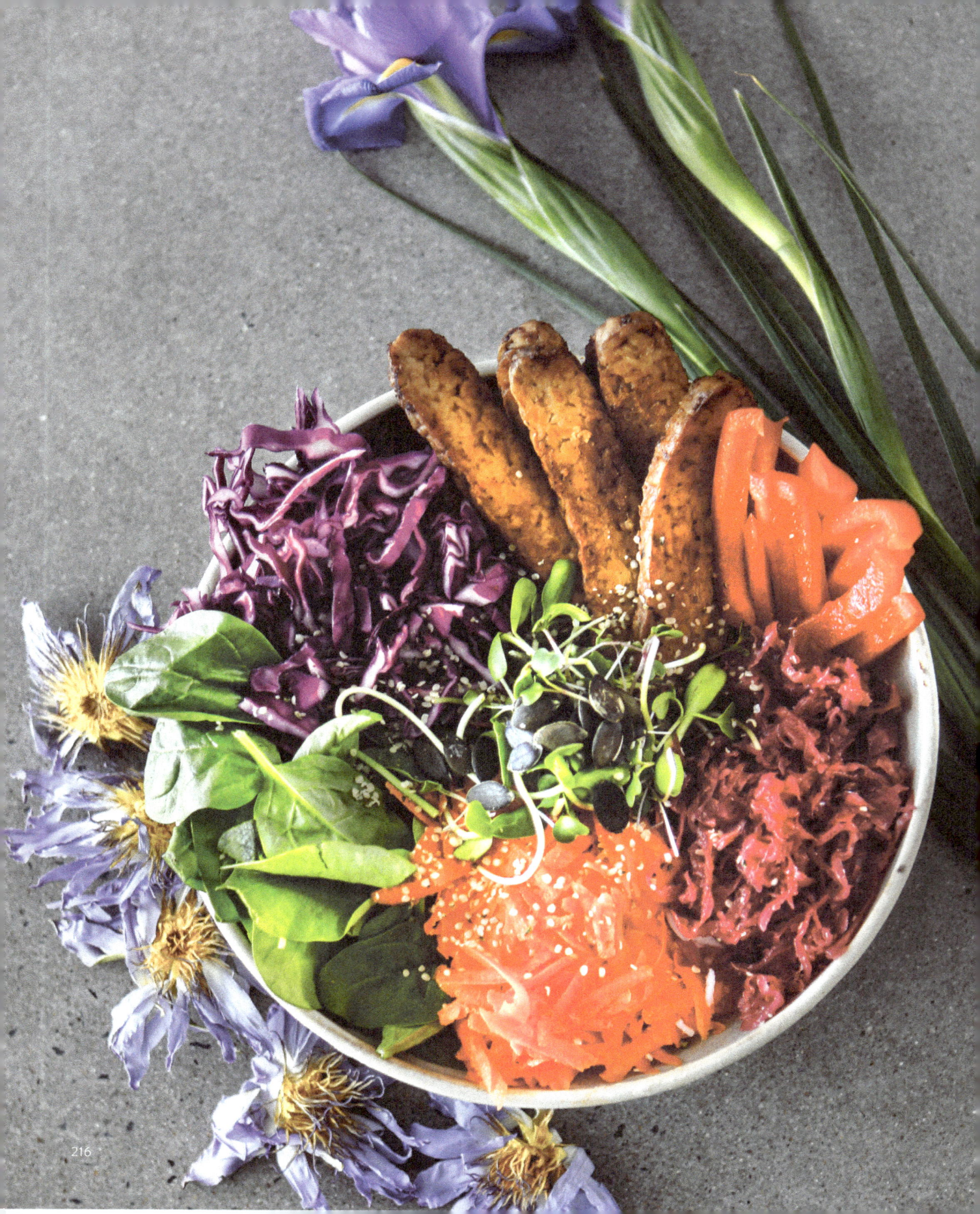

Vegan Tempeh Teriyaki Bowl

MAKES 2 BOWLS

INGREDIENTS

500 grams of Organic soy or chickpea tempeh

TERIYAKI

4 garlic cloves, diced

1 lime juiced

4 tablespoons of rice vinegar

2 tablespoons of maple or monkfruit syrup
or raw honey

⅓ cup of tamari or dark soy

2 tablespoons of sesame oil

1 teaspoon grated ginger or powder

2 teaspoon of kuzu or Agar Agar

SALAD

3 cups of rocket or purple/green cabbage

1 cup of Romaine lettuce or spinach leaves

1 purple or orange carrot, shredded or grated

1 red capsicum, diced

¼ cup of activated pumpkin seeds

¼ cup of hemp seeds

2 tablespoons of fermented vegetables or sauerkraut

METHOD

1. Blend the teriyaki marinade ingredients together in a food processor. Mix kuzu or Agar Agar in a little bit of cold water separately. Then heat marinade ingredients and add the kuzu or Agar Agar to thicken.

2. Place the thinly sliced tempeh into the teriyaki mix to marinate for at least 30 minutes.

3. When ready, quickly cook tempeh in a pan with a little oil on both sides or bake or dehydrate at under 46°C for 2 to 4 hours, if eating raw.

4. Place greens, carrot, capsicum, sauerkraut and seeds in a bowl and add the sliced teriyaki tempeh. Pour the leftover teriyaki sauce over the top. Sprinkle with pumpkin and hemp seeds, torn coriander and extra lime juice.

Superfood Powers

Tempeh is one of the healthiest, most beautifying foods on planet earth. It is an incredible source of isoflavones, B vitamins like B12, protein and antioxidants which help to protect against cancer, improve collagen production and hydrate dry and aged skin.

Meta Burn Bowl

SERVES 2

INGREDIENTS

2 pieces of Atlantic or red salmon (skin on)

MARINADE

4 tablespoons of toasted sesame oil

2 tablespoons of tamari

1 tablespoon of raw honey or monkfruit syrup

1 lemon, juiced

SALAD MIX

3 cups of kale, shredded

2 sticks of celery, diced

A handful of broccoli florets, diced

¼ head of red or green cabbage

½ cucumber, diced

2 tablespoons of organic pine nuts

META-BURN DRESSING

4 tablespoons of flaxseed or hemp oil, 4 tablespoons of Apple Cider Vinegar, 1 tablespoon of mustard seeds or paste, 1 lemon juiced, 2 red chilli peppers deseeded (blend all ingredients together in a processor adding oil if needed)

METHOD

1. Coat salmon in marinade ingredients and let this sit for at least 30 minutes.

2. Place salmon in a pan with a little olive oil and cook quickly on both sides or alternatively bake in the oven. Let this cool and then cut into small pieces.

3. Place chopped cabbage, cucumber, celery and other greens in a bowl with salmon.

4. Pour the meta-burn dressing over the top and sprinkle with pine nuts and basil leaves.

Superfood Powers

This beauty bowl is the ultimate weight loss and fat-burning beauty dish. The pine nuts contain a chemical that suppresses appetite; the dressing is a rich in omega 3 oils and lignans to burn stubborn fat; and the vegetables are natural weight loss kings. When you combine this with the beautiful Omega 3 fats found in the salmon, you have a perfect youth-promoting and fat burning beauty bowl.

Asian Poke 'Clear Skin' Bowl

SERVES 2

INGREDIENTS

2 pieces of Yellowfin tuna or another oily fish, chopped into 3 cm squares

½ cup of organic brown rice, cooked (optional)

1 orange, juiced

¼ cup of rice or coconut vinegar

4 tablespoons of toasted sesame oil

2 spring onions or scallions, chopped

¼ cup of tamari

SALAD

2 cups of watercress or rocket

4 small radish, sliced or grated

A handful of mung bean sprouts

Wakame flakes or another type of seaweed

A handful of black or white sesame seeds

½ avocado

METHOD

Cut the yellowfin tuna into squares and set aside.

Mix tamari, rice vinegar, orange juice, sesame oil and scallions and place the tuna in this mix, cover and put in the fridge for at least 2 hours to cook in the juices.

In two separate bowls, place some cooked brown or wild rice, rocket or watercress, sprouts and chopped avocado.

If you are following a keto diet, simply leave the rice out. When the tuna is ready put into the salad mix and sprinkle with coriander and black sesame seeds.

Superfood Powers

This dish contains plenty of Omega 3 oils, protein, selenium, zinc and Vitamin C to add a luscious glow to the skin, a bounce to the hair and a sparkle to the eyes.

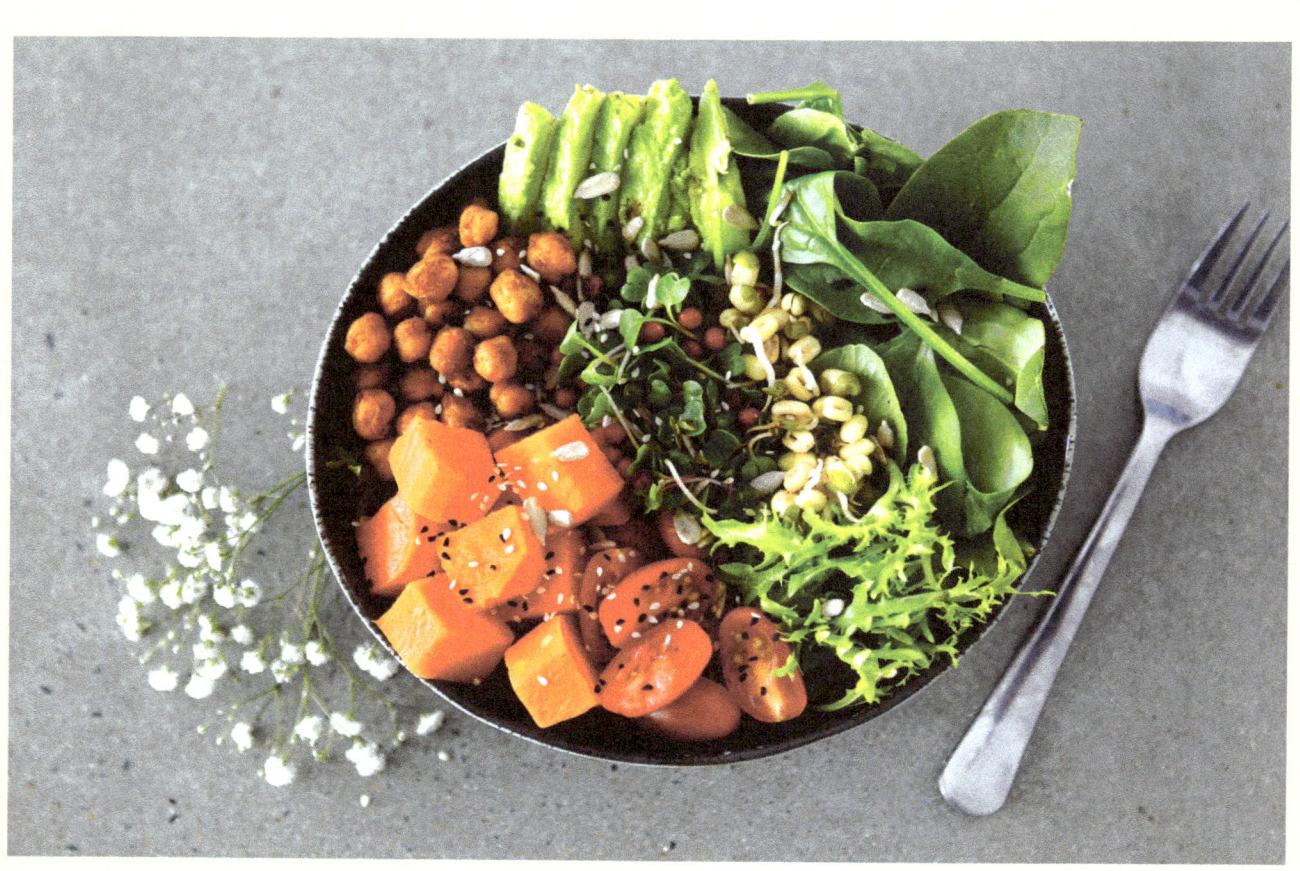

Chickpea Beauty Bowl
with Peppercorn Dressing

SERVES 1 TO 2

INGREDIENTS

SALAD

1 cup of chickpeas, rinsed and cooked (if in a hurry use organic canned chickpeas)

Chickpea and sweet potato spice mix – 1 teaspoon turmeric, 1 teaspoon oregano, 1 teaspoon paprika and 2 tablespoons of olive oil

2 sweet potatoes, peeled and sliced

3 cups of baby spinach leaves

3 cups of romaine or mixed lettuce

8 cherry tomatoes, halved

1 punnet of snow pea or alfalfa sprouts

½ avocado, diced

¼ cup of Sunflower seeds (preferably activated)

DRESSING

2 stalks of green peppercorns

1 lemon, juiced

2 tablespoons of chia or avocado oil

4 tablespoons of sesame oil (black or toasted)

1 tablespoon of raw honey or monkfruit syrup

2 tablespoons of yellow mustard paste or seeds

METHOD

1. If using dried chickpeas, soak in water for 12 hours or overnight to break down its anti-nutrients.

2. Drain and cook in a pan for 40 minutes until soft or in a pressure cooker with lots of water for 4 hours. Remove and dry.

3. Put spice mix into a bag and shake with chickpeas and sweet potato.

4. Spread chickpeas and sweet potato onto a lined tray and cook on a low heat in the oven until golden or dehydrate at 46 C for 4 hours if eating raw.

5. In two separate bowls, place spinach leaves, lettuce, cherry tomatoes, sprouts or snow peas and avocado. When sweet potato and chickpeas are ready, place in bowls sprinkling more chickpeas on top.

6. Blend dressing ingredients together and pour over this delicious vegan salad mix.

Superfood Powers

Even though chickpeas are quite high in carbohydrates, they are particularly rich in protein, B2, B6, potassium, zinc, iron and magnesium to calm nerves, beautify the hair and skin and to aid constipation.

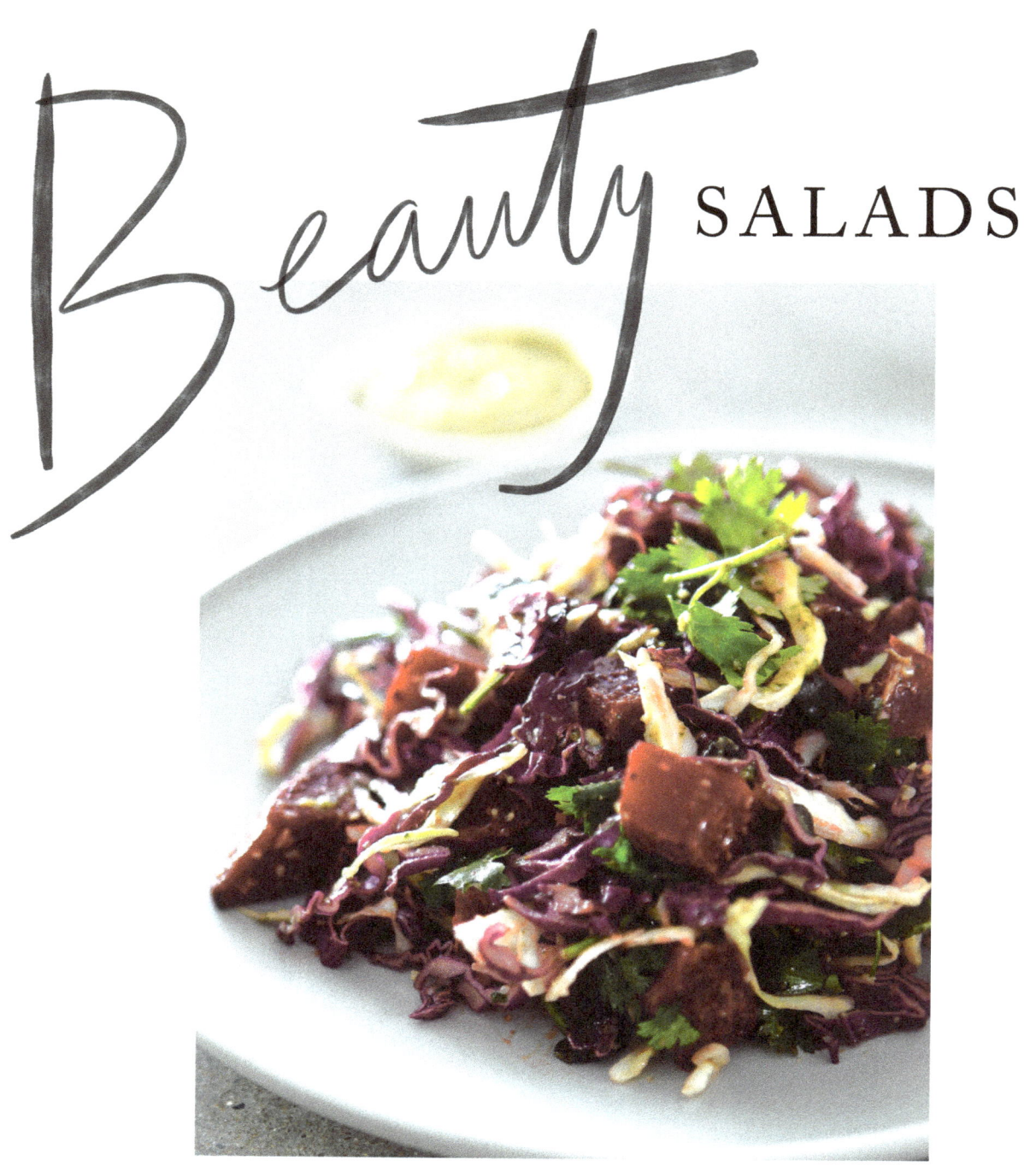

Beauty SALADS

Maui Kale Salad with a SECRET Dressing

INGREDIENTS

DRESSING

1 teaspoon of yellow mustard paste or seeds

4 tablespoons of toasted sesame oil

4 tablespoons of hemp oil or another Omega oil

2 tablespoons of Shiro or white miso paste

2 limes, juiced

¼ cup of sesame seeds

3 garlic cloves

A knob of ginger

4 tablespoons of brown rice vinegar

1 tablespoon of raw honey or maple syrup

A small handful of coriander

SALAD

Purple and white cabbage

Kale

Coriander

2 beetroots or 6 baby beets

¼ cup of activated pumpkin seeds

METHOD

1. Steam the baby beets or chopped beetroot and set aside.

2. Chop up kale and add to chopped purple and white cabbage and torn coriander.

3. Sprinkle the pumpkin seeds through this with the baby beets.

4. Now blend mustard, ginger, garlic, toasted sesame oil, sesame seeds, lime juice, Shiro miso, vinegar, coriander and honey.

5. Add a little more sesame oil or water if needed.

6. Pour this over the salad and mix through well. For an extra treat, mix a little goats' cheese through this salad.

Superfood Powers

Hawaii is my favourite place on planet earth (besides my home country and now Sri Lanka and the Maldives) and it isn't just the beautiful nature or the people, it is their incredible local food. This salad was inspired on one of our visits to Maui. We found a local Hawaiian restaurant and there I tasted one of the best kale salads in the world. I went back every day for the next five days to have this salad. The lovely chef wrote down his dressing for me. I have adapted it slightly but have still kept the original flavours. I hope you love this salad as much as I do!

Curried Enzyme Slaw

INGREDIENTS

SALAD

½ small purple cabbage, ribs removed and sliced thinly

½ small green cabbage, ribs removed and sliced thinly

1 Spanish onion, diced

1 red capsicum, diced

1 carrot, grated

1 bunch of fresh coriander, chopped

⅛ of pineapple, chopped into small pieces

A handful of walnuts

DRESSING

2 teaspoons of curry powder or 4 curry leaves

2 cloves of garlic, crushed

1 tablespoon of grated ginger

¼ cup of organic flaxseed or olive oil

1 lemon, juiced

1 teaspoon of Celtic sea salt

METHOD

1. To make the salad, combine cabbages, coriander, grated carrot, red capsicum and purple onion in a bowl.

2. Sprinkle walnuts through.

3. Add the chopped pineapple at the end.

4. To make the dressing, place all of the dressing ingredients into a food processor and blend until creamy. Toss the salad ingredients with the curry dressing.

Superfood Powers

This salad is packed full of Vitamin A, C and E, B Complex, minerals and skin-healing enzymes like bromelain. Pineapple helps to prevent skin pigmentation and encourages the production of hyaluronic acid, a substance that absorbs 100 times its weight in water to nourish and plump the skin.

Gingered Wakame Salad

SERVES 2 TO 3

INGREDIENTS

50 to 100 grams of wakame

4 tablespoons of tamari

1 lime, juiced

A bunch of coriander

8 to 12 snow peas, chopped

A handful of baby spinach leaves

1 red capsicum, diced

Broccoli sprouts

DRESSING

4 tablespoons of Apple Cider Vinegar (raw)

1 tablespoon of rice vinegar

1 to 2 tablespoons of tamari or Braggs amino acid seasoning

4 tablespoons of hemp, sesame or macadamia oil

1 lime or lemon, juiced

A small knob of ginger

METHOD

1. Soak the wakame in hot water until soft.

2. When soft, place in another bowl with tamari and lime juice. In separate bowls, place spinach leaves, chopped capsicum and snow peas with broccoli sprouts.

3. Meanwhile, blend the salad dressing ingredients and set aside. When the wakame is marinated nicely, take out and then add to the rest of the salad ingredients with the ginger dressing.

4. Place more broccoli or snow pea sprouts on top and sprinkle with sesame seeds

Superfood Powers

I am in love with seaweed, not just because it tastes delicious in a salad, but because of its incredible healing and longevity properties. Wakame is one of the best sources of chlorophyll, antioxidants and iodine. Iodine helps to speed up metabolism, stops hair loss, protects against all types of cancer and helps us to detoxify heavy metals, leaving a clean and oxygenated bloodstream.

Sweet Potato Salad with Wasabi and Lime Mayo

INGREDIENTS

Wasabi Mayo

3 garlic cloves

1 tablespoon of real wasabi
or horseradish paste

1 teaspoon of Celtic sea salt

Black pepper

1 lime, juiced

2 tablespoons of rice vinegar

2 tablespoons of hemp, chia,
flaxseed or sacha inchi oil

1 egg yolk (optional)

2 small chillies (optional – if you want spicier)

SALAD

2 small sweet potatoes

1 spanish onion, diced

2 spring onions, diced

A handful of watercress

½ red capsicum, diced

A handful of broccoli florets, diced

METHOD

1. Blend all of the mayo ingredients in a food processor and place in the fridge to set.

2. To make the salad, chop sweet potato into small cubes and steam or alternatively place in the oven at 180°C for 15 minutes or under the dehydrator at 45°C with a little olive oil, Celtic salt and paprika until ready.

3. Chop watercress or rocket and place in a bowl with capsicum, broccoli, red onion, spring onions and add sweet potato when cool. Pour the mayo over the top and serve with activated pumpkin seeds, sesame or macadamia nuts.

Superfood Powers

Sweet potato is a youth promoting superfood due to its ability to make hyaluronic acid. When you combine this with watercress and red capsicum you also have a perfect antioxidant salad that can speed up your metabolism, protect against skin cancer and maintain the health of your eyes.

Konjac Noodle Salad

INGREDIENTS

SALAD MIX

1 packet of konjac or shirataki noodles (if you cannot find these, use kelp, brown rice or zucchini noodles)

1 cup of bean sprouts

1 cup of snow peas, sliced

1 cup of chives or shallots, finely chopped

1 cup of Shiitake and or Enoki (Chop, soak in hot water for 20 minutes and then marinate in sesame oil, tamari and lime juice)

DRESSING

¼ cup of tamari

1 lime, juiced

1 tablespoon of rice vinegar

2 tablespoons of black sesame seeds

1 teaspoon of activated raw honey or monkfruit syrup

METHOD

1. Blend tamari, lime juice, rice vinegar, black sesame seeds and raw honey or monkfruit syrup. Set aside.

2. If using konjac noodles, rinse with water and cook for a few minutes in hot water and remove.

3. If you are eating only raw, spiralise any vegetable into a noodle and place on each plate with bean sprouts, snow peas and shallots. Quickly pan fry sauted mushrooms and add to salad.

4. Pour the yummy dressing over the top and place shredded coriander and roasted almonds on top.

Superfood Powers

Konjac or shirataki noodles contain virtually no calories, next to no carbohydrates and plenty of protein, minerals and glucomannan fibre. This fibre absorbs 200 times its weight in water, so it makes you feel full while enhancing weight loss and sugar balance.

Pomegranate Citrus Beauty Salad

SERVES 2 TO 3

INGREDIENTS

SALAD

¼ head of broccoli, chop up

1 avocado, sliced into squares

1 punnet of rocket leaves

½ head of Romaine lettuce (if you cannot find this, use mixed lettuce)

10 cherry tomatoes

Sunflower seeds (soaked and activated is better)

1 pomegranate

DRESSING

1 lime, juiced

1 orange, juiced

1 lemon, juiced

4 tablespoons of avocado oil

1 teaspoon of raw honey or coconut nectar

1 teaspoon of seeded mustard

METHOD

1. Blend together citrus juices, avocado oil, sweetener and mustard. Set this dressing aside.

2. Now toss together chopped broccoli, rocket, dill, avocado, tomatoes and lettuce. Sprinkle sunflower seeds through this mix.

3. Pour citrus dressing through the salad and mix well.

4. Cut open a pomegranate, bang on the back to remove the seeds and sprinkle through the salad mix. Serve on three plates and drizzle with dressing.

Superfood Powers

Citrus are very rich in minerals, Vitamin C and copper, which alkalises the body and boosts collagen production. Pomegranate is an anti-ageing hero. It prevents many forms of cancer, improves heart health, boosts metabolism, protects against skin ageing and increases the growth of hair and nails. This is a delicious salad for turning back the ageing clock.

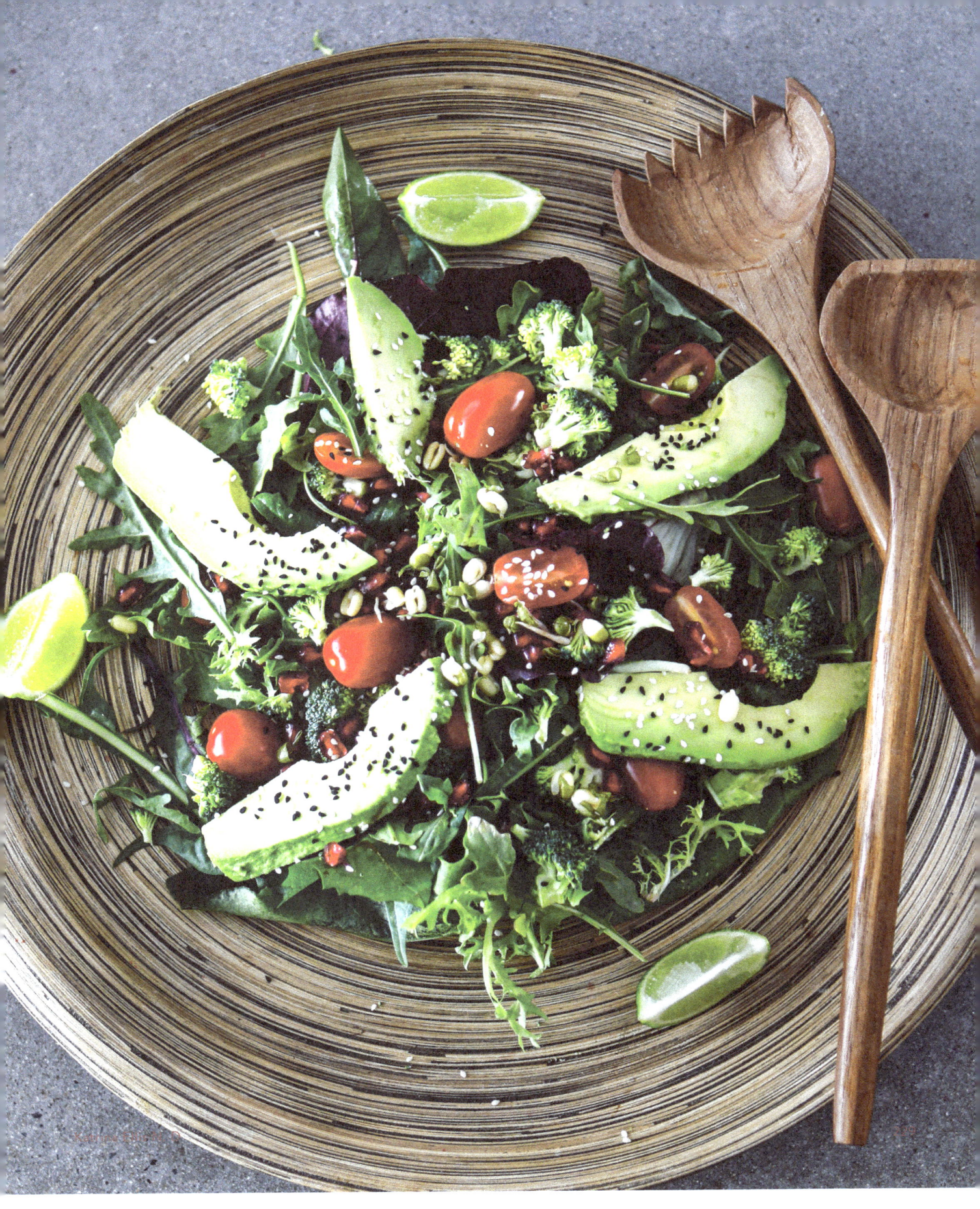

Thai Slaw with Nam Jim Dressing

SERVES 4

INGREDIENTS

SALAD

½ cabbage, shredded

1 carrot, grated

1 tomato, shredded

10 green beans, diced in 2 cm lengths

½ Spanish onion, diced

½ green papaya, shredded

Coriander, shredded

A handful of black sesame seeds

½ red capsicum, diced

DRESSING

3 red chillies, diced

4 garlic cloves, diced

2 cm chunk of ginger, diced

A handful of mint

2 teaspoons of fish sauce or tamari (if vegetarian)

1 teaspoon of yacon or monkfruit syrup or coconut nectar

3 limes, juiced

¼ cup of hemp, olive or sesame oil

METHOD

Mix all of the salad ingredients together and place in 3 or 4 bowls. In a mortar and pestle, grind chilli, garlic, ginger and mint. Add in natural sweetener, seasoning and lime juice. Mix together and slowly add in oil. Let this sit for a few minutes and then pour over the salad.

Superfood Powers

I added shredded green papaya to this Thai Coleslaw to pump up its cancer-protective and beautifying qualities. Green papaya contains a skin and cancer protective enzyme known as papain.

Radish, Shiitake and Radicchio Salad

SERVES 3 TO 4

INGREDIENTS

SALAD

6 small radishes, diced or shaved

6 fresh Shitake, diced (sauté in a pan with olive oil and tamari for a few minutes)

8 green beans, diced

1 small tub of rocket or radicchio

A handful of mixed lettuce

DRESSING

2 tablespoons of Shiro miso

3 limes, juiced

4 cm chunk of ginger

2 tablespoons of tamari

1 tablespoon of maple or monkfruit syrup or another natural sweetener

4 tablespoons of toasted sesame oil

METHOD

1. Chop up rocket and lettuce mix and place in 2 to 3 bowls.

2. Mix through green beans and radish and add sautéed shitake mushrooms.

3. Process or mix miso, lime juice, ginger, tamari and natural sweetener and pour over the salad mix.

4. Dress with black sesame seeds.

Superfood Powers

Radish would have to be one of my fav beauty foods and one of the best liver-cleansing vegetables on the planet. The rich amount of Vitamin C, antioxidants, phosphorous, zinc and B complex found in this salad helps to provide protection against free radicals while hydrating the skin.

Oriental Quinoa Salad

SERVES 3 TO 4

INGREDIENTS

1 cup of quinoa

2 cups of water

1 red pepper, thinly sliced

1 small zucchini, julienned

1 carrot, julienned

2 cups of Romaine or another lettuce, thinly sliced

DRESSING

2 tablespoons of tahini

1 tablespoon of crushed chilli or chilli paste

1 teaspoon of tamari, fish sauce
or Bragg's amino acid seasoning

2 tablespoons of sesame oil

1 tablespoon of rice vinegar

A small chunk of ginger

METHOD

1. Use a julienne or a spiraliser to turn the zucchini and carrots into thin, noodle strips.
    Finely chop the lettuce and mix through with chopped red pepper and spring onions.

2. Rinse quinoa in cold water, then add to a pan with twice as much water, bring to
    the boil and simmer for 15 minutes or until fluffy.

3. When quinoa cools, mix through lettuce mix.

4. In a food processor, blend dressing ingredients adding a little more water if needed.
    Place quinoa mix into 3 to 4 bowls and pour dressing over the top.

5. Dress with crushed almonds, sprouts and lime juice.

Superfood Powers

Quinoa is a protein rich seed that contains an abundant amount of magnesium, iron, manganese, copper and vitamins
which improves skin health, energy production, reduces inflammation and makes your hair grow as fast as grass.

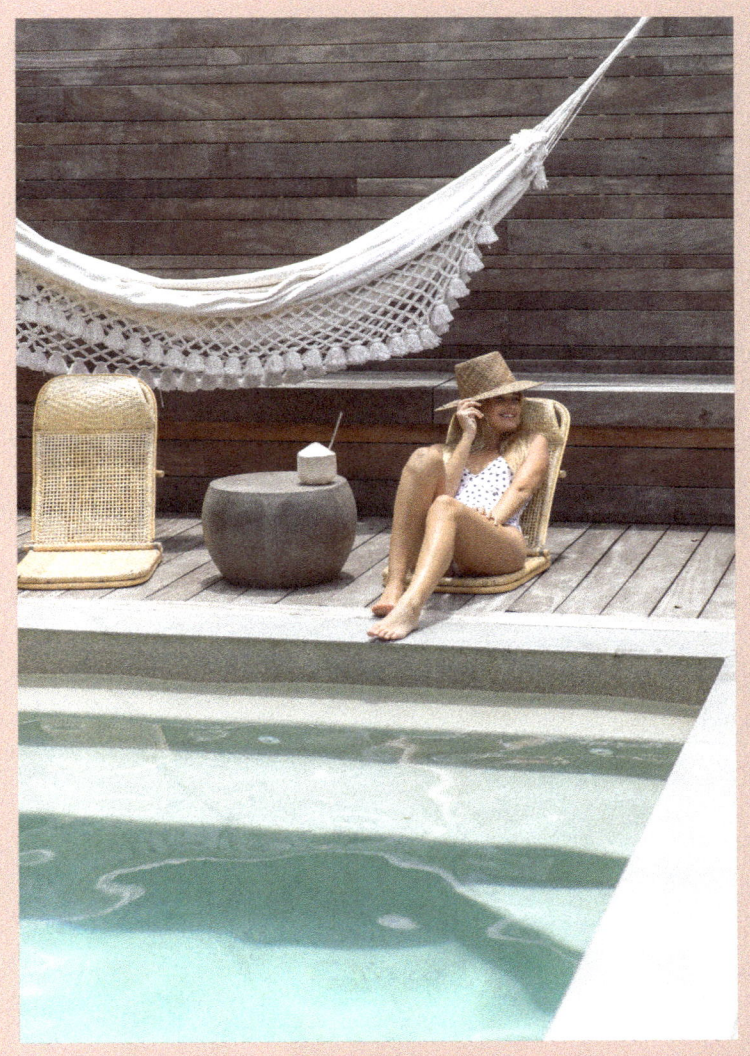

Minted Larb Gai

SERVES 3 TO 4

INGREDIENTS

6 tablespoons of premium fish sauce
or Bragg's amino acid seasoning

2 limes, juiced

1 to 2 teaspoons of maple or monkfruit syrup,
coconut nectar or raw honey

4 small red chillies, diced

½ cup of coriander, shredded

½ cup of mint, shredded

3 shallots, finely chopped

½ red onion, finely chopped

500 grams of minced chicken or turkey
(if vegan use quinoa mince (see page 242)

½ cup of water

1 tablespoon of toasted rice powder

METHOD

1. Throw minced chicken, turkey or quinoa mince into a pan with a little sesame oil and water and start cooking, using a spatula to break up. Make sure it is in its natural juices. If it is drying out add more water. When cooked transfer to a bowl with chopped shallots and red onion.

2. Mix together fish sauce (or Bragg's if vegetarian), lime juice, natural sweetener and chopped chilli. Pour a little through the chicken mix and slowly add the toasted rice powder.

3. When the flavor is perfect, mix through coriander and mint leaves. Serve in lettuce cups or on a plate with torn coriander, chilli and lime.

Superfood Powers

Larb Gai is a traditional Thai chicken salad dish. There are now many different variations made on this recipe including using turkey and vegan mince. Commercial fish sauce is very high in sodium, so I use a natural fish sauce that contains only anchovies and sea salt. If vegan replace with Bragg's amino acids, tamari or a fermented bean paste. Mint, coriander and chilli can all improve digestion, wipe out fungus and bacteria, reduce inflammation and even help offer protection against colon, lung and skin cancer.

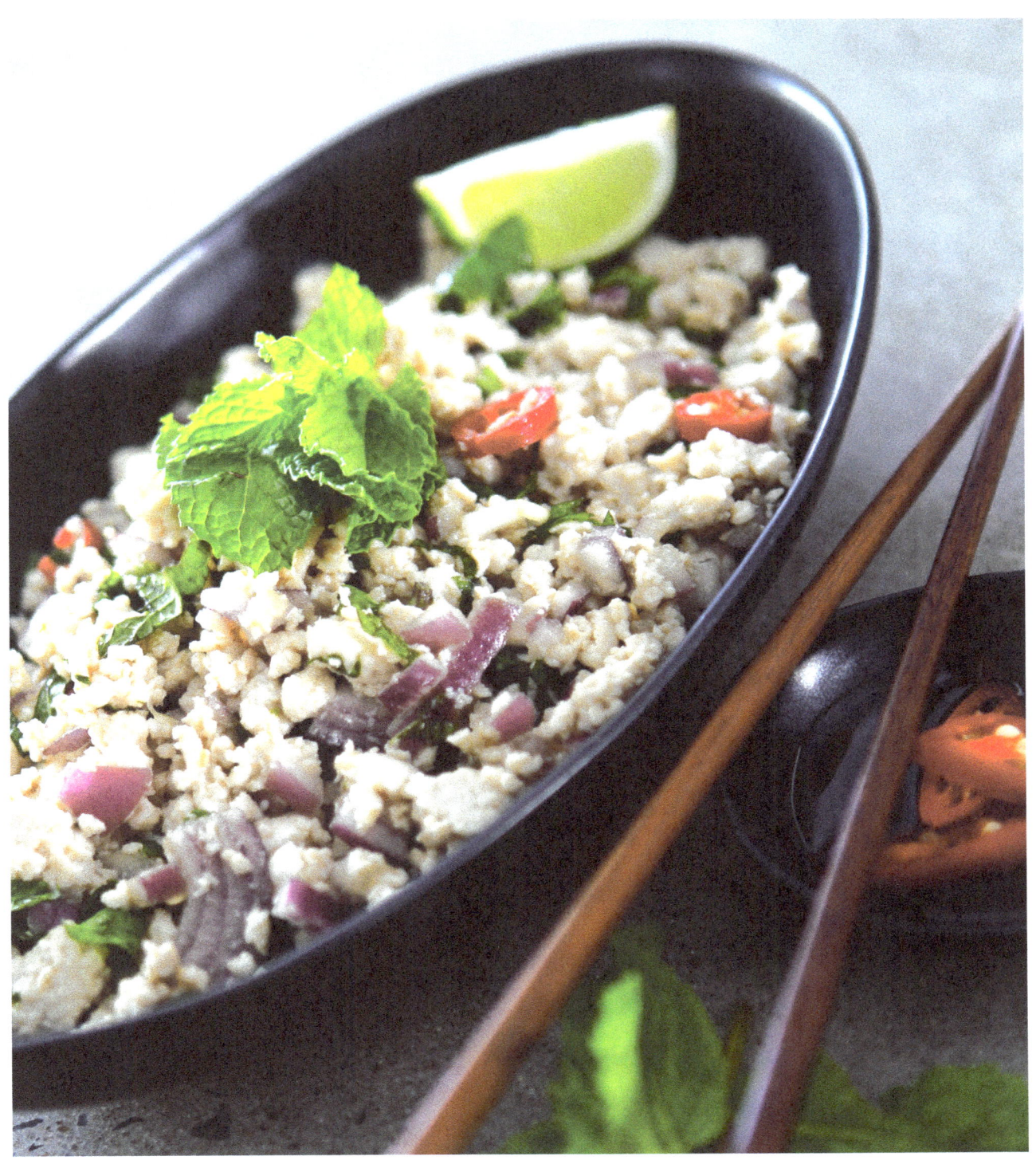

When you
Nourish
you Flourish

Vietnamese Poached Organic Chicken Salad

SERVES 4

INGREDIENTS

Poaching Mix

4 chicken breasts

1 litre of chicken or vegetable stock, broth or water (recipe in 'Soups')

1 knob of ginger, grated

2 cloves of garlic, finely sliced

1 tablespoon of sesame oil

4 cinnamon quills

Black pepper

SALAD

1 carrot, shredded

A handful of mint

A handful of coriander

½ wombok or Chinese cabbage

A handful of bean sprouts

A handful of snow peas

Crushed almonds (great if dehydrated, activated or toasted)

DRESSING:

2 tablespoons of Tamari or fish sauce

2 limes, juiced

1 tablespoon of brown rice vinegar

1 teaspoon of maple or monkfruit syrup or stevia

METHOD

1. Place all poaching ingredients into a pot with the chicken. Bring to the boil, then reduce heat and let simmer for 60 minutes with the lid on. While you are waiting for the chicken, prepare the salad and the dressing.

2. Shred wombok and carrot and mix together with bean sprouts and torn coriander and mint.

3. Blend salad dressing ingredients and put aside.

4. Remove the poached chicken, use a fork to shred this and place into bowls with salad mix. Pour dressing over the top and finish with toasted, crushed almond pieces. If you are a vegetarian, tempeh or tofu can be made just like the chicken.

Superfood Powers

Chinese cabbage is rich in indoles which help balance hormones, prevent cancer and remove harmful toxins through the liver. Cinnamon helps to regulate blood sugar, kills harmful bacteria and fungus and supports the health of neurons in the brain. It is one of the best natural weight loss spices known. When you combine this with ginger, garlic and black pepper you have a pure thermogenic super treat.

MOORISH *Vegan* MAINS

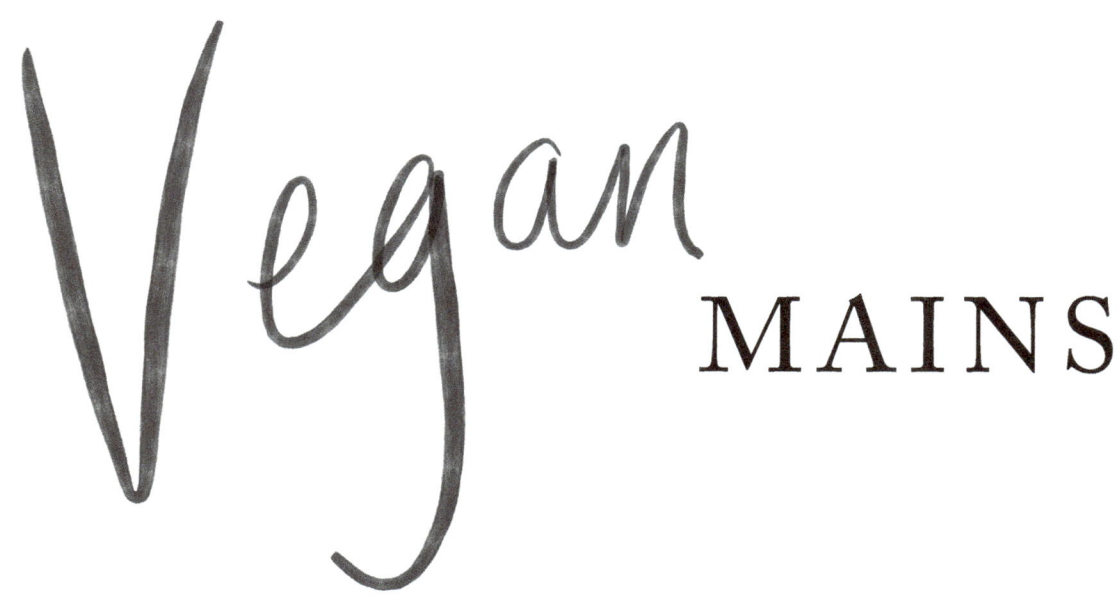

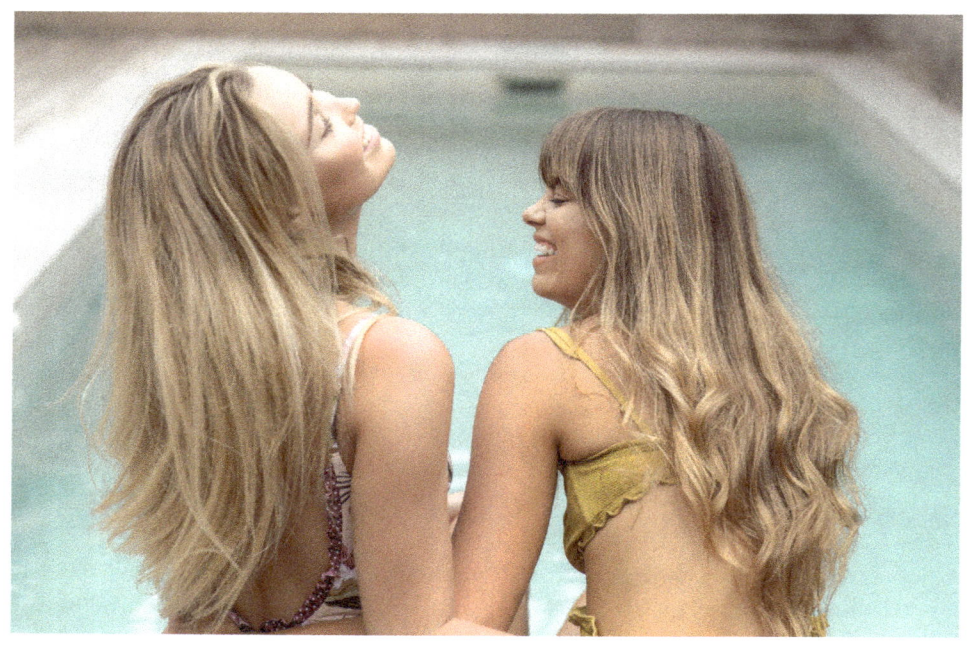

The Alchemy of Beauty

Raw Vegan Tacos with Mint Salsa

SERVES 2

INGREDIENTS

VEGAN NUTTY MINCE

½ cup of almonds

½ cup of walnuts

½ cup of hulled hemp seeds

2 tablespoons of hemp seed oil

1 teaspoon of cumin

2 garlic cloves or 1 teaspoon of garlic powder

1 tablespoon of tamari

1 tablespoon of Bragg's amino acid seasoning

2 limes, juiced

CONDIMENTS ON TOP

A handful of coriander

A handful of fresh sprouts

½ red capsicum, diced

A handful of black olives

METHOD

1. To make the taco mince, place all of the ingredients into a food processor and blend or pulse, leaving a little bit chunky. If you prefer not to eat 100% raw, cook nutty mince quickly in a pan with a little oil or under a grill to make crunchy.

2. Place 1 scoop of the taco mince into each cabbage or lettuce leaf and add chopped olives, sprouts, sliced red capsicum and rocket. Put a dollop of Beauty Sambal Sauce or tomato mint salsa onto each burrito cup. (See page 168).

Superfood Powers

This dish is a pure essential fatty acid superfood treat. Almonds, walnuts and hemp seeds are incredible sources of Omega 3, 6 and 9 fatty acids which help nourish and hydrate the skin, hair and nails. They are also packed with minerals, antioxidants and vitamins like Vitamin E and B complex. What a yummy skin and metabolism boosting dish!

Cauliflower Nasi Goreng

SERVES: 2 TO 3 PEOPLE

INGREDIENTS

1 brown onion, diced

2 cm chunk of ginger, finely diced

3 cloves of garlic, finely diced or minced

1 teaspoon of shrimp paste (or fermented bean paste if you are vegan)

3 tablespoons of kecap manis (healthy version below) or oyster sauce

1 lime, juiced

2 tomatoes, shredded

A handful of coriander

4 tablespoons of peanut or sesame oil

MAIN

½ cauliflower

¼ green cabbage, diced

½ red capsicum, diced

2 spring onions or scallions, diced

½ carrot, diced into small cubes

METHOD

1. Add a little cold-pressed, organic peanut or sesame oil to a pan. As it begins to heat add garlic, ginger, pepper, onion and shrimp or fermented bean paste. Mix well as it cooks.

2. In a food processor, pulse the cauliflower until it looks like rice. Now add to the pan, with chopped capsicum, cabbage, carrot and spring onions.

3. Add healthy kecap manis or oyster sauce, lime juice, black pepper and Himalayan salt to season. Add the shredded tomatoes in at the end.

4. Make a circle in the middle of the wok and break three eggs in and as the egg cooks, chop into squares with spatula and mix through.

5. Serve nasi goreng on three plates with torn coriander, egg and a squeeze of lime. Yum.

Superfood Powers

I love rice, but unfortunately most rice (especially white rice) is high in carbohydrates which can cause glucose intolerance and weight gain. Brown, red and black rice are definitely better choices due to their rich fibre and nutrient content, but still not great if you are following a ketogenic diet. This yummy version of nasi goreng uses cauliflower instead of rice. Cauliflower is a cruciferous superhero. It protects against all types of cancers, helps to detoxify you of harmful toxins and improves brain health. This dish can be made completely raw too by simply mixing all of the ingredients together and leaving the eggs out.

Healthy Kecap Manis

Traditional Indonesian kecap manis is high in sugar, sodium and lots of preservatives like MSG. Here is a healthy version of this delicious sauce:

INGREDIENTS

¼ cup of tamari or shoyu

¼ cup of molasses, yacon syrup or erythritol

1 star anise

4 garlic cloves, minced

1 piece of fresh ginger, minced

METHOD

In a pan, heat up all of the ingredients until the molasses dissolves. If you wish to thicken, use a little kuzu or Agar Agar.

You can keep this in the fridge and use in your dishes.

Korean San Choy Bau Cups

QUINOA MINCE OR BEEF

These can be made completely vegan or with grass-fed beef or even organic chicken or turkey mince.
They are absolutely divine and super healthy.

INGREDIENTS

8 to 10 butter lettuce leaves or similar

2 garlic cloves

1 knob of ginger

2 limes, juiced

1 tablespoon of gochujang sauce

2 tablespoons of olive or peanut oil

1 tablespoon of maple syrup, coconut nectar or stevia

2 tablespoons of tamari or fish sauce

QUINOA MINCE

½ cup of quinoa, 2 cloves of minced garlic, 2 deseeded and finely diced red chilli, a bunch of diced coriander, 2 tablespoons of tamari, ½ teaspoon of Celtic sea salt, 1 lime squeezed

PICKLED VEGETABLES

2 tablespoons of rice vinegar, 2 teaspoons of coconut sugar or maple syrup, ½ teaspoon of Celtic sea salt – mix together in a bowl. Add radishes, carrot, cabbage, cucumber or chilli, cover and refrigerate for 1 hour. You now have yummy pickled vegetables.

GRASS-FED RIB EYE

sliced into thin slices

METHOD

1. Place lettuce cups onto each plate. Add pickled vegetables to each cup.

2. Use a food processor to blend garlic, ginger, lime juice, natural sweetener, tamari or fish sauce and gochujang sauce. If you want it hotter, add some chopped chilli at the end.

3. If you eat meat, marinate your grass-fed organic beef in this mix for 15 to 30 minutes.

4. If you are using quinoa mince, rinse the quinoa and add to a pot with extra water, bring to the boil and then simmer for around 15 minutes or until the quinoa looks fluffy. Drain and let dry. Mix through the other ingredients. To make the mince crunchy, spread on a tray and toast in the oven for twenty minutes or dehydrate. Now you have a yummy vegan mince. Place the vegan mince into the lettuce cups with pickled vegetables and top with coriander, bean sprouts and drizzle with the Korean sauce.

5. If you are using the beef, quickly pan fry the beef keeping tender and add to the lettuce cups with the same topping and drizzle with this yummy sauce. Add picked vegetables. Enjoy.

Superfood Powers

This dish is a perfect and satisfying weight loss dish that provides all the perfect ingredients to make hyaluronic acid for a plumper skin. The quinoa mince is rich in protein, minerals and flavonoids, which enhances your metabolism, skin vitality and hair growth.

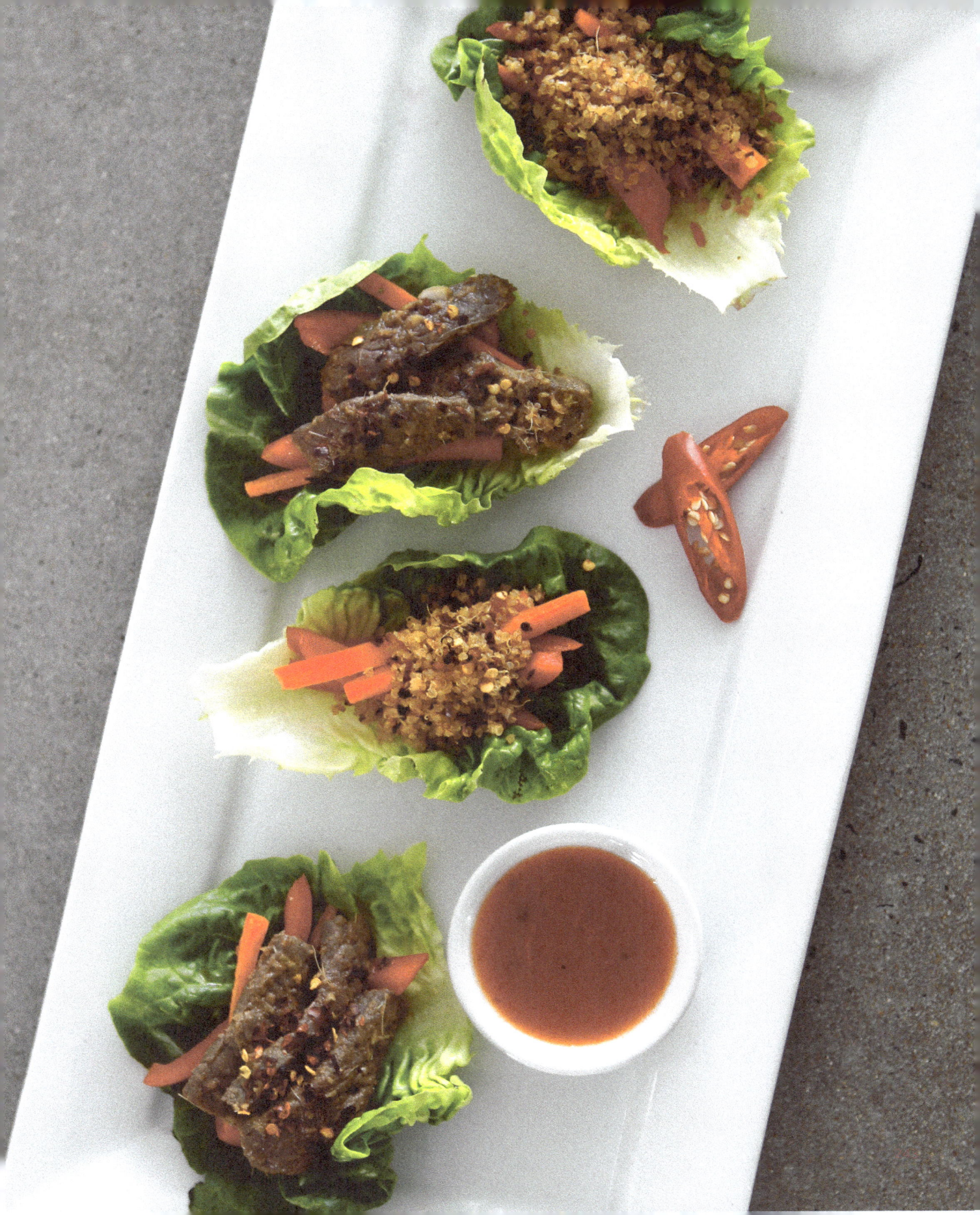

Eating well is Self love

Malaysian Satay Kelp Noodles

SERVES 3 TO 4

INGREDIENTS

1 packet of kelp or Konjac Noodles (or vegetable noodles if eating raw)

2 carrots, diced

2 shallots or scallions, diced

1 cup of cabbage, shredded

10 greens beans, diced

A handful of broccoli florets, diced

¼ cup of black sesame seeds

2 limes, cut into wedges

DRESSING

3 tablespoons of almond butter
or 1 cup of organic almonds (soaked)

2 tablespoons of tamari

2 tablespoons of apple cider or rice vinegar

2 small red chillies, deseeded and finely chopped

3 tablespoons of sesame oil

1 tablespoon of maple syrup, raw honey
(or monkfruit syrup if eating ketogenic)

1 clove of garlic

1 knob of ginger

Hot water

METHOD

Process almond butter, tamari, chilli, ginger, vinegar, garlic, natural sweetener and hot water in a food processor to create this delicious satay sauce. If you are eating 100% raw, simply place chopped vegetables into bowls with zucchini noodles and mix the satay sauce through. If using kelp noodles, soak in hot water for ten minutes until soft and mix through the mix.

If you want this dish cooked, put chopped vegetables into a wok with a little peanut or sesame oil and stir the satay sauce through as you heat vegetables. Serve on plates with torn coriander and toasted almonds. This satay sauce is also the perfect marinade for tempeh. Marinate the tempeh for 30 minutes in this sauce and bake, dehydrate or quickly cook and serve with the vegetables.

Superfood Powers

This dish is packed with Vitamins A, C, E and D, zinc, magnesium, manganese, copper and healthy oils to nourish the beauty of your skin, eyes and hair

Nasu Dengaku with a Twist

I first tried this dish when I visited Japan and loved it straight away. I have created a much healthier version of this delicious dish with some ultimate beauty-enhancing qualities.

SERVES 3 TO 4

INGREDIENTS

4 to 6 eggplants, skinned and chopped into squares

4 tablespoons of olive oil

3 spring onions

1 tablespoon of miso

2 tablespoons of mirin

2 tablespoons of sesame oil

1 tablespoon of coconut sugar, monkfruit syrup or raw honey

Sake (optional) – make with the glaze

METHOD

1. Slice your eggplants in half. Score their flesh and brush with a little olive oil.

2. Place on a baking tray and cook at 180°C until flesh is tender or, if you following a raw diet, place in a dehydrator and cook until tender.

3. To make the glaze, combine mirin, miso and natural sweetener in a saucepan, adding the sesame oil as well. Remove the eggplants and brush the glaze onto these.

4. Place back in the oven and heat for around 4 minutes. The coating should be bubbling or continue to dehydrate with the glaze on top.

5. Serve with sesame seeds and chopped coriander.

Superfood Powers

Eggplants are rich in chlorogenic acid to guard against skin cancer and premature skin ageing. They are also rich in water and enzymes to help improve hair and nail growth.

Temple Tempeh with Garlic

SERVES 2 TO 3

INGREDIENTS

500 ml of hot water

500 grams of organic firm tofu or tempeh, chopped into small squares

6 tomatoes

1 head of bok choy or pak choi

2-3 garlic cloves, crushed

2 lemongrass sticks, finely chopped

2 limes, juiced

4 tablespoons of tamari

2 tablespoons of mirin or brown rice vinegar

2 tablespoons of chopped coriander

Temple Mix – 1 part Celtic salt, 1 part black pepper, 1 part garlic powder, 2 parts maple or monkfruit syrup

METHOD

1. Heat a large wok and add hot water, salt and vinegar and bring to the boil.

2. Add the tofu or tempeh and cook for 5 minutes. Then remove the tofu or tempeh and put on a board to cool.

3. If you want your tofu/tempeh crispy, cook with a little olive oil in a pan in batches and then set aside.

4. In another wok, add the tomatoes, lemongrass, tamari, lime juice, garlic and temple mix to make a delicious sauce.

5. Add the bok choy or any Asian greens in at the end. Sprinkle with chopped coriander.

This dish goes great with brown rice or cauliflower rice, if eating ketogenic.

Superfood Powers

I absolutely love tempeh – but when I mention the word to clients they grimace at the thought. This is simply because most people do not know how to marinate or cook tempeh properly. This dish should improve your love for tempeh. Tempeh is packed with protein, Vitamin K2 and B12 to help improve the beauty of the skin, and the health of your telomeres, slowing down skin ageing.

Japanese Curry

Curries are not native to Japanese cultures. In fact, Japanese people mostly use packet mixes from a box. I have created a much healthier version that still has that yummy Japanese curry taste, without the added preservatives and sodium.

INGREDIENTS

1 onion, diced

2 tablespoons of grated ginger

2 tablespoons of garlic, minced

2 tablespoons of olive oil

1 sweet potato, diced

¼ head of cauliflower, diced

1 carrot, diced

1 stick of celery, diced

Protein – organic chicken, tofu, tempeh or similar

1 tablespoon of curry powder

1 tablespoon of turmeric powder

1 teaspoon of Celtic salt

1 tablespoon of mirin or brown rice vinegar

2 cups of water

2 tablespoons of millet flour, Kuzu or Agar Agar
(to thicken the mix)

METHOD

1. In a pan sauté onion, ginger and garlic with olive oil until tender.

2. Add the vegetables and protein source and continue to sauté. Slowly add water and then stir in curry powder, turmeric, mirin, Celtic salt and more water.

3. Cook the vegetables in this liquid, adding tamari and mirin. When the vegetables are ready, add the natural thickener.

4. If you want to sweeten, use a little maple syrup, coconut nectar, monkfruit or stevia. Now you have a delicious and healthy version of a Japanese curry.

Superfood Powers

This is not the most nutritious dish, compared to some of my other creations, yet it is still high in Vitamins A, C, magnesium, manganese, zinc and anti-inflammatory ingredients found in the curry and turmeric. The cauliflower and sweet potato improves this dish's nutritional potential, helping to guard you against several forms of cancer and improving the hydration and elasticity of your skin.

Winter Greens Marinated in White Miso Sauce

SERVES 2 TO 3

INGREDIENTS

2 tablespoons of white miso paste

2 tablespoons of sesame seeds

2 tablespoons of brown rice vinegar or mirin

2 limes, squeezed

1 tablespoon of raw honey or monkfruit syrup
(if eating keto)

2 garlic cloves, minced

2 tablespoons of tamari

4 tablespoons of roasted sesame oil

4 florets of broccoli or broccolini

250 grams of organic tofu or tempeh or mushrooms,
diced into small cubes (optional)

4 spring onions, diced

1 carrot, diced

A handful of wombok or bok choy

METHOD

1. Chop up all of the vegetables. Mix together mirin, natural sweetener, lime juice, garlic, tamari, sesame oil and white miso paste.

2. Place vegetables and tofu, tempeh or mushrooms a wok with a little peanut oil, and add the miso sauce.

3. Cook quickly before greens wilt and serve on 3 plates with brown or cauliflower rice, quinoa or alone.

Superfood Powers

I love miso so much, especially Shiro miso! Miso is a fermented soybean paste that is incredibly healthy. It is a natural prebiotic that improves digestion, encourages the removal of toxins from your body and protects you against radiation. Broccoli and bok choy are amazing indole-rich vegetables that guard against several forms of cancer while adding a beautiful glow to the skin.

GIFTS FROM THE Sea

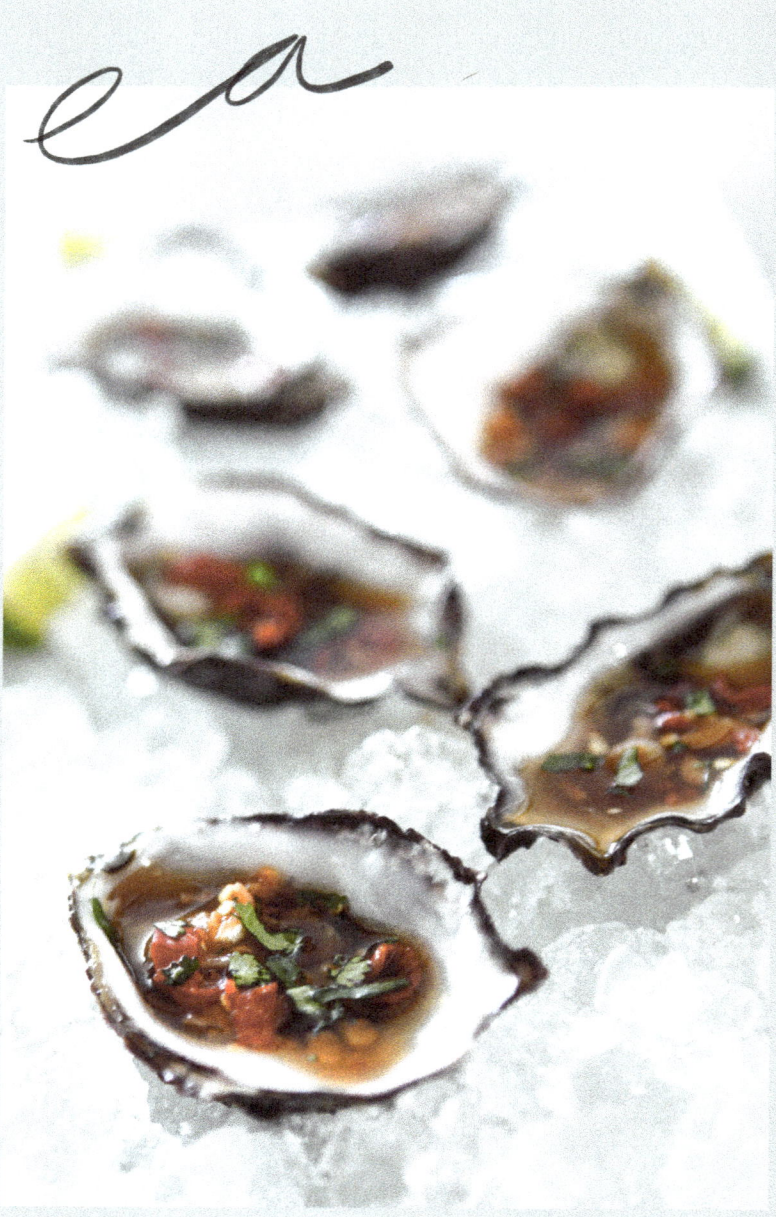

Oysters in Chilli, Coriander and Tamari Marinade

SERVES 2 (DEPENDING ON HOW MUCH YOU LOVE OYSTERS)

INGREDIENTS

12 local, fresh oysters – or as many as you like

2 fresh limes, juiced

4 tablespoons of tamari or fish sauce

6 red chillies, deseeded and finely diced

4 tablespoons of brown rice vinegar

1 teaspoon of coconut nectar, monkfruit or maple syrup

3 garlic cloves, minced

1 bunch of coriander, finely chopped

METHOD

1. This is a very simple dish to create, but super healthy and festive for dinner parties.

2. Chill the oysters on ice. Simply mix lime juice, sugar, tamari, minced garlic and rice vinegar in a bowl. Add the finely chopped coriander and chilli pieces to make a pretty sauce. Pour a little of this mix into each oyster cup.

3. Serve with the chilled oysters. Eat straight away.

Superfood Powers

Oysters are one of the healthiest skin foods on the planet. They are incredibly rich in zinc, protein and other nutrients which boosts libido, energy, mood and collagen repair. They are also packed with Omega oils enhance the beauty of your hair, skin and nails.

Evie-Ray's Crispy-skinned Salmon with Chermoula Rub

SERVES 3 TO 4

INGREDIENTS

4 pieces of salmon fillets with the skin on

2 tablespoons of first cold pressed olive oil

1 teaspoon of Himalayan/Celtic sea salt

CHERMOULA RUB

1 cup of parsley

1 cup of coriander leaves

2 cloves of garlic

1 teaspoon of cumin

1 teaspoon of coriander seeds

½ teaspoon of paprika

½ teaspoon of cayenne

1 tablespoon of lemon juice

1 tablespoon of olive oil

½ cup of sheep's, Greek or another type of yoghurt

METHOD

1. In a food processor, process parsley, coriander, garlic, paprika, cayenne, cumin, oil and lemon juice. Stir in the yoghurt and add some Celtic salt for flavour.

2. Coat the salmon with Celtic sea salt and olive oil. Place in a pan with the skin down and cook for around 3 minutes or until you can see a crispy skin.

3. Then turn over and cook for another couple of minutes on the other side. Place on each plate and serve with torn coriander and chermoula rub.

4. For extra beauty potential, finely dice garlic cloves, chilli and coriander and quickly cook in a pan until crispy and sprinkle on top of each plate.

Superfood Powers

Chermoula is traditionally used as a rub for chicken or fish dishes, but it can also make a fantastic dip or sauce. It is incredibly healthy as parsley contains nutrients which strengthens the bones and teeth, flushes excess fluid from the body, improves kidney function and guards against sun-related skin ageing. Salmon is one of the healthiest fishes on planet earth, especially if it is wild and free to roam in clean waters. Salmon's omega 3 oils help to nourish the skin, hair and nails, reduce inflammation and protect against disease.

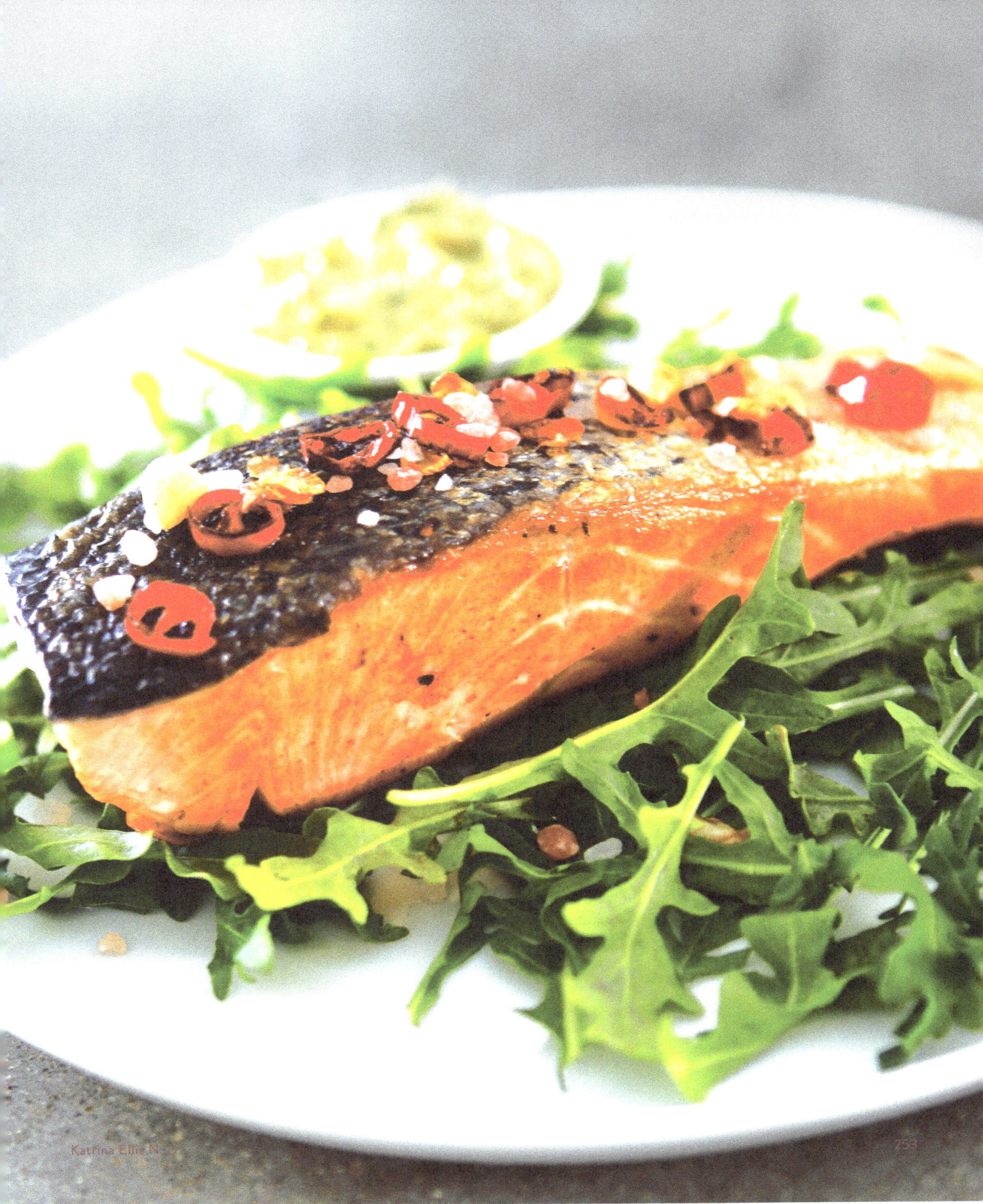

Snapper with Middle Eastern Spices

SERVES 4

INGREDIENTS

4 Goldband snapper or sea bass fillets

SPICE MIX

30 grams of roasted hazelnuts

30 grams of sesame seeds

1 tablespoon of garlic powder

1 tablespoon of cumin seeds

2 teaspoons of coriander seeds

2 teaspoons of smoked paprika

¼ teaspoon of turmeric

1 whole lime, squeezed

2 teaspoons of olive oil

1 teaspoon of Celtic sea salt

METHOD

1. If you have a Thermomix, heat the seeds for 3 minutes or alternatively place in a pan and cook for a few minutes. The seeds should begin to pop. Then place them in a mortar and pestle and grind them down.

2. Add this to a food processor with crushed hazelnuts, sesame seeds, Celtic salt, garlic, paprika and turmeric.

3. Now add the oil and lime to this mix to make a paste. Rub the fish with the paste and place in the fridge for twenty minutes.

4. Then put the fish on a baking dish and cook for 15 minutes or until tender, or place in pan and cook quickly with a little oil or ghee on each side. Serve with torn coriander and sesame seeds.

Superfood Powers

I love the spices in this dish as they help to protect against parasites, viruses and bacteria while boosting immunity and aiding weight loss. Hazelnuts contain all the nutrients you need to make serotonin, the body's happy hormone, and when you combine this with the DHA in fish you have an endorphin boosting-meal.

Marinated Sea Bass in Lime Salsa

SERVES 2 TO 4

INGREDIENTS

2 to 4 fresh ocean sea bass or snapper fillets

A pinch of Celtic sea salt

2 cloves garlic, minced or crushed

1 green chilli, minced

2 limes

Fresh coriander

Salsa

4 limes

½ onion

¼ teaspoon of olive oil

2 tomatoes

A handful of coriander leaves

1 red pepper

METHOD

1. To make the salsa, put lime juice and flesh, onion, olive oil, tomatoes, pepper and coriander in a processor. Keep slightly coarse. Let this sit for two hours.

2. Crush garlic, chilli and coriander together and rub along the fish slices.

3. Pour the juice and zest of limes on the fish with a little Celtic sea salt. Leave this to marinate.

4. Bake in the oven for twenty minutes or until ready or steam fish in a banana leaf with the marinade on top.

5. When fish is ready, spoon the salsa on top.

Superfood Powers

This salsa is packed full of Vitamin A, C and phytochemicals like lycopene, all designed to protect you against the damage of the sun's harmful UV rays. What a yummy way to provide a natural sunscreen.

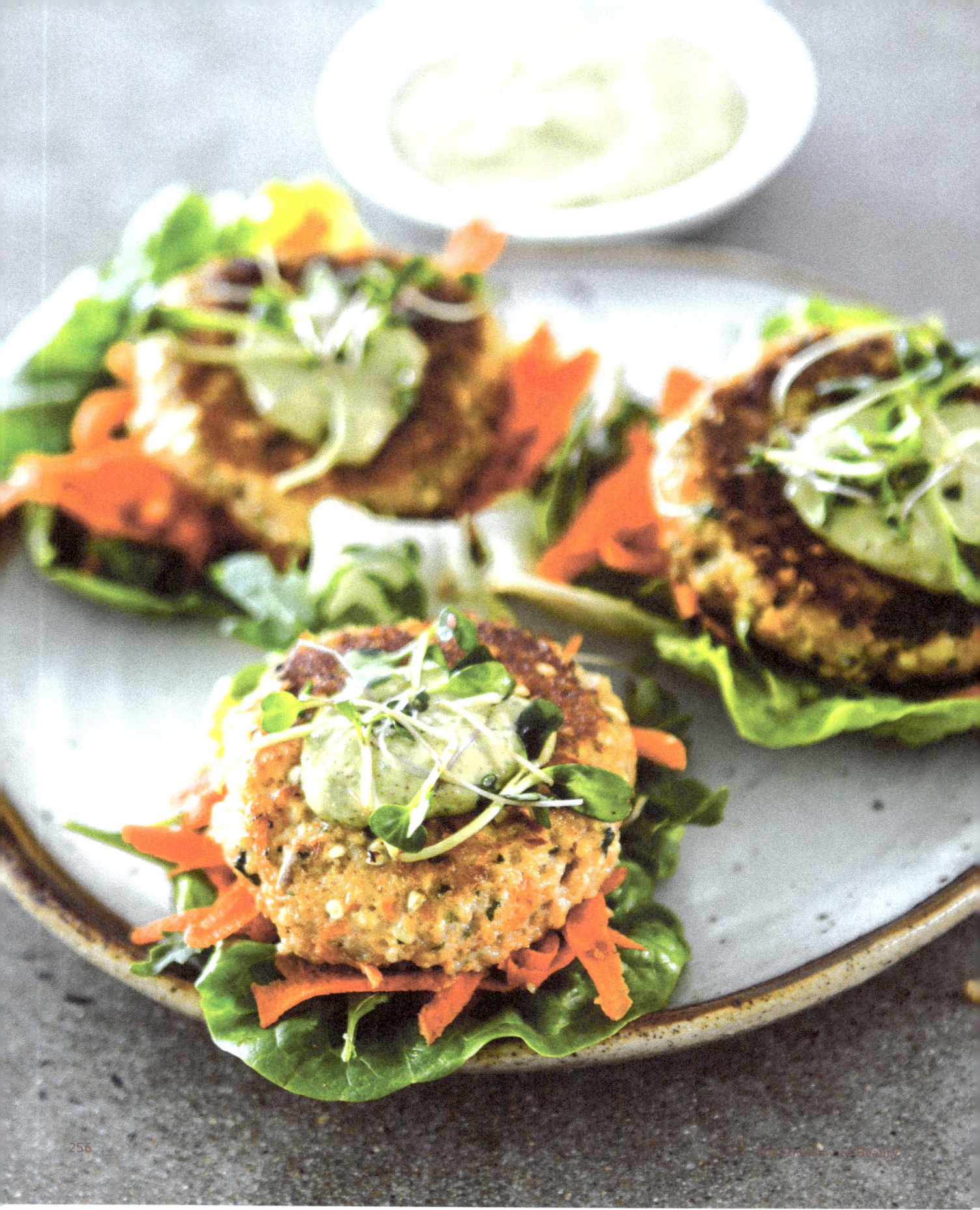

Thai Snapper Burgers with Green Tahini Sauce

SERVES 3 TO 4

INGREDIENTS

500 grams of snapper or mackerel fillets

½ to 1 cup of toasted buckwheat (if you don't have, use cooked buckwheat)

6 shallots, finely chopped

1 small zucchini, grated

1 purple carrot, grated (if you don't have use orange)

2 garlic cloves, crushed

1 organic egg

¼ cup of parsley

¼ mint or dill

2 Kaffir lime leaves

2 coriander leaves

2 chillies, chopped

1 teaspoon of Celtic sea salt

GREEN TAHINI SAUCE

¼ cup of tahini

A large handful of parsley

A large handful of coriander

1 lemon, juiced

2 cloves of garlic

2 tablespoons of olive oil

METHOD

1. In a food processor, pulse the fish to make a nice paste.

2. Add zucchini, herbs, carrot, onion, egg, garlic, chilli, coriander and salt and pulse until combined.

3. Mix in the toasted buckwheat. Roll into balls, flatten and place in the fridge on a tray for one hour.

4. If you want your snapper burgers crunchy you can roll them in rice crumbs.

5. To make the green tahini sauce, blend all of the ingredients together in a food processor. Cook the burgers either on a baking tray in the oven, on a dehydrator or in a little oil or ghee in a pan.

6. When ready, serve in lettuce cups with green tahini sauce drizzled over the top. I often eat these as a high protein snack during the day.

Superfood Powers

Fish is a fantastic source of Omega 3 fatty acids. These oils protect you against the inflammation that drives cancer, skin dehydration, ageing, arthritis and memory problems. The sauce is rich in antioxidants and minerals like magnesium and calcium, which calms your nerves, encourages beauty sleep and strengthens your bones and teeth.

Salmon or Tuna Tartare

SERVES 2 TO 3

INGREDIENTS

500 grams of fresh ocean salmon
or sashimi grade tuna

2 limes

2 shallots, chopped

2 tablespoons of parsley

1 cucumber

2 tablespoons of dill

2 tomatoes, diced

Lettuce cups

Celtic sea salt

METHOD

1. Cut fish into tiny cubes and mix with lime juice, shallots and parsley.

2. Dice tomatoes finely and add to the mix, along with dill.

3. Season the fish mixture with Celtic sea salt and fresh pepper. Chill in the fridge for 1 hour.

4. When ready, serve in lettuce cups or on cucumber ribbons.

Superfood Powers

Salmon and tuna are both fantastic sources of essential fatty acids, protein, Vitamin A and C, zinc and other minerals which improve skin hydration, energy, weight loss, inflammation and hormone balance.

Coconut and Lime Halibut Ceviche

MAKES 2 TO 3 GLASSES

INGREDIENTS

500 grams of halibut or mahi mahi

2 fresh limes, juiced

2 to 3 scallions, diced

½ cup of coconut cream

A handful of coriander, chopped

A handful of mint, chopped

1 avocado, cubed

Celtic sea salt

METHOD

1. Make sure any veins are removed from the fish and that it is cleaned beautifully.

2. Chop the fish into small 2 cm cubes. Juice the limes and add to coconut cream with the Celtic sea salt.

3. Place the fish into this mix and put into the fridge for 1 hour (some people do this for only 30 minutes, but you can marinate it for up to 2 hours). It will begin to turn white as it cooks in the juices.

4. In the meantime, finely dice the spring onions, coriander and mint and cube the avocado.

5. When the fish is ready mix together and divide into four cups or plates. Drizzle with lime juice and dress with chopped chilli.

Superfood Powers

Ceviche is incredibly healthy as it retains all of the ingredients' essential fatty content to nourish the hair, skin and nails. When you combine this dish with coriander, coconut cream and avocado you have a natural oil-rich treat that will make your skin glow with vitality.

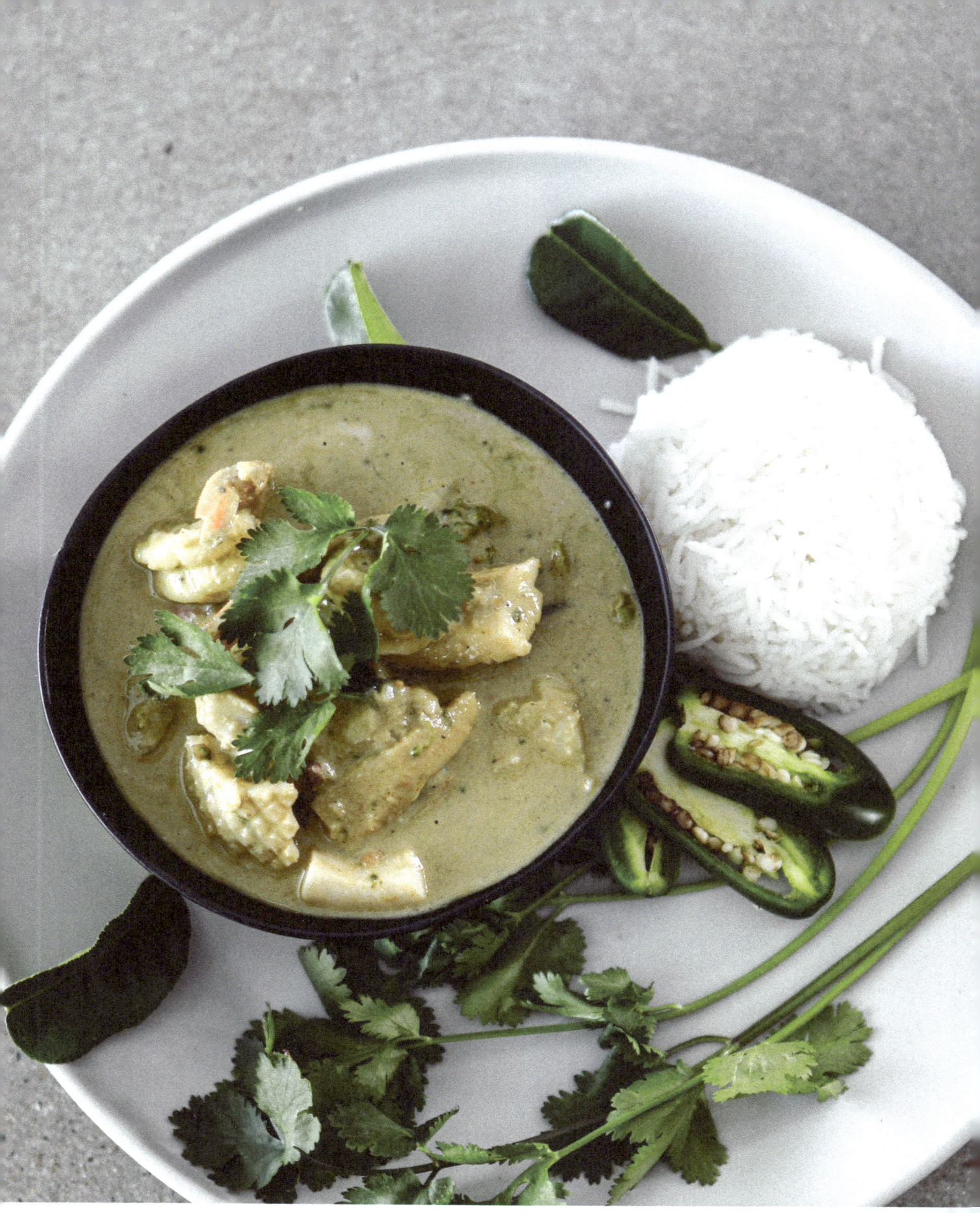

Thai Green Fish Curry

SERVES 3 TO 4

INGREDIENTS

400 grams of local whiting fillets

1 onion, diced

2 garlic cloves

8 green beans

400 ml of coconut milk or cream

1 tablespoon of fish sauce or tamari

GREEN CURRY PASTE

4 teaspoons of coriander seeds

2 teaspoons of peppercorns (green if you can get)

2 teaspoons of cumin seeds

2 spring onions or 1 red onion

1 coriander bunch, use the roots and stems

8 to 10 green chillies, deseeded and diced

2 tablespoons of galangal

4 garlic cloves

2 tablespoons of lime zest

2 tablespoons of shrimp paste

1 to 2 stalks of lemongrass, diced

METHOD

PASTE

Firstly make the paste. If you have a Thermomix, dice onion and garlic and then turn to 1 and sauté for 3 minutes. Then add the rest of the ingredients and place on 7 or 8 for 15 seconds or until you form a beautiful, green paste. This paste can be stored in the fridge for months. If you have a normal food processor, sauté onion and garlic in oil and when soft, add with the rest of the ingredients to the blender and puree until you get the perfect paste.

FISH CURRY

To make the fish curry, put a tablespoon of peanut oil into a pan and sauté the onion and garlic. When soft, add 2 tablespoons of your green curry paste, vegetable stock and coconut cream or milk. Simmer and add fish (cut into pieces), green beans, carrots and red capsicum. If you want this a little sweeter, add 1 tablespoon of maple syrup, stevia or coconut sugar (traditionally in Thailand they use palm sugar). Simmer on a low heat for ten minutes or until everything softens.

Place steamed jasmine, or brown rice, into bowls and serve the curry with torn coriander, Thai basil and bean sprouts. If you are a vegetarian, feel free to add any other protein source to this beautiful curry and if eating ketogenic use cauliflower rice or simply leave out.

Superfood Powers

I love a green curry and I love the spiciness of this one. Green curry paste is incredibly rich in capsaicin, a flavonoid that speeds up your metabolism, encourages the removal of toxins and heavy metals, and guards against the free radical damage that causes skin ageing and cancer.

Prawn Tamarind

SERVES 3 TO 4

INGREDIENTS

12 banana prawns, peeled and deveined

1 tablespoon of sesame, peanut or rice bran oil

1 tablespoon of crushed garlic

1 tablespoon of crushed shallots

TAMARIND SAUCE

2 tablespoons of tamarind paste or 20g of tamarind pulp

4 tablespoons of hot water

2 tablespoons of fish sauce or tamari

2 stalks of lemongrass, chopped finely

1 tablespoon of coconut sugar or maple syrup

METHOD

1. Mix tamarind, fish sauce or tamari, water, natural sweetener and lemongrass in a blender.

2. To cook the prawns, heat in a wok with crushed garlic and shallots, turn them over.

3. When they start to cook, add the tamarind mix. Garnish with spring onions and coriander.

Superfood Powers

Just like oysters, prawns are incredibly rich in zinc, magnesium, calcium, iron, Vitamin A, iodine and B vitamins, which help to help nourish the skin, hair and nails and to uplift the mood, improve sleep and relax the muscles.

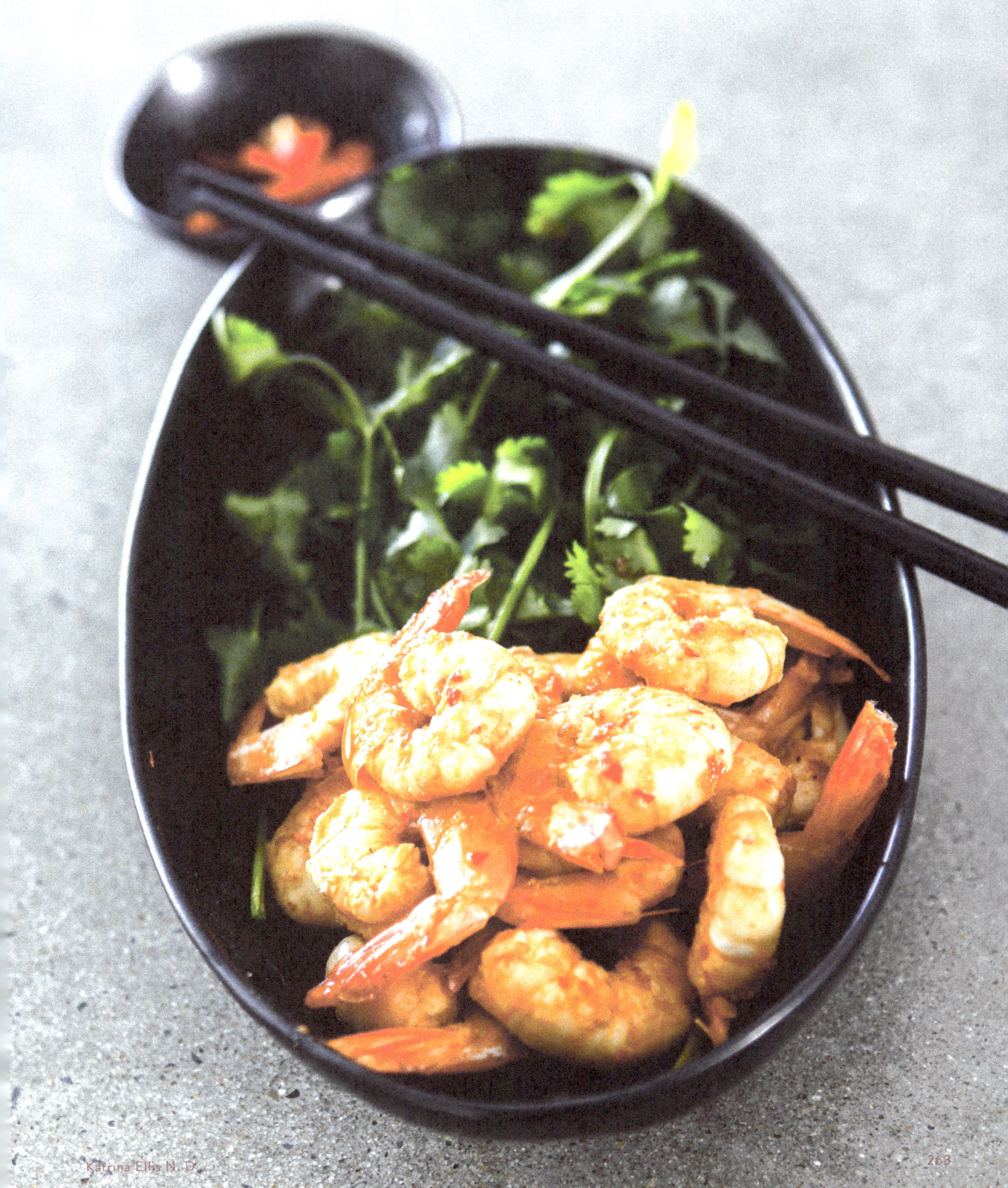

Steamed Snapper in Garlic, Chilli and Lime

SERVES 4

INGREDIENTS

4 local Goldband snapper fillets or the whole fish (scaled)

6 garlic cloves, diced finely

1 knob of ginger, minced

6 small red chilli peppers, diced

1 tablespoon of coriander

3 tablespoons of fish sauce or tamari

1 teaspoon of coconut nectar

¼ cup of lime juice

¼ cup of chicken or vegetable stock or broth

METHOD

1. Firstly crush the garlic, ginger and chilli in a mortar and pestle, adding a little lime to make a paste.

2. Cut small slashes into the fish and place the mix into these slits. In a bowl, blend garlic, chilli, coriander, tamari, natural sweetener, lime, ginger and stock to make the sauce.

3. Pour half of this sauce over the fish and steam in a banana leaf or in a steamer, until cooked. When the fish is ready, place evenly onto plates with torn coriander, fried garlic and chilli and extra ginger and lime sauce.

Superfood Powers

Snapper is high in Vitamin A and protein, zinc and healthy omega oils. If you want an even healthier fish, feel free to swap the snapper for an oilier fish like mackerel, herring, halibut or another.

Gingered Lime Prawns

SERVES 3

INGREDIENTS

12 banana prawns (or tempeh if you are a vegetarian)

2 to 4 tablespoons of fish sauce or tamari,
shoyu or Bragg's aminos

3 tablespoons of brown rice vinegar

2 limes, juiced

4 garlic cloves

4 small red chillies, diced

3 tablespoons of toasted sesame oil

3 cm chunk of ginger

METHOD

1. Peel and devein the prawns, leaving the tails on.

2. Blend all of the marinating ingredients together in a food processor to make a delicious sauce.

3. The prawns can either sit in this mix overnight, or for a few hours.

4. Cook prawns in a heated wok or pan on both sides (don't over cook them) and serve with stir fried miso greens, or a delicious salad.

Almond, Garlic and Cumin-crusted Snapper

SERVES 2

INGREDIENTS

2 fillets of snapper or another fish

1 cup of organic almonds

2 garlic cloves

1 teaspoon of cumin

A pinch of Celtic sea salt

1 tablespoon of olive oil

1 teaspoon of garlic powder

Black pepper

METHOD

1. Blend almonds, garlic, cumin, salt, olive oil and pepper in a food processor until you get a nice crumb. Place in a bowl and mix with a bit more olive oil.

2. Coat your fish with this almond mix (it also tastes great with macadamia nuts) and bake in the oven for 15 minutes or in a pan with a healthy oil or ghee.

3. Serve with fresh lemon juice and salad.

Superfood Powers

Almonds are incredibly healthy with their rich mineral, vitamin, antioxidant and Omega oil content. When you combine this with cumin and garlic cloves, you have a great anti-bacterial, immune boosting dish that provides some incredible beauty and healthy promoting gifts.

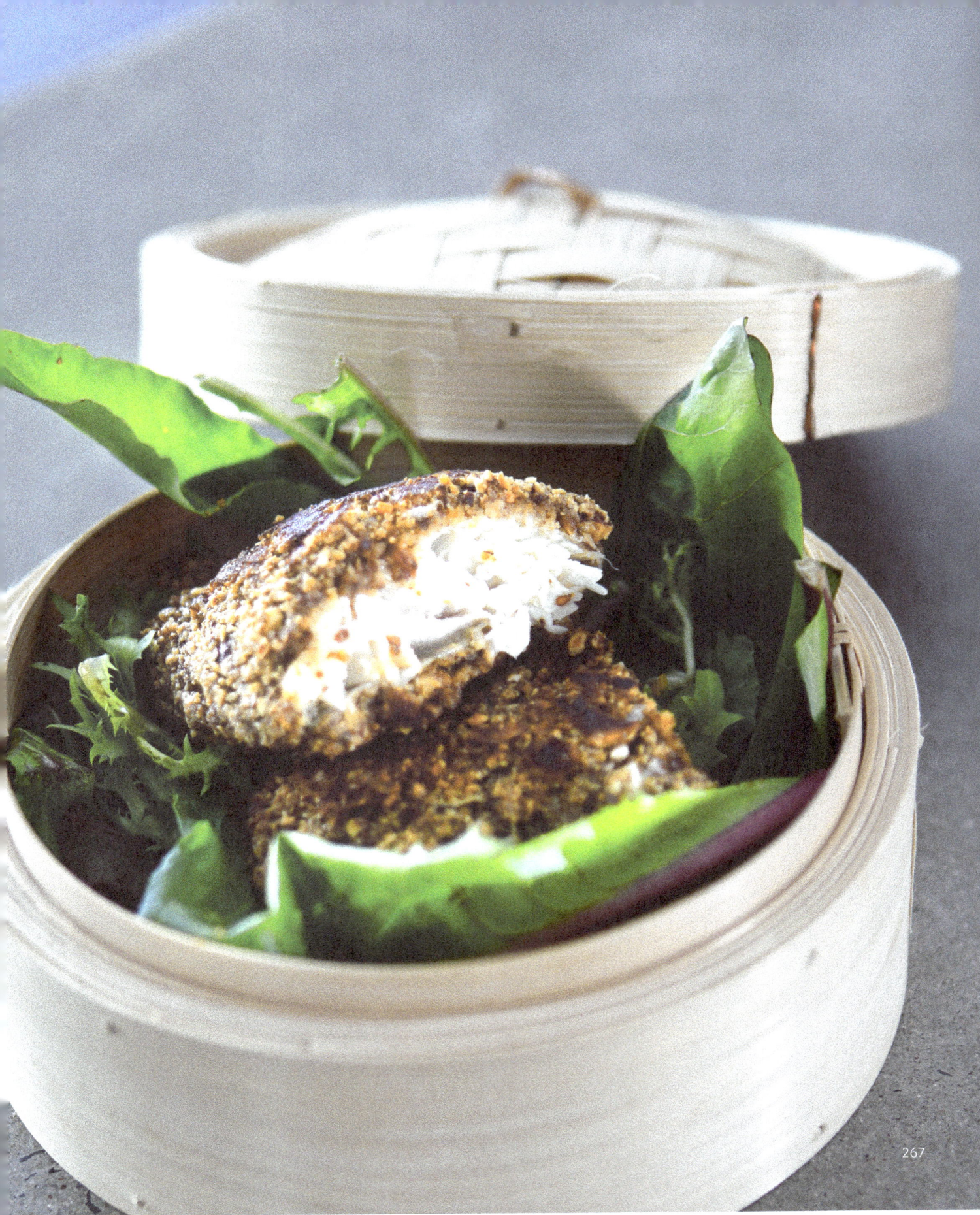

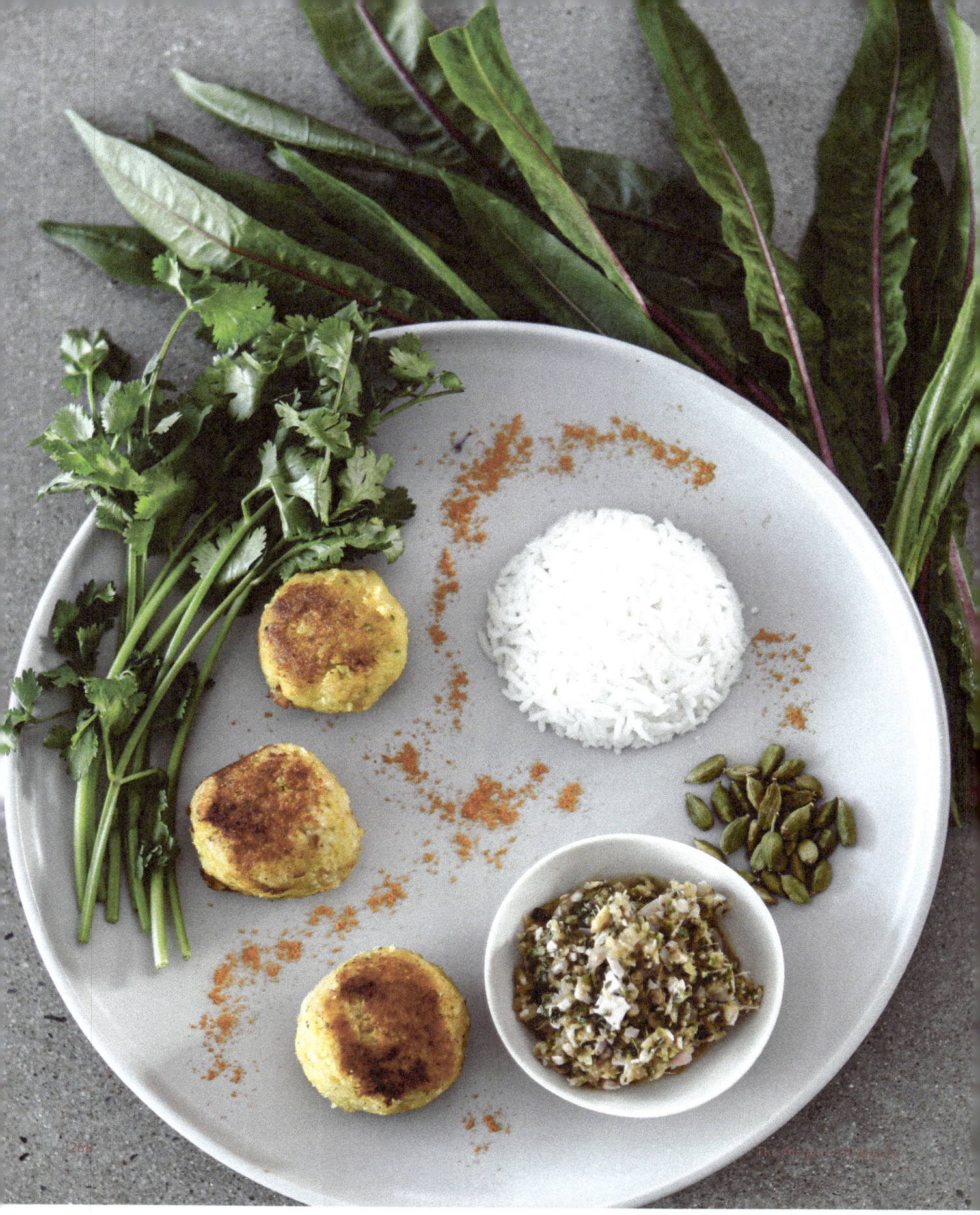

Spiced Sri Lankan Fish Balls with Sambal

SERVES 3 TO 4

INGREDIENTS

400 grams of snapper, kingfish or another white fish

½ cup of rice bread crumbs

3 sweet potatoes

1 teaspoon of cumin seeds

1 teaspoon of mustard seeds

1 tablespoon of ginger powder

1 tablespoon of turmeric powder

½ teaspoon of black pepper

2 green chillies, chopped

1 teaspoon of cardamom seeds

1 teaspoon of cumin

METHOD

1. Cut the snapper or other fish into squares.

2. Cut and steam sweet potato. You can also use parsnip, swede or normal potato.

3. Heat the cardamon and mustard seeds in a pan until they pop and add cold to a food processor or Thermomix with the fish, ginger, cumin, turmeric, chilli and black pepper.

4. Add rice crumbs, flaxseed or almond meal to bind nicely and more spices if you want extra flavour. If you wish you can add a raw egg to bind it, but it doesn't always need this.

5. Quickly pan fry with a healthy oil. If you want a crunchy outside, roll in quinoa or rice crumbs and then fry.

Superfood Powers

This would have to be one of my favourite dishes. When I first visited the Maldives, a beautiful Sri Lankan chef taught me the art of making this traditional dish. These fish balls are so easy to make and are super delicious. The sambal in the condiments section is a perfect accompaniment with these fish balls.

Lemongrass Yellow Prawn Curry

SERVES 2 TO 3

INGREDIENTS

12 green banana prawns

4 shallots, chopped

1 red capsicum, diced

8 green beans

YELLOW CURRY PASTE

2 curry leaves or 1 tablespoon of curry powder

1 tablespoon of turmeric

1 teaspoon of ground coriander

3 yellow chillies, sliced
(or red chilli if you can't find these)

3 garlic cloves, diced

1 stalk of lemongrass, diced

4 shallots, diced

½ teaspoon of shrimp paste
(or a fermented bean paste if vegan)

1 knob of galangal or ginger, diced

1 tablespoon of tomato puree

2 tablespoons of fish sauce or tamari

2 tablespoons of coconut sugar or monkfruit syrup

Coconut milk

METHOD

PASTE

To make the yellow curry paste, simply blend all of the curry ingredients together in a food processor until you get a nice mix, adding coconut milk if needed.

Store this in a jar in the fridge for up to 2 weeks. This is a quick version. The longer version involves roasting the spices and then blending them to make a paste.

CURRY

1. To make this delicious curry, saute onion and garlic in a pan until soft, add 2 tablespoons of yellow curry paste and then the coconut milk or cream.

2. Slowly add the vegetables and begin to cook. Peel and devein the green banana prawns (I leave the tails on) and throw into the curry mix at the end.

3. Cook for around ten minutes. Now you have a delicious yellow prawn curry!

This curry can be made vegan by replacing prawns with sweet potato, Shiitake mushrooms or any other vegetable.

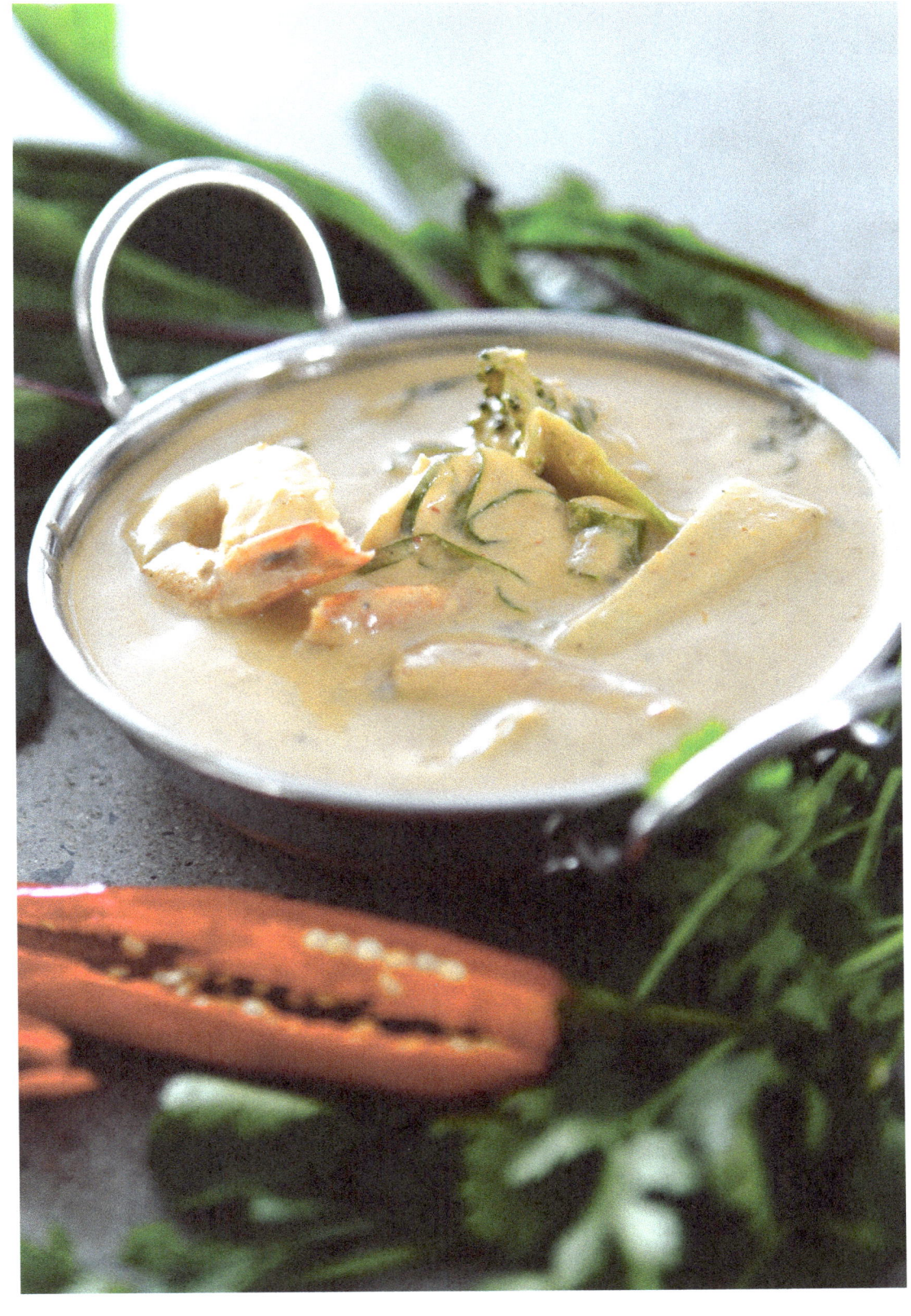

Sweet

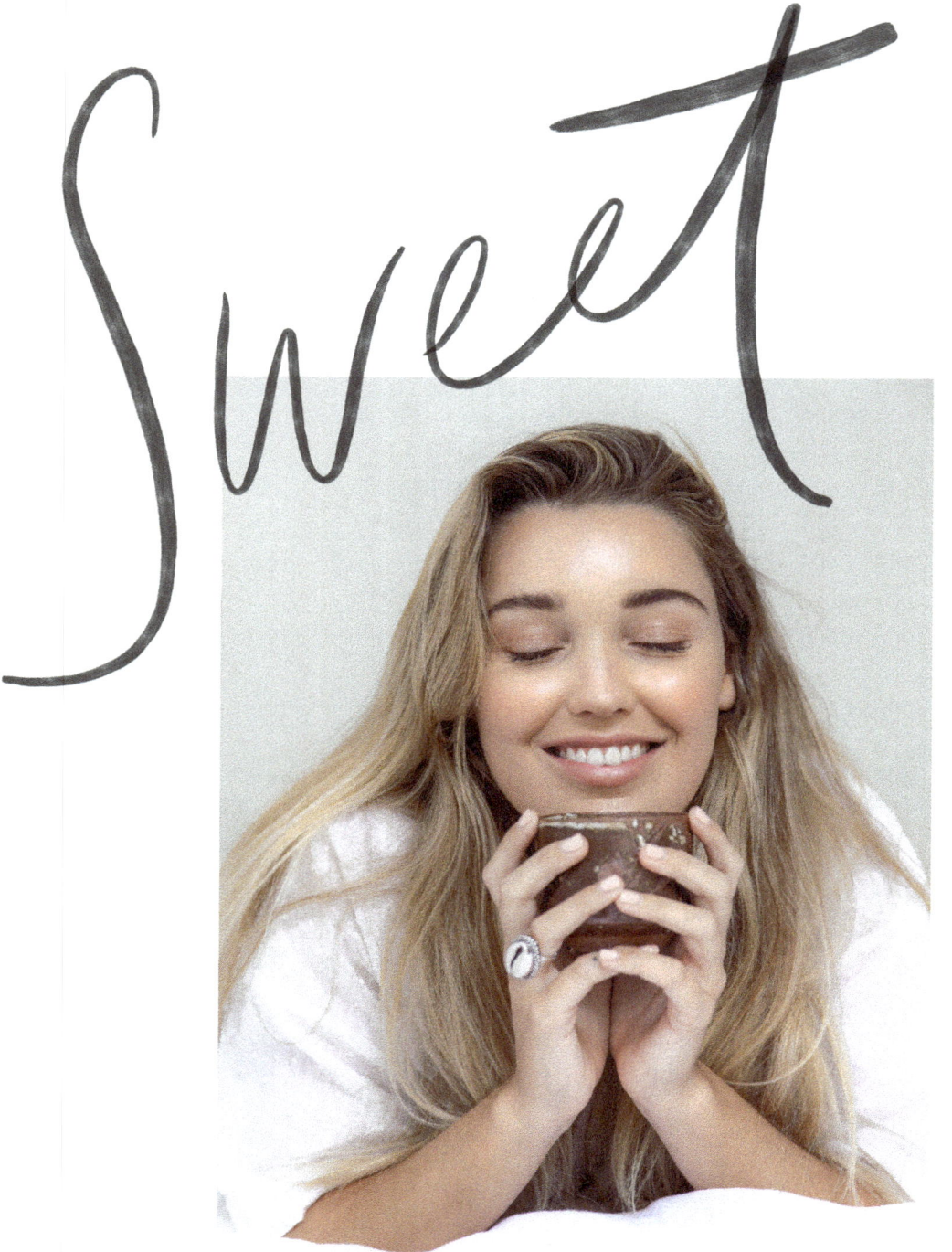

TREATS

The Alchemy of Beauty

Matcha Raw Cheesecake

MAKES 1 SMALL CAKE

INGREDIENTS

2 cups of raw almonds

½ cup of flaxseed meal

1 cup of coconut flakes

8 Medjool dates, chopped

¾ cup of coconut cream

3 cups of macadamia or cashews, soaked

2 teaspoons of matcha powder

½ cup of coconut or avocado oil

½ cup of maple or monkfruit syrup, raw honey or coconut nectar

METHOD

1. To make the base blend almonds, flaxseed meal and coconut flakes in a food processor, slowly adding in the dates.

2. Press this mixture into a glass pan and place in the fridge to set.

3. Soak nuts for at least 2 hours, blend with sweetener, oil and cream.

4. Add the Matcha in at the end.

5. Pour this mix over the base. Place in the fridge to set.

Superfood Powers

Matcha is a powdered green tea that is 150 times higher in natural polyphenols than most green tea, making it an incredible health promoting superfood. Matcha helps to burn fat, improves your digestion, protects against skin cancer and boosts energy.

Kaia's Raw Caramel Slice

MAKES 1 SMALL TRAY

BASE

¾ cup of almonds

1 cup of medjool dates

½ to 1 cup of coconut oil

CARAMEL LAYER

2 cups of cashews or macadamia (pre-soaked)

½ cup of maple, monkfruit or yacon syrup

⅓ cup of water

CHOCOLATE LAYER

¼ cup of coconut oil or cacao butter (melted)

¼ cup of maple or monkfruit syrup or medjool dates

¼ cup of cacao powder

1 teaspoon of vanilla

A pinch of Himalayan or Celtic salt

METHOD

1. Place all of the base ingredients into a food processor and blend.

2. Press mixture into a tray with your fingers, flattening as you go.

3. Place in the freezer for 1 hour to set. Now place all of the caramel layer ingredients into your food processor, adding water to get the right texture.

4. Pour this layer over the top of the base and place back in the freezer for 1 hour.

5. Finally, melt the coconut oil and blend with sweetener, cacao, vanilla and Celtic sea salt for the chocolate layer.

6. Pour over the top of the set caramel layer. Place in the fridge or freezer and wait for another hour to set. It will be ready to serve.

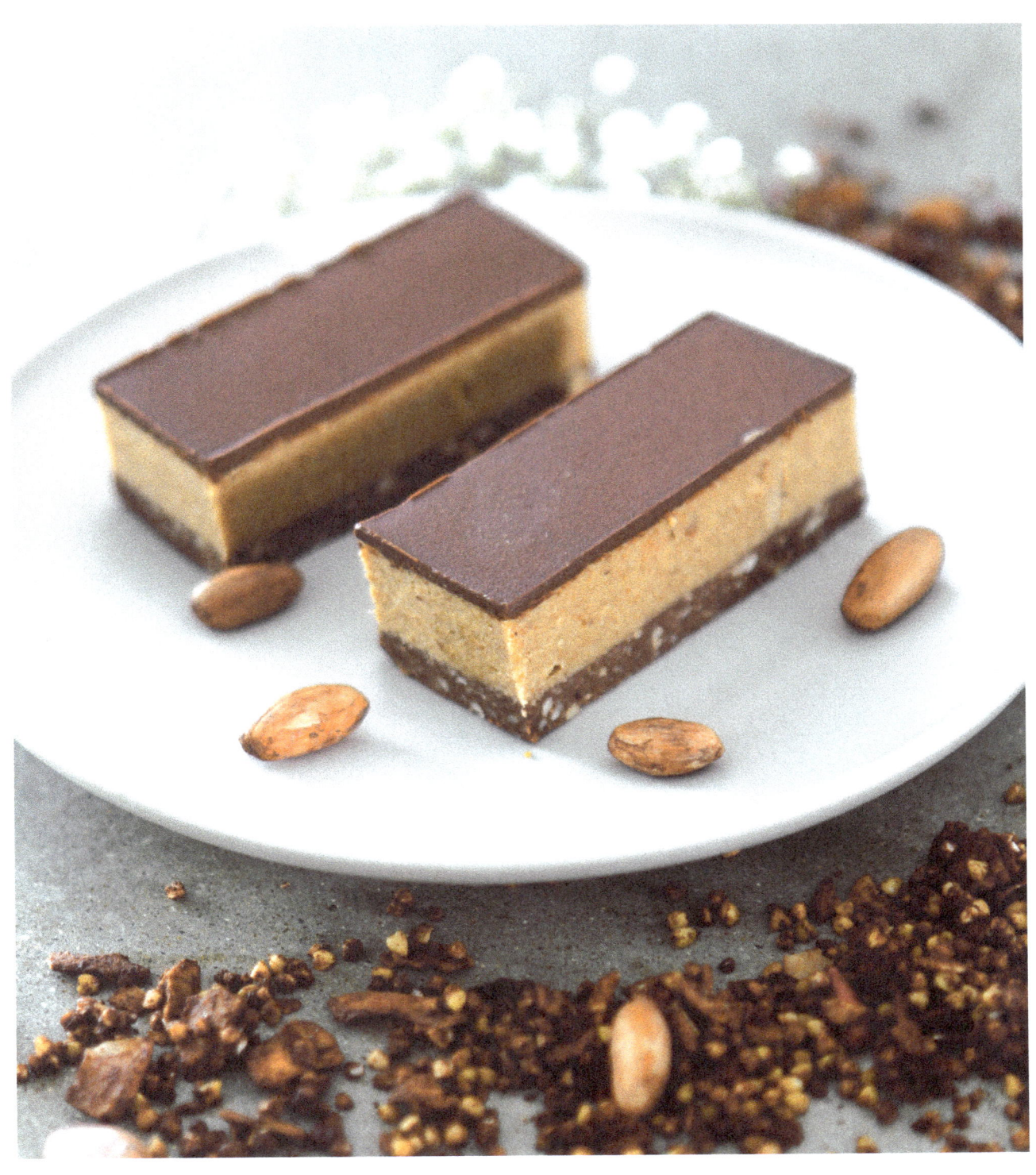

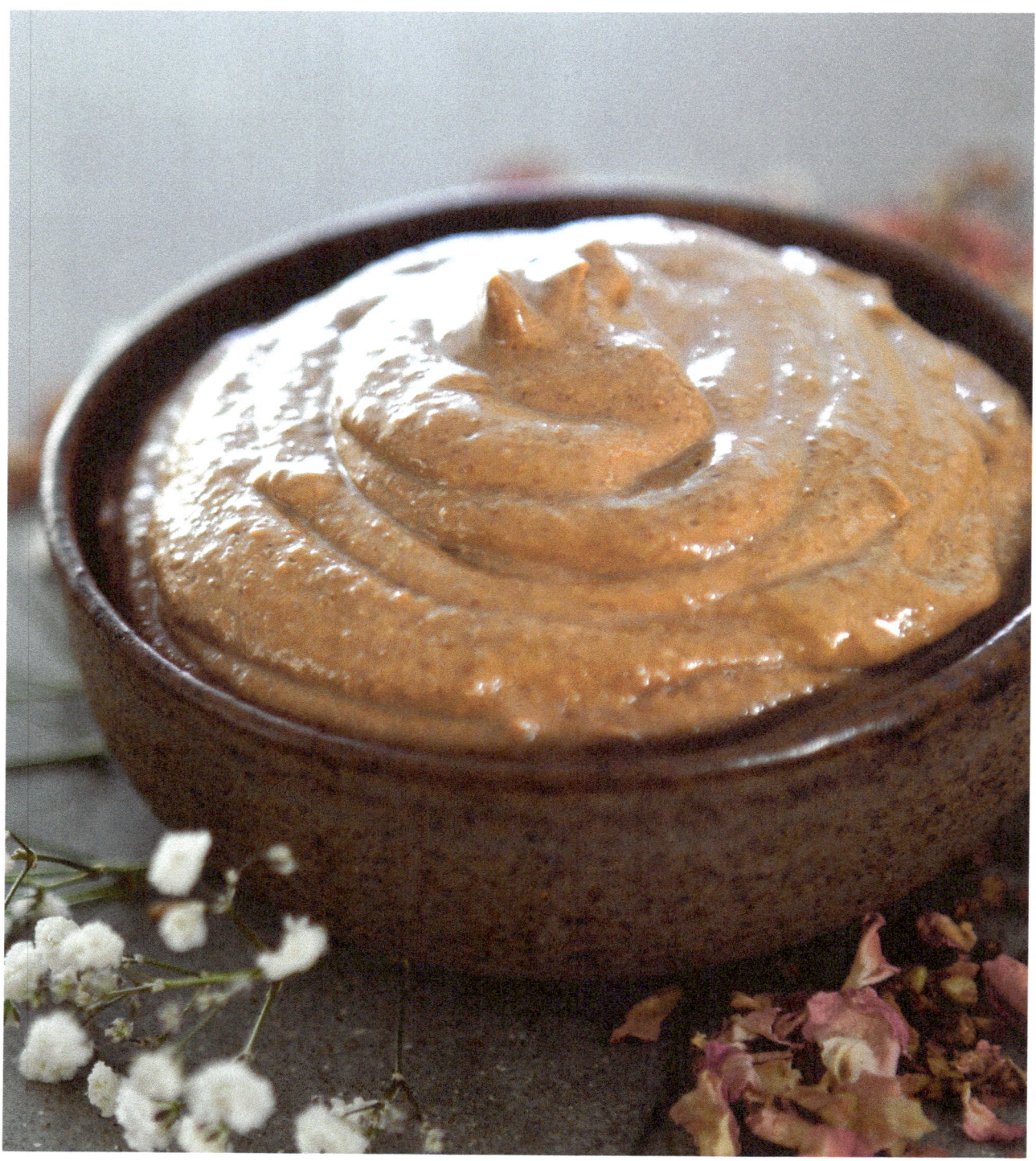

The Alchemy of Beauty

Teff Antioxidant Choc Mousse

MAKES 2 LARGE GLASSES

INGREDIENTS

2 large ripe avocados

¼ to ½ cup of maple syrup or another natural sweetener

¾ cup of coconut cream or coconut meat

½ cup of cooked teff

¼ cup of cacao or carob powder

1 teaspoon of vanilla essence

Chopped pistachios, cacao nibs and fresh mint

METHOD

1. Put ½ cup of teff into a pan with around 2 cups of water, bring to the boil and simmer for around 15 to 20 minutes.

2. Remove from heat and strain with water. It should be nice and fluffy. Now place into a food processor or Thermomix with avocado and coconut cream and blend.

3. Slowly add the rest of the ingredients until you get a nice, smooth consistency.

4. Pour into 2 glasses and either eat straight away or set in the fridge. Sprinkle some coconut flakes and cacao nibs on top or anything else you wish.

Superfood Powers: Teff is a gluten free protein rich grain often eaten in African cultures. For a little grain it is incredibly rich in nutritional value. It contains 8 amino acids, including lysine, which helps your body repair old cells and replace them with new ones. Because of its rich mineral content, it can strengthen bones, teeth and connective tissues too.

Raw Cacao Orange Cheesecake

MAKES 1 TIN

CRUST

1 cup of almonds (soak for 2 to 4 hours)

¼ cup of cacao powder

1 cup of dates

FILLING

4 oranges, juiced (plus lots of rind)

2/3 cup of maple, monkfruit or yacon syrup

2 ½ cups of cashews (soak for 2 to 4 hours)

½ cup of coconut butter

METHOD

1. Combine all of the crust ingredients in a food processor and blend It should stick together nicely. Add a little water if it doesn't. Place in the fridge to set for one hour.

2. Now grate the zest of the oranges. Squeeze the juice out of the oranges. Place cashews, syrup, coconut butter and orange juice and zest into a food processor and blend until smooth.

3. Pour over the crust and let this set in the fridge for 4 hours or alternatively, freeze. Feel free to replace oranges with mango, blueberries or raspberries for different taste and healing qualities.

Superfood Powers

Oranges are a fantastic source of Vitamin C and over 60 different flavonoids including limonene which helps to protect against several forms of cancer including melanoma and premature skin ageing.

Carob and Goldenberry Probiotic Slice

MAKES 1 SMALL TIN

INGREDIENTS

2 to 3 teaspoons of your favourite multi-strain probiotic powder

½ cup of grated coconut or fresh coconut meat

½ cup of goldenberries

¾ cup of carob powder (if you don't like carob use cacao at ½ cup)

½ cup of sunflower seeds (pre-soaked for 2 hours)

½ cup of pumpkin seeds (pre-soaked for 2 hours)

1 cup of almonds (pre-soaked for 2 hours)

¼ cup of maple syrup, Yacon or another natural sweetener

4 Medjool dates

3 tablespoons of coconut oil

METHOD

1. In a food processor blend berries, maple syrup, seeds, nuts and dates.

2. Melt coconut oil and mix with grated coconut and carob powder. Blend both mixes together.

3. Pour into a greaseproof dish, flatten down and place into the fridge to set. When it is firm, cut into slices.

4. To pump up the nutritional profile of this slice add a super berry, collagen or vegan protein powder.

Superfood Powers

Carob is often forgotten in the world of superfoods. It is a natural anti-bacterial, anti-viral and antioxidant that is brilliant for tummy upsets, particularly loose bowel motions. It is a good source of selenium, (a powerful antioxidant that guards against skin ageing) and contains over twenty polyphenols which help to guard against cancer too.

Raw Choc Hazelnut Creams

MAKES 4 BIG CREAMS

BASE

1 cup of almond meal

½ cup of almonds

2 tablespoons of cacao powder

¼ cup of cacao butter or coconut oil

½ cup of Yacon, monkfruit or maple syrup,
raw honey or Medjool dates

MIDDLE

2 to 3 soft bananas

1 teaspoon of stevia leaf powder or 4 tablespoons
of maple or monkfruit syrup

½ to 1 cup of soaked hazelnuts

1 teaspoon of vanilla essence

TOP LAYER

½ cup of cocoa powder

½ cup of cacao powder

1 avocado

½ cup of maple, monkfruit or yacon syrup
or a few drops of stevia

1 teaspoon of pure vanilla extract

1 tablespoon of Lucuma powder

4 tablespoons of cacao butter
or coconut oil (melted – optional)

METHOD

1. Blend all of the base ingredients in a food processor or Thermomix. It should have a dough-like consistency. Press into a small pan and let this chill in the fridge or freezer for one hour.

2. Now blend all of the middle layer ingredients together in a processor until you get a nice creamy texture. Pour this over the base layer and put back into the fridge or freezer to set.

3. Finally, blend all of the ingredients of the top layer together in a food processor until you get a creamy consistency. If you want this to set harder, add the cacao butter or coconut oil.

4. Place on top of the hazelnut layer and let this set in the fridge or freezer for another hour.

5. Now take out and cut into circles or squares and you have the healthiest, most delicious, triple-layered hazelnut creams ever.

Superfood Powers

Banana and hazelnuts are both rich sources of minerals, Vitamin E and essential fatty acids, which nourish the skin, hair and nails and help you make lots of serotonin to stay happy and stress-free.

Pistachio and Blueberry Chocolate Squares

MAKES 1 TRAY

INGREDIENTS

1 cup of pistachios (pre-soak for two hours)

½ cup of fresh blueberries

1 big, ripe avocado

1 tablespoon of mesquite powder (if you can't find use lucuma)

4 tablespoons of cacao powder

½ cup of cacao butter or coconut oil

½ cup of shredded coconut or coconut cream

5 tablespoons of raw honey, maple, monkfruit or Yacon syrup or dates

¼ cup of purified water

METHOD

1. Process pistachios, blueberries, avocado, cacao powder, coconut, mesquite, natural sweetener and enough water to make slightly creamy, but still thick.

2. Warm up cacao butter and pour into the mix and blend some more. Use a little butter or oil in a square tin and then pour the mix in.

3. Place in the freezer and when hard, cut into chocolate shaped pieces. Take out of the freezer and keep in the fridge.

Superfood Powers

Blueberries are a true superfood as they contain huge amounts of Vitamin C and anthocyanins to boost immunity, protect against disease and to improve the beauty of your skin, hair and eyes.

Raw Lavender and Raspberry Ice-Cream

SERVES 4

INGREDIENTS

2 cups of cashews (pre-soak for 2 hours)

2 young coconuts (take the meat from this) or 2 cans of coconut cream

1 cup of water

1 cup of maple syrup or another natural sweetener

2 tablespoons of vanilla extract

¼ cup of coconut oil

A few drops of lavender essential oil or 1 teaspoon of lavender extract, or 3 teaspoons of dried lavender

½ cup of fresh raspberries

METHOD

1. Blend all of your ingredients in a blender, adding the oil last. You can replace coconut oil with olive sacha inchi or avocado oil. I also like to add the raspberries at the end so they are not too crushed.

2. Place in an ice-cream maker or in the freezer, stirring every hour or so.

3. This is absolutely delicious and so easy to make. I really love adding probiotic powders to my ice-creams too.

Superfood Powers

This is a delicious, natural alternative to chemical filled ice-cream. When you add lavender you have a pure skin treat that helps with calming irritated skin, soothing eczema and dryness and balancing sebum production. It is also great for enhancing beauty sleep and calming the nerves. It is very floral, so if you do not like the lavender flavor, simply leave out or replace with an oil you love.

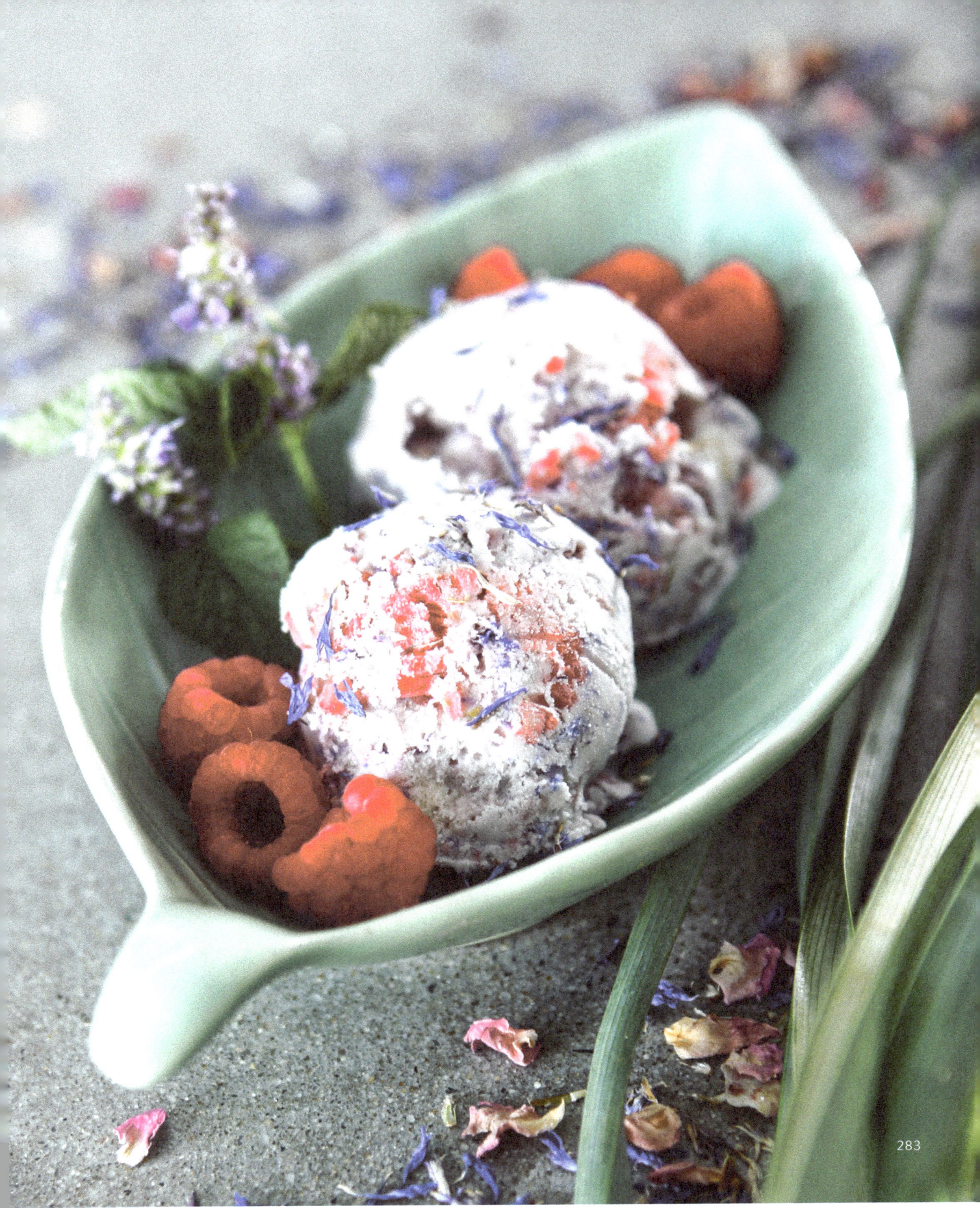

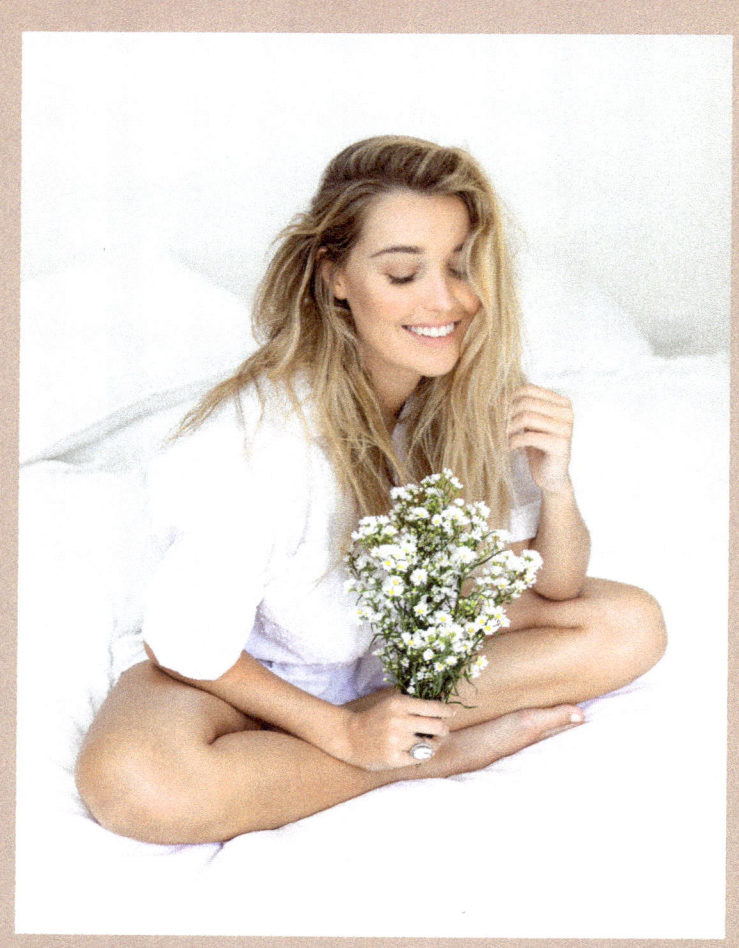

Substituting Nuts and Coconut in Recipes

I am asked everyday if there are alternatives for using nuts or coconut in recipes. Nuts are often a first choice for health cooks because of their rich mineral and omega oil content. But for anyone with a nut or coconut allergy, there are some great substitutes.

MY BEST SWAPS INCLUDE:

FLOURS
Hemp flour, banana flour, millet flour or buckwheat

FOR THICKENING
tapioca starch, kuzu root or Agar Agar

FOR SWEETENING
monkfruit syrup, stevia, Medjool dates

IN CAKES
olive, rice bran or avocado oil

NUTS CAN BE REPLACED WITH SEEDS OR GRAINS
pumpkin, sunflower, chia and hemp seeds

MILKS
hemp, cashew, quinoa or sesame milk

Collagen Protein Pots

MAKES 4 POTS

INGREDIENTS

1 cup of hazelnuts (pre-soaked for 2 to 4 hours)

½ cup of pumpkin or sunflower seeds

¼ cup of hulled hemp seeds

¼ cup of chia seeds (pre-soak with water)

¼ cup of pumpkin seed or vegan protein powder

2 tablespoons of coconut oil

¼ cup of maple, raw honey, monkfruit syrup
or 5 drops of stevia

2 tablespoons of organic cacao or carob powder

2 to 4 tablespoons of collagen powder
(vegan options available)

METHOD

1. Soak chia seeds with some water and leave
    for 30 minutes.

2. In another bowl mix together hemp seeds, collagen and
    carob or cacao powder.

3. In a food processor or Vitamix, blend the rest of the
    ingredients. Put all the mixes together and blend.

These can be put into pots to set in the fridge and eaten as
a skin snack or as a breakfast treat.

Superfood Powers

As I've mentioned before, hazelnuts are a superb source of essential fatty acids, Vitamin E and minerals, which help enhance the production of collagen. When you add a collagen powder and hemp seeds to this mixture, you have a perfect skin-boosting pot that can help to plump up skin, heal the gut and reduce inflammation.

Dragon Fruit Pink Popsicles

SERVES 8

INGREDIENTS

½ dragon fruit

1 to 2 cups of hulled hemp seeds

2 cups of macadamia or cashews (pre-soak to soften)

¼ cup of maple, monkfruit or yacon syrup
or 8 medjool dates

¼ cup of coconut water or cream
(if you want creamier popsicles)

METHOD

1. Blend all of the ingredients well until you get a creamy texture. Place into ice-block moulds and freeze. Now you have the prettiest pink popsicles in town.

Superfood Powers

Dragon fruit is a rich source of antioxidant vitamins that can help to reduce sun-induced skin damage, acne and dehydration. It contains 90% water, huge amounts of fibre and is low in calories, making it a perfect sugar-free treat for those on weight loss or ketogenic diets.

Mango and Berry Yoghurt Pops

MAKES 4 TO 6 POPSICLES

INGREDIENTS

1 large mango

1 cup of blueberries

1 cup of raspberries

1½ cups of Greek, sheep or coconut yoghurt

1 to 2 tablespoons of a super berry powder
(Açai, Macqui, goji etc)

METHOD

These are very easy to make and super nutritious. If you do not eat yoghurt, you can use fresh mango juice instead or swap this yoghurt with coconut, sheep's or nut yoghurt.

1. Blend one large mango and mix with ½ cup of yoghurt, and pour into ½ of the bottom of the popsicle mould. Place in the freezer to set.

2. Then blend blueberries with some more yoghurt and a super berry powder and pour in another ⅓'s worth of the mould and set in the freezer.

3. Finally, mix the last bit of yoghurt with raspberries and pour that in. Now you have a beautiful triple-layered berry popsicle.

4. If you do not have time, just blend all of the ingredients together and place into ice-block moulds.

Superfood Powers

These beautiful popsicles are packed with cancer-fighting and youth-promoting polyphenol flavonoids. They help to beautify the skin, protect the capillaries and veins against damage, brighten the eyes and improve the health and condition of the hair. Greek yoghurt is full of live bacteria, which improves your digestive health and the beauty of your skin.

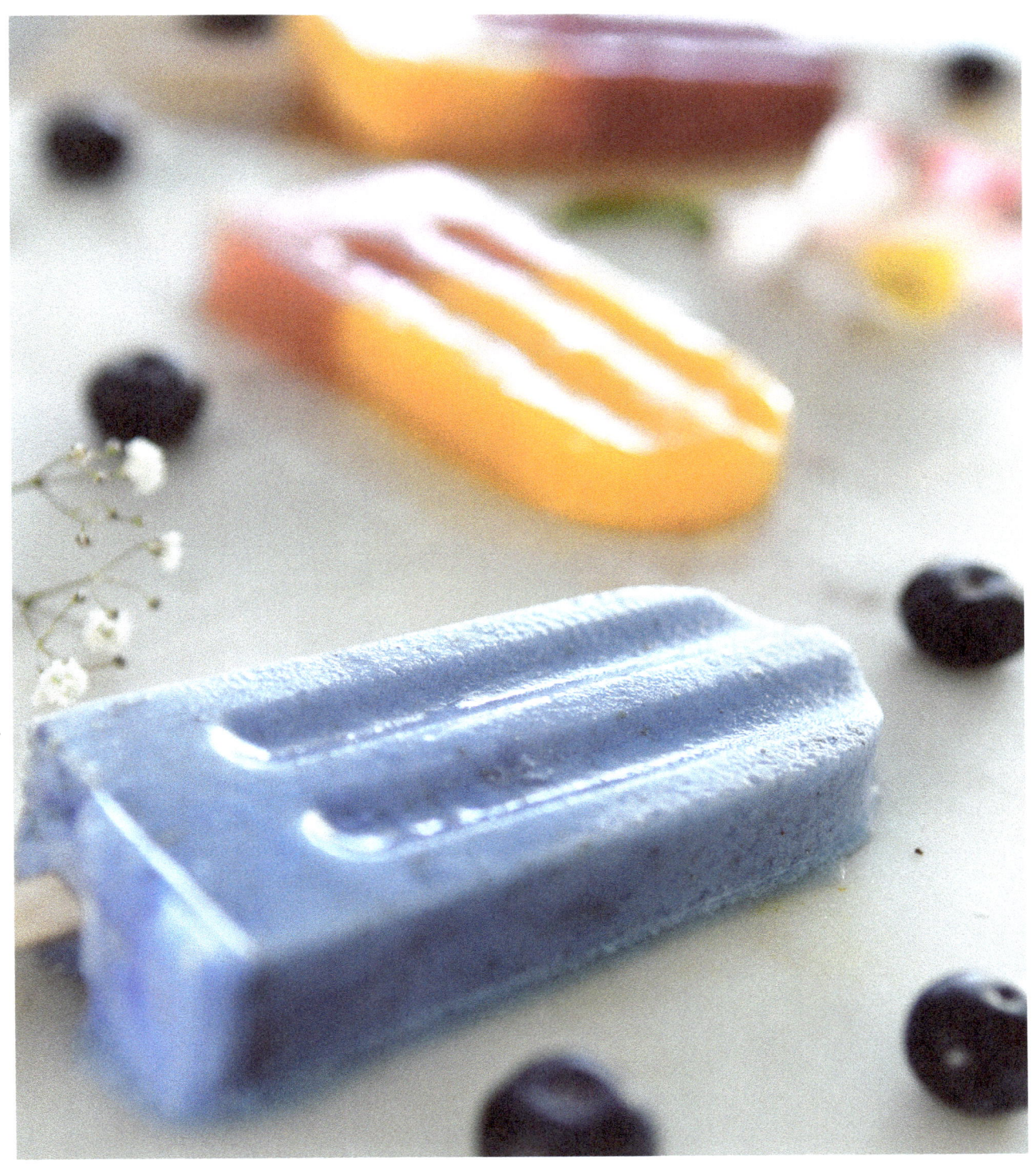

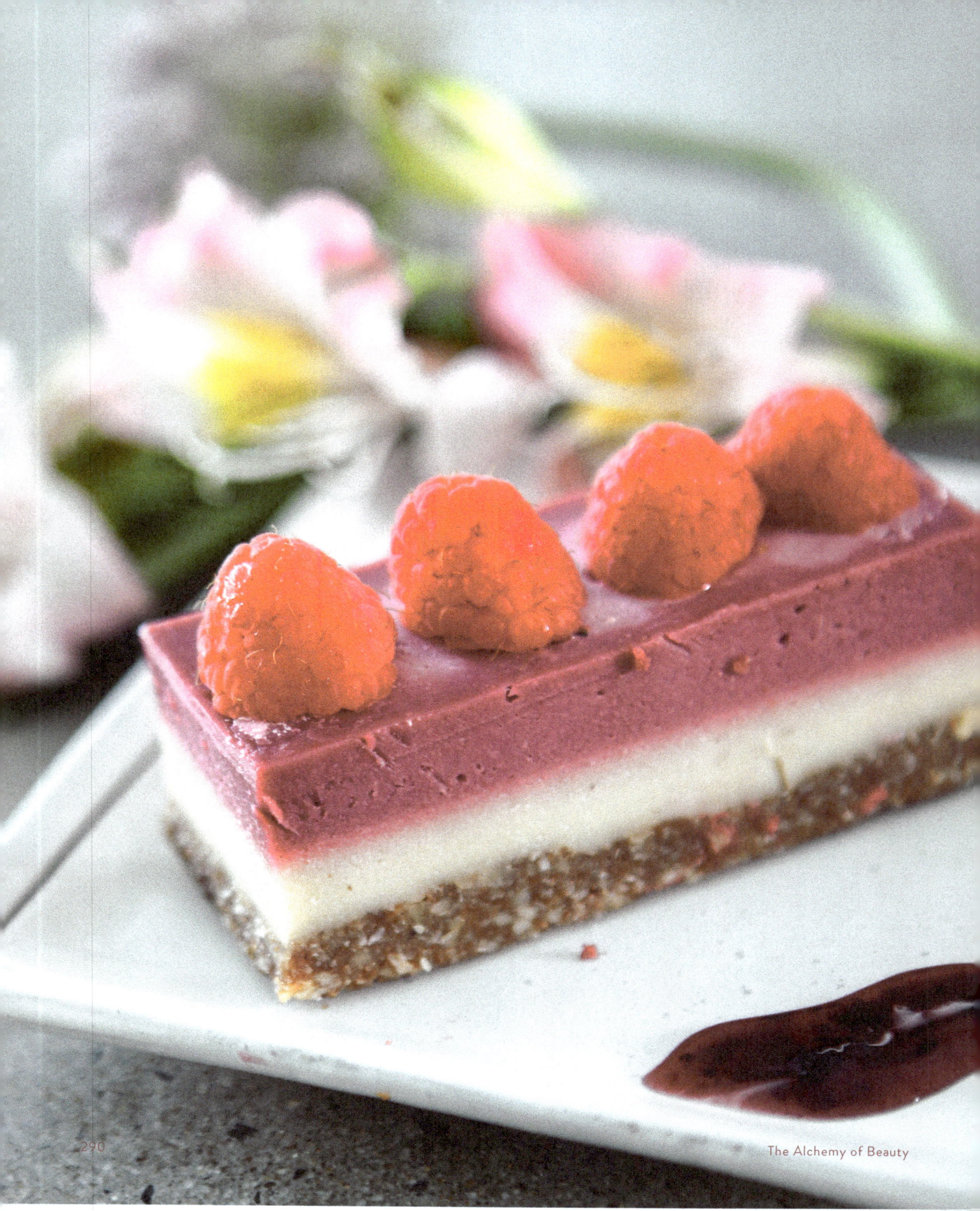

The Alchemy of Beauty

Raw Super Berry Cheesecake

MAKES 1 TIN

CRUST

1 cup of organic almonds (soak for 4 hours)
or almond flour (if you are in a hurry)

½ cup of organic hemp seeds, hulled

½ cup of maple syrup or coconut nectar

¼ cup of organic coconut flakes

½ cup of medjool dates

FILLING

2/3 cup of maple syrup or coconut nectar

3 cups of organic cashews
(soaked for 4 hours or overnight)

½ cup of coconut oil or butter (optional)

½ cup of maple syrup or coconut nectar

1 lemon or lime, juiced

A dash of celtic salt

Water

TOP LAYER

500 grams of frozen organic berries (strawberry,
blueberry, raspberry or another)

1 lemon, juiced

2 tablespoons of chia seeds

2 tablespoons of maple syrup or coconut nectar

METHOD

1. To make the base, combine all of the ingredients in a food processor, vitamix or thermomix. It should create a dough like consistency. Press into the baking dish and keep in the fridge to set for one hour.

2. Now place cashews, natural sweetener, lemon or lime, celtic salt and coconut butter or oil into a food processor and continue to blend until smooth. Add water if you need smoother. Pour over the crust and place in the freezer to set.

3. To make the berry layer, simply blend frozen berries, sweetener, lemon juice and chia seeds. If you do not have chia, you can use agar agar or xanthum gum. Now pour this delicious berry layer over the cheesecake and place back in the freezer to set.

Superfood Powers

Berries are one of the best sources of flavonoid rich antioxidants and Vitamin C to help protect against several forms of cancer including skin cancers and melanoma. When you combine berries with omega rich nuts and seeds you have a powerful youth-promoting cheesecake that you should never feel guilty devouring.

QUICK BEAUTY TABLES

Collagen-Boosting Superheroes

ASPARAGUS	GREEN, LEAFY VEGGIES LIKE KALE, SPINACH, ROMAINE LETTUCE, SWISS CHARD	PINEAPPLE
BERRIES – BLUEBERRIES, RASPBERRIES, GOJI, AÇAI		PUMPKIN SEEDS
BONE BROTHS	HOT PEPPERS: CHILLI, CAYENNE, PAPRIKA, JALAPENO	RED VEGETABLES : BEET, RED PEPPERS,
CABBAGE: ALL COLOURS AND TYPES	NUTS: BRAZIL, ALMONDS, WALNUTS	SEAWEEDS
CARROTS	OILY FISH: SALMON, TUNA, MACKEREL, HERRING, SARDINES	SWEET POTATOES
CRUCIFEROUS VEGETABLES LIKE BROCCOLI, RADISH, CAULIFLOWER, BRUSSELS SPROUTS	OLIVES	SOY: ORGANIC AND FERMENTED, IE. NATTO, TEMPEH
FLAXSEEDS	ORANGE VEGETABLES : CARROT, SWEET POTATO	
GARLIC	OYSTERS	TOMATOES
GREEN TEA	LEMONS, LIMES, GRAPEFRUIT	WALNUTS

Hyaluronic Acid-Boosting Superheroes

Hyaluronic acid is a carbohydrate that is naturally present in the skin and joints, and acts as a cushion. It moisturises and plumps up the skin leaving it hydrated, squishy and wrinkle-free. This is also great for dry skin, eczema, dermatitis and psoriasis. The foods that make this yummy substance include:

BONE BROTHS

ORANGES WHICH ARE HIGH IN NARINGENIN AND STOPS HA BREAKDOWN

VITAMIN A OR CAROTENE FOODS INCLUDING SWEET POTATO, SQUASH, PUMPKIN, CARROTS, PEACHES, BROCCOLI, SPINACH

FERMENTED SOY IE. NATTO, TEMPEH

ORGAN MEATS INCLUDING GRASS-FED, LIVER

GRAPE SKINS AND RED WINE HIGH IN RESVERATROL CONTENT

PHYTOPLANKTON

VITAMIN C FOUND IN BERRIES, CITRUS (LEMON, LIME, GRAPEFRUIT, ORANGE), KIWIFRUIT AND OTHERS.

GRAPEFRUIT

ROOT VEGETABLES INCLUDING TARO, YAMS, SWEET POTATO

MAGNESIUM, FOUND IN BANANA, STRAWBERRY, TOMATO, SPINACH, GREEN BEANS, BROCCOLI, ASPARAGUS, SWEET POTATO, LETTUCE, CARROTS, PINEAPPLE, KIDNEY BEANS, LENTILS, PINTO BEANS

SEAWEEDS

WATER

TOMATOES WHICH ARE HIGH IN NARINGENIN AND STOP HA BREAKDOWN

ZINC FOUND IN PUMPKIN SEEDS, OYSTERS, ALMONDS, OILY FISH, ORGANIC CHICKEN, GRASS-FED MEAT

Keratin-Boosting Superheroes

Keratin is a protein that adds strength to hair, skin and nails.
Certain foods can boost the production of this. They include:

ASPARAGUS	GRASS-FED MEAT	PUMPKIN
BONE BROTHS	GUAVA	SWEET POTATOES
BRUSSELS SPROUTS	KALE	APRICOTS
CANTALOUPE	LEGUMES	CARROTS
CAULIFLOWER	MANGO	QUINOA
EGGS	MUSHROOMS	SALMON
GARLIC	ONIONS	SPINACH
GELATIN	PAPAYA	

Sun-Protection Superheroes

If you want amazing natural protection against the sun's harmful UV rays, then look no further than the food you eat. Certain nutrients in foods can provide you with a strong SPF factor to guard against free radical damage and reduce the possibility of skin cancer. These include:

ALMONDS	HAZELNUTS AND OIL	SEAFOOD, PINK
BEETROOT	KALE	SESAME SEEDS AND OIL
CARROTS	LEMON AND LIMES	SPINACH
COFFEE WHICH IS RICH IN B3 AND PREVENTS SKIN CANCER	OLIVES AND OLIVE OIL	STRAWBERRIES
	PAPAYA, RED	SWISS CHARD
FISH EGGS	POMEGRANATE	TOMATO (ESPECIALLY COOKED, TOMATO PASTE, TOMATO POWDER)
GRAPEFRUIT	RED PEPPERS	TOMATOES, SUN-DRIED TOMATOES
GREEN TEA	SALMON, WILD CAUGHT, RED OR PINK	TURMERIC
GUAVA		WATERMELON

Melanin-Stimulating Foods

Melanin is the pigment that helps to determine our skin and hair colour.
When we are exposed to sunlight, we produce more melanin. Foods that
help to increase melanin include:

ALMONDS	LIMA BEANS	RAW DAIRY
AVOCADO	MELON	SESAME SEEDS
BANANA	OILY FISH	SHELLFISH
CARROTS	ORGAN MEATS	TOMATO
CHOCOLATE	OYSTERS	WHOLE GRAINS
EGG YOLK	PEANUTS	

Luscious Hair
and Nail Superheroes

AÇAI	GRASS-FED MEAT	OILY FISH (SALMON, SARDINES, HERRING, HALIBUT, TUNA ETC)
ALFALFA	GREEK YOGHURT	PARSLEY
ALMONDS	GREEN TEA	QUINOA
ASPARAGUS	HEMP SEEDS, HEMP OIL	RED PEPPER
AVOCADO	HORSETAIL	ROSEMARY
BARLEY GRASS	KALE	SOYBEANS
BLUEBERRIES	LECITHIN	SPINACH
BROWN RICE	LENTILS	SPROUTS
CELERY	MSM	STRAWBERRIES
CHAMOMILE	NETTLES	SWEET POTATOES
COCONUT OIL	NUTS AND SEEDS (ESPECIALLY ACTIVATED)	WALNUTS
EGGS, FOR BIOTIN		WHEATGRASS

"

She was beautiful, but not like
those girls in the magazines.

She was beautiful, for the way she thought.

She was beautiful, for the sparkle in her eyes
when she talked about something that she loved.

She was beautiful, for her ability to make
someone smile even if she was sad.

No she wasn't beautiful, for
something as temporary as her looks.

She was beautiful,
deep down to her soul.

"

F Scott Fitzgerald

Lightning Source UK Ltd.
Milton Keynes UK
UKHW051459310720
367474UK00003B/53